Dysexecutive Syndromes

Alfredo Ardila · Shameem Fatima ·
Mónica Rosselli
Editors

Dysexecutive Syndromes

Clinical and Experimental Perspectives

Springer

Editors
Alfredo Ardila
Sechenov University
Moscow, Russia

Albizu University
Miami, FL, USA

Mónica Rosselli
Florida Atlantic University
Davie, FL, USA

Shameem Fatima
COMSATS University Islamabad
Lahore, Pakistan

ISBN 978-3-030-25076-8 ISBN 978-3-030-25077-5 (eBook)
https://doi.org/10.1007/978-3-030-25077-5

This Springer imprint is published by the registered company Springer Nature Switzerland AG
The registered company address is: Gewerbestrasse 11, 6330 Cham, Switzerland

Introduction

The term "executive function" is relatively new in the cognitive and behavioral neurosciences. Nonetheless, since the nineteenth century, it has been documented that frontal lobe damage can result in a wide range of cognitive and behavioral disturbances. Phineas Gage represents the best-known report of impairments potentially associated with frontal lobe pathology (Harlow, 1868). Toward the end of the nineteenth century, Oppenheim (1890, 1891) associated personality disturbances with orbital and mesial frontal lobe pathology. The "frontal lobe syndrome" was conceptualized during the early twentieth century by Feuchtwanger (1923). He proposed that frontal lobe pathologies were associated with disturbances that were not directly related to memory, language, speech, or sensorimotor deficits. Goldstein (1944) suggested that the capacity of the frontal lobe includes "the abstract attitude", mental flexibility, and understanding of the contextual situation of behavior. Luria (1969, 1980) referred to three functional units in the brain: (1) arousal-motivation (limbic and reticular systems); (2) receiving, processing, and storing information (postrolandic cortical areas); and (3) programming, controlling, and verifying activity (frontal lobes). Luria suggested that the third unit has an executive role. Lezak (1983) emphasized the fluid nature of executive functioning and observed that both cognitive and emotional aspects were involved.

In recent years, cognitive neuroscience, particularly neuropsychology, has used the term "executive functions" as an umbrella term to describe several interrelated higher cognitive processes such as inhibitory control, working memory, behavioral temporality, cognitive flexibility, planning, self-regulation, monitoring, and similar behavioral and cognitive functions. These functions play a significant role in the successful production of goal-oriented behaviors as well as in the successful performance of daily activities. Executive or cognitive control is a related term that refers to a complex set of cognitive processes working in a top-down functioning mechanism (Diamond, 2013). Cognitive control is an essential life skill that helps in problem-solving, attention holding and control, learning, decision-making, planning, and regulating behaviors (Chung et al. 2014).

Regarding neuroanatomical correlates, the neuropsychological literature has described that executive functions are closely related to frontal lobe activity.

Indeed, the term executive function has been used interchangeably with frontal lobe functioning. With the advent of advanced neuroimaging techniques, it has been found that successful performance of executive abilities is not only dependent on intact frontal lobe structure and functions but is also mediated by dynamic and functional connections between frontal regions, retro-Roladic, and subcortical areas of the brain (Ardila, Bernal, & Rosselli 2017; Chung et al. 2014; Collette et al. 2006; Bonelli & Cummings 2007; Marvel & Desmond 2010). The smooth and effective behavioral expression of intact executive functions depends on the functional integration and effective connections between cortical and subcortical regions.

During the last decades, a myriad of books dedicated to the analysis of executive functions have been published (e.g., Anderson, Jacobs & Anderson 2010; Eslinger & Flaherty 2018; Miller & Cummings 2017; Rabbitt 2004; Roberts, Robbins & Weiskrantz 1998; Tirapu-Ustárroz, García Molina, Ríos-Lago & Ardila 2012). It is time to publish a book devoted to the analysis of the dysexecutive syndromes or executive dysfunctions. Baddeley (1986) coined the term "dysexecutive syndrome" to refer to the dysregulation of executive functions usually resulting from frontal lobe damage. The syndrome is represented in emotional, motivational, and behavioral problems as well as in cognitive deficiencies related to executive skills such as planning, mental flexibility, inhibition, and working memory. The symptoms of the syndrome can be seen in many clinical conditions, including neurodegenerative diseases such as frontotemporal dementia.

"Executive dysfunction" is described as a disturbance in the efficiency of higher regulatory executive functions (Elliott 2003) which may result in neurocognitive deficits and behavioral symptoms. The terms "executive dysfunction" and "frontal lobe dysfunction" have been some times used interchangeably based on clinical evidence from patients with brain injuries to frontal regions. However, evidence from more recent studies based on imaging techniques, including fMRI and PET scan, has suggested that executive dysfunction is not only associated with frontal lobe abnormalities, but also with the dysfunctional connections between frontal, retro-Rolandic, and subcortical brain regions (Bonelli & Cummings 2007; Chung et al. 2014).

Executive dysfunctions are also associated with a wide range of psychopathologies, including neurodevelopmental and traumatic brain injuries. The symptoms from neurodevelopmental disorders may include problems with inhibitory control, impulsivity, planning difficulties, working memory deficits, problems with sustained and selective attention, and deficits in mental flexibility. These clinical conditions include autism spectrum disorder, attention deficit hyperactivity disorder, fetal alcohol spectrum disorders, Tourette syndrome, and phenylketonuria (Jurado & Rosselli 2007).

Additionally, executive function deficits are also observed in many psychiatric disorders such as depression and schizophrenia (Johnson 2012). Soraggi-Frez et al. (2017) and Caixeta et al. (2017) provided evidence of executive function deficits, particularly related to working memory, in patients with bipolar disorder. In these psychiatric conditions, executive function deficits are attributed to either frontal lobe abnormalities or dysfunctional fronto-subcortical networks. Berger et al. (2016) provided evidence for impaired fronto-parietal activation in schizophrenics compared to healthy controls using an electrophysiological pattern of activation. These deficits present a challenge to patients in adapting to the social and workplace requirements and even in adherence to treatment plans. Therefore, there is a need to assess executive function deficits and their link with psychopathology in psychiatric patients for the management of clinical symptoms and social adjustment. Moreover, neurophysiological and cognitive impairments are associated with substance use. Evidence shows that alcohol, opiate, and stimulant abusers show impaired performance on various executive function tasks (Barry & Petry 2008; Verdejo-Garcia et al. 2006).

This book has been divided into six parts. Part I (Theoretical Approaches) represents a theoretical framework for the analysis of the diverse dysexecutive syndromes. Two issues are reviewed: the commonality and diversity of executive disturbances, and the executive function brain organization. Part II (Developmental Executive Dysfunction) consists of two chapters reviewing the most common executive dysfunction syndromes found during childhood development: attention deficit hyperactivity disorder and autism spectrum disorders. One chapter is dedicated to analyzing the impairments that children with attention-deficit hyperactivity disorder have in tasks tapping inhibition, working memory, and sustained attention, and to describe their deficits of self and emotional regulation processes. The subsequent chapter analyzes impairments in planning, cognitive flexibility, and working memory related to the spatial domain in children with autism spectrum disorders. The following part (Acquired Executive Dysfunction) is devoted to executive dysfunctions observed in the cases of neurological conditions such as traumatic head injury, substance abuse, and subcortical diseases. The executive deficits that distinguish normal from abnormal aging are the topic of another chapter in this section, presenting evidence of age-related changes in executive functions and comparing these with the functional decline in the cases of vascular disease and degenerative disorders such as the frontal variant of Alzheimer's disease. Finally, an analysis of the executive function deficits in the use of information technology is included in this section. Individuals of all ages use technology in everyday life; however, for some, it can also be an agent of diverse negative consequences, particularly in the domain of executive function. These consequences are analyzed in this chapter. Part IV (Executive Dysfunction and Personality Disorders) includes the personality disorders associated with executive dysfunction, particularly in convicted individuals who have exhibited extreme violent and criminal behaviors and in others, such as ex-combatants, who have been exposed to violence in war environments for extended periods of time. Some neuropsychiatric disorders are associated with executive dysfunction, such as depressive disorders and HIV infection, and this is the topic of Part V (Executive Dysfunction in Neuropsychiatric Disorder). Interestingly, a biochemical disorder such as depression and an infectious disorder such as HIV have the potential to impair similar brain mechanisms that are also affected in attention deficits and other executive control problems. Part VI (Assessment of Executive Dysfunction) examines assessment issues in executive dysfunction. In the first chapter, the evaluation procedures and the most common executive function tests are described. The last two chapters of this section are devoted to the assessment of executive dysfunction in bilingual subjects and the corresponding cross-cultural questions. The active use of two languages seems to generate brain changes that are reflected in the performance of neuropsychological tests, particularly in those assessing executive function. An analysis of the complex interaction between bilingualism and executive functions across the lifespan is presented, and its implications for the assessment of bilingual individuals are discussed. In other chapters of this section, differences in executive function test performance are analyzed across individualistic (Western) and collectivistic (Asian) cultures. In addition, the assessment of basic cognitive functions, higher executive functions, and nonverbal abilities is reviewed across cultures and includes the adaptation of new executive function tests for Asian countries.

We are convinced that this book significantly extends the analysis of executive functions and dysfunctions, from a fundamental and clinical perspective.

Finally, we want to express our most sincere gratitude to Springer, and especially to Katherine Chabalko and Lilith Dorko for their support and understanding in the process of publishing this book.

Alfredo Ardila
Shameem Fatima
Mónica Rosselli

References

Ardila, A., Bernal, B., & Rosselli, M. (2017). Executive functions brain system: An activation likelihood estimation meta-analytic study. *Archives of Clinical Neuropsychology, 33*(4), 379–405.

Anderson, V., Jacobs, R., & Anderson, P. J. (Eds.). (2010). *Executive functions and the frontal lobes: A lifespan perspective*. Psychology Press.

Baddeley, A. (1986). *Working memory*. Oxford: Oxford University Press.

Barry, D. & Petry, N. M. (2008). Predictors of decision-making on the Iowa Gambling Task: Independent effects of lifetime history of substance use disorders and performance on the Trail Making Test. *Brain and Cognition, 66,* 243–252.

Berger, B., Minarik, T., Griesmayr, B., Stelzig-Schoeler, R., Aichhorn, W., & Sauseng, P. (2016). Brain Oscillatory Correlates of Altered Executive Functioning in Positive and Negative Symptomatic Schizophrenia Patients and Healthy Controls. *Frontiers in Psychology, 10.*

Bonelli R. & Cummings J. L. (2007). Frontal-subcortical circuitry and behavior. *Dialogues in Clinical Neuroscience, 9,* 141–151.

Caixeta, L., Soares, V. L. D., Vieira, R. T., Soares, C. D., Caixeta, V., Ferreira, S. B., et al. (2017). Executive Function Is Selectively Impaired in Old Age Bipolar Depression.

Chung, H. J., Weyandt, L. L., & Swentosky A. (2014). The Physiology of executive functioning," in S. Goldstein, & J. A. Naglieri (Eds.). *Handbook of Executive Functioning*. pp. 13–27. New York, NY: Springer Science and Business Media.

Collette, F., Hogge, M., Salmon, E., & Van der Linden, M. (2006). Exploration of the neural substrates of executive functioning by functional neuroimaging. *Neuroscience, 139,* 209–221.

Elliott, R. (2003). Executive functions and their disorders. *British Medical Bulletin,* 65, 49–59.
Eslinger, P. J., & Flaherty, C. (2018). Executive Functions and Behavior Across the Lifespan. *The Wiley Handbook on the Aging Mind and Brain*, 253–269.
Harlow, J. M. (1868). Recovery from the passage of an iron bar through the head. *Massachusetts Medical Society Publications*, 2, 327–346.
Feuchtwanger, E. (1923). *Die Funktionen des Stirnhirns*. Berlin: Springer.
Goldstein, K. (1944). The mental changes due to frontal lobe damage. *Journal of Psychology,* 17, 187–208.
Johnson, M. H. (2012). Executive function and developmental disorders: the flip side of the coin. *Trends in Cognitive Sciences, 16,* 454–457.
Jurado, M. B. & Rosselli, M. (2007). The elusive nature of executive functions: a review of our current understanding. *Neuropsychological Review, 17,* 213–233.
Lezak, M. D. (1983). *Neuropsychological assessment* (2nd ed.). New York: Oxford University Press.
Luria, A. R. (1969). Frontal lobe syndromes. In P. J. Vinken & G. W. Bruyn (Eds.). *Handbook of clinical neurology* (Vol. 2, pp. 725–757). Amsterdam: North Holland.
Luria, A. R. (1980). *Higher cortical functions in man* (2nd ed.). New York: Basic.
Marvel, C. L. & Desmond, J. E. (2010). Functional topography of the cerebellum in verbal working memory. *Neuropsychological Reviews, 20,* 271–279.
Miller, B. L., & Cummings, J. L. (Eds.). (2017). *The human frontal lobes: Functions and disorders*. Guilford Publications.
Oppenheim, H. (1890). ZurPathologie der Grosshirngeschwülste. Arch PsychiatrieNervenkrankh, 21:560–587.
Oppenheim, H. (1891). ZurPathologie der Grosshirngeschwülste. Arch PsychiatrieNervenkrankh, 22:27–72.
Rabbitt, P. (Ed.). (2004). *Methodology of frontal and executive function*. Psychology Press.
Roberts, A. C., Robbins, T. W., & Weiskrantz, L. E. (1998). *The prefrontal cortex: executive and cognitive functions*. Oxford University Press.
Soraggi-Frez, C., Santos, F. H., Albuquerque, P. B., & Malloy-Diniz, L. F. (2017). Disentangling Working Memory Functioning in Mood States of Bipolar Disorder: A Systematic Review. *Frontiers in Psychology, 26.*
Tirapu-Ustárroz, J., García Molina, A., Ríos-Lago, M., & Ardila, A. (2012). Neuropsicología de la corteza prefrontal y las funciones ejecutivas. *Barcelona: Viguera.*
Verdejo-Garcia, A., Bechara, A., Recknor, E. C., & Perez-Garcia, M. (2006). Executive dysfunction in substance dependent individuals during drug use and abstinence: An examination of the behavioral, cognitive and emotional correlates of addiction. *Journal of the International Neuropsychological Society, 12,* 405–415.

Contents

Editors and Contributors

About the Editors

Alfredo Ardila received his Ph.D. from the Moscow State University in the field of neuropsychology. Currently, he is Professor at the Sechenov University in Moscow, Russia, and at the Albizu University in Miami, USA. His primary research interests include the brain organization of cognition, historical origin of human cognition, aphasia, bilingualism, and executive functions. He has received several awards and honors, such as the Latin American award in neurosciences and the Hispanic Neuropsychological Society Lifetime Achievement in Cultural Neuropsychology Award.

Shameem Fatima received her Ph.D. from the University of Punjab in the field of Applied Psychology with a specialization in neuropsychology. Currently, she is an Assistant Professor at the COMSATS University Islamabad, Lahore campus. Her primary research interests include executive functions, neuropsychological assessment, forensic psychology, and neuro-developmental disorders. She has obtained many awards including but not limited to the Punjab University Talent Award in 2000, the 5th HEC Outstanding Research Award, and the CUI Lahore Best Researcher Award in 2017.

Mónica Rosselli received her Ph.D. in biomedical sciences (neuropsychology) from the National Autonomous University of Mexico. She is currently Assistant Chair and Professor in the Department of Psychology at Florida Atlantic University in Davie, Florida (USA) where she heads the Neuropsychology Laboratory. She serves as an investigator in various capacities for longitudinal studies funded by the Florida and National Institutes of Health, including the 1Florida Alzheimer's Disease Research Center. Her research interests are in the areas of bilingualism, neuropsychological assessment, neurocognitive development, cross-cultural neuropsychology, and geriatric neuropsychology. She was recognized in 2013 with the Hispano-American Neuropsychology Award.

Contributors

F. Taylor Agate Department of Psychology, University of Victoria, Victoria, BC, Canada

Alfredo Ardila Sechenov University, Moscow, Russia;
Albizu University, Miami, FL, USA

Fernanda Arruda Department of Psychology, Florida Atlantic University, Davie, FL, USA

Deven M. Christopher Department of Psychology, Florida Atlantic University, Davie, FL, USA

Karla Ximena Díaz Galván Laboratorio de Psicofisiología y Neuropsicología, Facultad de Psicología, Universidad Nacional Autonoma de Mexico, Mexico City, Mexico

Shameem Fatima COMSATS University Islamabad, Lahore, Pakistan

Mauricio A. Garcia-Barrera Department of Psychology, University of Victoria, Victoria, BC, Canada

Olga Inozemtseva Instituto de Neurociencias, CUCBA; Departamento de Estudios En Educación, CUCSH, Universidad de Guadalajara, Guadalajara, Mexico

Justin E. Karr Department of Physical Medicine and Rehabilitation, Harvard Medical School, Spaulding Rehabilitation Hospital, Home Base, A Red Sox Foundation and Massachusetts General Hospital Program, Boston, MA, USA

Merike Lang Department of Psychology, Florida Atlantic University, Davie, FL, USA

Judy D. Lobo Department of Psychology, University of Miami, Miami, FL, USA

Asucena Lozano Gutiérrez Laboratorio de Psicofisiología y Neuropsicología, Facultad de Psicología, Universidad Nacional Autonoma de Mexico, Mexico City, Mexico

Roger C. McIntosh Department of Psychology, University of Miami, Miami, FL, USA

Edgar Mejía Núñez Instituto de Neurociencias, Universidad de Guadalajara, Guadalajara, Mexico

Feggy Ostrosky Shejet Laboratorio de Psicofisiología y Neuropsicología, Facultad de Psicología, Universidad Nacional Autonoma de Mexico, Mexico City, Mexico

David Pineda Grupo Neuropsicología y Conducta—GRUNECO, Facultad de Psicología, Universidad de San Buenaventura, Medellín, Colombia

Mónica Rosselli Department of Psychology, Florida Atlantic University, Davie, FL, USA

Humera Sharif University of Lahore, Lahore, Pakistan

Colette M. Smart Department of Psychology, University of Victoria, Victoria, BC, Canada

Carlos Tobón Grupo Neuropsicología y Conducta—GRUNECO, Facultad de Medicina, Universidad de Antioquia UdeA, Medellín, Colombia

Valeria L. Torres Department of Psychology, Florida Atlantic University, Davie, FL, USA

Idaly Vélez-Uribe Department of Psychology, Florida Atlantic University, Davie, FL, USA

Ryan E. Wong Department of Psychology, University of Victoria, Victoria, BC, Canada

Part I
Theoretical Approaches

Chapter 1
Unity and Diversity of Dysexecutive Syndromes

Mauricio A. Garcia-Barrera

1.1 Introduction

There is no other cognitive construct in Neuropsychology that holds so much mystery as the so-called **executive function**, and it is not a surprise that the elusive nature of this cognitive function (as brilliantly characterized by Jurado & Rosselli, 2007) has generated an ever-growing amount of research, theoretical and empirical, across disciplines. But why is such function so attractive to us? Perhaps it is its omnipresent involvement in human (and some animal) non-routine activities, or likely it is how ubiquitous its dysfunction is after developmental and acquired brain injury. Possibly, it is just because science thrives on the unknown and the inscrutable. Understanding a concept as complex as executive function requires an executive mind, a developed metacognitive ability, a mind that thinks about itself. In talking about consciousness and metacognition, Nelson (1996, p. 114) recalls the words of the American philosopher, Dennett (1991), who pointed out that "Even if mental events are not among the data of science, this does not mean we cannot study them scientifically.... The challenge is to construct a theory of mental events, using the data that scientific method permits" (p. 71). Although this position was later criticized as materialistic and overly crediting the scientific approach, those words could serve as an omen of our current state of affairs regarding the nature of executive function.

Thus, what is executive function? Short answer: we don't know. Long-answer: we don't really know, but I would make an attempt to briefly summarize in this chapter what we do know, with a particular interest in describing how, from the definition of the term, we have come to understand that either the parts or the whole of this higher-order, cognitive control capacity can become dysfunctional, a phenomena some recognize as a "dysexecutive syndrome".

M. A. Garcia-Barrera (✉)
Department of Psychology, University of Victoria, Victoria, BC, Canada
e-mail: mgarcia@uvic.ca

A. Ardila et al. (eds.), *Dysexecutive Syndromes*,
https://doi.org/10.1007/978-3-030-25077-5_1

1.2 Executive Function: A Construct

There are several references in the literature to an executive type of regulation of cognition and behavior, with one of the most influential in Neuropsychology being the description of unit III by Luria (1973). He defined it as the component of his model of the hierarchical organization of the working brain responsible for the programming, regulating, and verifying mental activity. In his own words:

> Man not only reacts passively to incoming information, but creates *intentions*, forms *plans* and *programmes* of his actions, inspects their performance, and *regulates* his behaviour so that it conforms to these plans and programmes; finally, he *verifies* his conscious activity, comparing the effects of his actions with the original intentions and correcting any mistakes he has made. (Luria, 1973, pp. 79, 80. Italics from original text)

At this time, Pribram (1973, 1976) introduced the terms "executive of the brain" referring to the role of the frontal lobes in monkeys, and later introduced the term "executive functions" referencing the functions of the frontal lobes in humans. However, the term "executive functions" appears to have been officially introduced to the Neuropsychology field in 1982, by Muriel D. Lezak, a term evolving from what she called in her earlier writings "executive capabilities", referring to "those mental capacities necessary for formulating goals, planning how to achieve them, and carrying out the plans effectively" (Lezak, 1982, p. 281).

Executive function is best defined as a psychological **construct**, that is, a variable useful to explain phenomena that are not directly observable; in this case, it is a concept about an invisible function constructed from what can be observed, such as behavior, or inferred, such as the processes of the mind (Uttal, 2001). The term "function" comes from mathematics, defined as a relation between inputs and allowable outputs. Zelazo, Carter, Reznick, and Frye (1997) pointed out, in the context of executive function, the term "function" refers to a complex activity with a regular outcome, which can be effected on a range of alternative ways. The crux of the problem of any definition of executive function is the elucidation of this particular complex activity or "function". In attempting to address it, several questions have emerged, including: is this a unitary function or a diverse range of functions? Is this function (or are these functions) measurable? What are the neural structures supporting executive function(s)?

One of the most compelling definitions of executive function to date is proposed by Jurado and Rosselli (2007), who stated that,

> In a constantly changing environment, executive abilities allow us to shift our mind set quickly and adapt to diverse situations while at the same time inhibiting inappropriate behaviors. They enable us to create a plan, initiate its execution, and persevere on the task at hand until its completion. Executive functions mediate the ability to organize our thoughts in a goal directed way and are therefore essential for success in school and work situations, as well as everyday living. (p. 214)

There is, however, a plethora of other definitions for executive function. As early as 1996, there were already over 33 different definitions documented (Eslinger, 1996). In a comprehensive systematic analysis of empirical studies, Baggetta and Alexander

(2016) demonstrated that of 106 published papers that met their selection criteria, the authors of those papers cited 83 different sources to support their approach to the concept (most of them cited less than 6 times within the sample). Furthermore, Baggetta and Alexander also identified that only 59% of the published papers included in their review presented an explicit definition of executive function, which they defined as instances in which the authors addressed its main characteristics and the area the construct was supposed to influence. The areas of influence were grouped into four central themes: (1) goal-directed behaviors, (2) action and thoughts, (3) cognition, and (4) self-regulation of behaviors, cognition, and emotions. The rest 41% published papers incorporated implicit definitions, which were characterized as those including an implied meaning via specific select words or phrases (conceptual), citations of other author's (referential), their combination (conceptual-referential), and via the tasks used to assess executive performance and behavior (measurement). This range of approaches is consistent with the idea of executive function as an elusive construct. The synthetic definition that Baggetta and Alexander (2016) proposed states:

> Executive function is a set of cognitive processes that: (1) guides action and behaviors essential to aspects of learning and everyday human performance tasks; (2) contributes to the monitoring or regulation of such tasks; and (3) pertains not only to the cognitive domain, but also socioemotional and behavioral domains of human performance. (p. 24)

Built in the two aforementioned definitions are some underlying principles of both unity (i.e., "a set") and diversity (i.e., plural terms such as executive abilities, functions, cognitive processes), some executive components are referenced (i.e., shifting, inhibiting, planning); there is a sense of purpose (i.e., adaptation, goal-directed behavior, guidance, monitoring), and measurable outcomes of executive functioning are listed (i.e., academic achievement, work success, socioemotional performance). Having these two working definitions as a starting point, the issues of the unity versus diversity of the construct, its measurability, and its localization seem more approachable. The following sections deal with those issues in some more depth.

1.3 The Unity and Diversity of Executive Function

For several decades, examination of the nature of frontal lobe functioning served as a foundation for our knowledge about executive function. Experts in the fields of neurosciences, cognitive sciences, and neuropsychology, regularly met to discuss their insights about the obscure functions of the frontal lobes. One of the regulars of these meetings was Hans-Lukas Teuber, Professor and Head of the Psychology Department (now Department of Brain and Cognitive Sciences) at Massachusetts Institute of Technology. He is considered to be one of the founders of the field of Neuropsychology. One of those meetings occurred at the University of Pennsylvania in 1962. Captured within the memories of the Pennsylvania Symposium "Frontal granular cortex and behavior" (Warren & Akert, 1964) is Teuber's lecture "The

Riddle of Frontal Lobe Function in Man." Despite the fact that the title includes "function" in singular, Teuber (1964) made evident his hesitation between assigning a unitary concept to frontal lobe function and supporting the idea of dissociation. The document captures this exchange occurring during the discussion session:

> Dr. ROSVOLD: Did I understand you to say, Dr. Teuber, that we don't have a unitary concept of frontal lobe function and we are not likely to develop one?
>
> Dr. TEUBER: What I probably said was that I started out by trying to find a unitary concept, but as I moved along, it became clear that no single-factor hypothesis could carry one far enough to cover all the manifestations of frontal lesions. And yet the thing that is so tempting to me after this symposium is to think that there may be a family resemblance among symptoms, even among those which seem in part dissociable .... (Warren & Akert, 1964, p. 442)

Teuber continued to be intrigued by this debate, and in 1971 he delivered a lecture during a satellite event to the Pennsylvania Symposium held in Jablonna (a small village in east-central Poland), titled "Unity and Diversity of Frontal Lobe Functions" (worth noting the plural). During this lecture, Teuber furthered his hypothesis that the common feature that unifies frontal lobe functions may be "corollary discharges" from prefrontal areas that are neither motor nor sensory, and consisting of the firing of two sets of signals: the output top-down signal to effector organs, and a simultaneous discharge from frontal lobes to posterior areas, which presets the sensory system for the anticipated consequences of actions (Teuber, 1972). He made the point that this may be the unifying mechanism to a range of diverse frontal lobe functions and dysfunctions clinically observed after damage to anterior cortex in human and animal cases.

These ideas have more than a simple historical value. They marked the path for several decades of research on the frontal lobes and executive functions that followed. The debate "unity **versus** diversity" progressed from the logic "unity **or** diversity" to the logic "unity **and** diversity." However, it took several years for the debate to be settled. Homuncular, top-down attention-based regulatory agencies such as the Supervisory Attentional System (SAS) by Norman and Shallice (1986) for the selection of action programs within information processing systems, and Baddeley's Central Executive (CE; Baddeley, 1996) for the control of attention (focus and switch) over information to be processed within working memory systems, were quite influential in bringing back the idea of a unitary mechanism. With the arrival of the new millennium, these hypotheses were further developed, acknowledging the possible dissociation of CE and SAS into components (Baddeley, 2002; Shallice, 2002, respectively). However, several models within cognitive neurosciences continue to pursue similar unitary approaches to prefrontal cognitive control function (e.g., Banich, 2009; Miller & Cohen, 2001).

Miyake and his colleagues (2000) revisited the unity and diversity theme, with two new elements that, likely unexpectedly, revolutionized the field of research on executive functions. First, they adjudicated the "unity and diversity" principle to executive functions (worth noting the plural) rather than to frontal lobe functions; and second, they used a latent variable analytical approach including combined confirmatory factor analysis (CFA) and structural equation modeling (SEM) components, which offered a new pathway to the examination of at least three (authors acclaimed) "core" executive functions: inhibition of prepotent responses ("**inhibition**"), mental set shifting ("**shifting**"), and updating and monitoring of working memory representations ("**updating**"). This seminal study, conducted on a sample of 137 undergraduate students from the University of Colorado, was published in Cognitive Psychology. In the two decades since its publication, this article has set a new citation record with 10,000 citations (in comparison, Beck, Ward, Mendelson, Mock, & Erbaugh, 1961, "An inventory for measuring depression" has accumulated close to 6000 citations per decade since publication).

Why is Miyake et al.'s (2000) approach so popular? The proposal that the structure of a construct that is latent and elusive in nature, could be somewhat modeled via CFA meets the needs of several researchers, and answered a call for a better operationalization and measurement of this complex aspect of human cognitive and socioemotional functioning, or at least it accounted for the cognitive piece. A particular feature of CFA is that it accounts for the effects of task impurity, that is, the non-executive abilities involved in task performance, an issue commonly observed in tasks measuring executive functions (Burgess, 1997). Another feature of CFA is that it has the potential to reduce the effects of common method variance, as the selection of indicators and their relationships to factors are set a priori. The three-component model has been emulated using a range of tasks and in different age groups (e.g., Friedman et al., 2006, 2008; Lehto, Juujärvi, Kooistra, & Pulkkinen, 2003; Vaughan & Giovanello, 2010). Other studies have used a range of executive components and tasks, and in samples representing the lifespan, with CFA solutions ranging from one factor (e.g., Brydges, Reid, Fox, & Anderson, 2012; de Frias, Dixon, & Strauss, 2006; Ettenhofer, Hambrick, & Abeles, 2006; Hughes, Ensor, Wilson, & Graham, 2010; Wiebe, Espy, & Charak, 2008) to five (e.g., Fournier-Vicente, Larigauderie, & Gaonac'h, 2008).

Ever since the publication of Miyake et al.'s (2000) paper, inhibition, updating, and shifting have become to represent the most accepted and studied executive components. Interestingly, these authors stated that, "... we are not claiming that the three investigated executive functions are the only executive functions. [...] there are other important relatively basic functions that need to be added to the current list" (pp. 89, 90). However, only a few researchers have taken this caution into account. In several iterations of their approach and using the same sample, Friedman and colleagues (2008, 2009, 2011, 2016) have evolved their original three-component model to a nested-factor model in which all indicators load to a "general factor," while indicators for shifting and updating co-load onto their specific factors (shifting and updating), the exception being inhibition whose variance was fully explained by the general factor, further demonstrating the unity and diversity of the cognitive components of executive function.

More recently, my team (Karr et al., 2018) completed a critical, comprehensive, and systematic review of the empirical literature that examined the structure of executive functions using the latent variable approach on performance-based tests. Further, and using all available data from 46 samples ($N = 9756$) from eligible papers, we conducted a re-analysis of the data by systematically testing seven competing derivations of Miyake's model: (1) a unidimensional (one factor) model, (2) a bi-dimensional model with shifting and updating merged, (3) a bi-dimensional model with inhibition and updating merged, (4) a bi-dimensional model with shifting and inhibition merged, (5) Miyake's original three-factor model including inhibition, updating, and shifting, (6) a nested-factor model with a common executive function bi-factor and specific factors for shifting and updating, and (7) a complete bi-factor model with both, a common executive function bi-factor and the three specific factors for inhibition, shifting, and updating. Among our findings, we demonstrated that no model consistently converged and met the minimal fit criteria for acceptance across all samples (Karr et al., 2018). Specifically, we showed that rates of model acceptance (a model converges and meets fit criteria) and model selection (a model not only converges but shows superior fit to competitive models) were overall quite low. For instance, the nested factor was the most successful among adults (i.e., the model with a common executive function bi-factor and specific factors for shifting and updating), with rates of acceptance ranging from 41 to 42% and selection rates ranging from 8 to 30%, whereas in children, the most successful model was unidimensional, with rates of acceptance ranging from 32 to 36% and selection rates ranging from 21 to 53% (Karr et al., 2018). Our latent variable re-analysis of the published data demonstrated greater support to the idea of unity of executive functions among child and adolescent samples, whereas the principle of "unity and diversity" was more likely to be observed among adult samples. This finding supports the hypothesis of differentiation of executive functions across the lifespan (Müller & Kerns, 2015).

Overall, these findings suggest that although latent variable continues to be a promising approach for the examination of executive functions, research studies need more thoughtful a priori designs, with more powerful sample sizes, reliable instruments, and better examination of construct validity (e.g., alternative models including other important executive functions). Furthermore, despite the success of Miyake and his research team's approach, the low replicability rates of the three-component model demonstrated by Karr et al.'s (2018) systematic study confirms that the jury is still out on the structure of the executive function construct.

1.4 Executive Functions

Despite great progress in the conceptualization of executive function as a "unity and diversity"-based umbrella term that incorporates several components (Baggetta & Alexander, 2016; Jurado & Rosselli, 2007; Müller & Kerns, 2015), and the psychometric demonstration of a latent structure that may support that conceptualization (Karr et al., 2018; Miyake et al., 2000), there remains an important issue to be addressed, and it is the proliferation of terms assigned as specific executive functions. Unfortunately, there are too many taxonomies and a growing list of components, creating low construct validity and scientific skepticism.

Following a sophisticated (and quite clever) approach, Packwood, Hodgetts, and Tremblay (2011) demonstrated the need to apply the principle of parsimony (or "Occam's razor") to the examination of executive functions; that is, the idea that a phenomenon should be explained by the simplest and most economical theory, with the least number of explanatory or causal variables (Epstein, 1984). When it comes to executive functions, we are far from parsimony. Packwood et al. (2011) conducted a targeted and systematic review of the literature that yielded a selection of 60 papers that met their criteria, and from these publications 68 different executive terms were extracted. This review was followed by a latent semantic analysis (LSA) and a hierarchical cluster analysis (HCA). The LSA estimated the strength of the semantic association between different executive functions, based on their definitions, in such a way that terms that are semantically similar were grouped together based on a similarity score between −1 (opposite meaning) and 1 (identical meaning). The LSA yielded a final term count of 50 after the elimination of semantic redundancies. Five executive functions were identified as the most commonly distinguished in the literature: **Planning** (48%), **working memory** (42%), **inhibition** (42%), **set shifting** (32%), and **fluency** (27%). This result clearly shows the impact of Miyake et al.'s tripartite model.

Moreover, the HCA was used to reduce the number of executive function tasks identified in the literature, as a significant overlap was made evident in their review. The HCA evaluated similarities between task descriptions, using the statements of the authors of the selected papers about what the tasks were measuring. The HCA reduced the original 98 tasks to 18 clusters, which were aligned with 32 of the 50 executive functions identified via the LCA. Therefore, Packwood and her colleagues identified 18 "measurable" executive functions based on their analyses. A large reduction, yet, is still far from achieving parsimony. In this context, they proposed defining executive function as "… a system responsible for the acquisition of task context and the implementation of rules used to guide behavior, regardless of the specific behaviors or response required by a given task (e.g., inhibition of a prepotent response, set shifting)" (Packwood et al., 2011, p. 465). They invite us to focus our research efforts on understanding the dynamics (e.g., executive functioning) rather than the players (i.e., executive functions), as the dynamics are dictated by neural mechanisms that we may be closer to comprehend, whereas the players are only assumed based on the abilities we believe tasks measure, observed only via behavioral outcomes. Wisely, they also reminded us that the interaction of a number of functions might give rise to a large number of alternative behavioral responses, so we may be wasting time by focusing on finding the isolated functions.

Can these multiple functions be conceptually reduced to a more parsimonious taxonomy? Perhaps. Several approaches illustrate this effort. The original tri-factor approach (i.e., **updating**, **shifting**, **inhibition**) proposed by Miyake and his colleagues (2000), including its later versions (e.g., bi-factorial approach including a common executive factor, Friedman & Miyake, 2017), are examples of an effort to achieve parsimony (Karr et al., 2018). Stuss, Shallice, Alexander, and Picton (1995) proposed an approach differing from latent variable analyses (i.e., psychometric) and focusing on brain lesions (i.e., clinical). It is a "going back to the origins" position (e.g., Phineas Cage case, Pribram's and Luria's work), in which the effort was concentrated on the examination of brain–behavior relationships. Stuss and his colleagues emphasized the need to examine the possible fractionation of executive function by studying frontal lobe function in patients with solely focal, single, frontal lobe lesions. They proposed a conceptualization of executive function that includes an aspect of unity (the "root") and diversity ("the branches"). The "root" is represented by attention, the cognitive foundation of all other processes. The "branches" correspond to three processes: (1) **energization**, associated with bilateral superior medial regions, it is the process of initiation and sustaining behavioral responses, particularly in the absence of external triggers or motivators; (2) **task setting**, associated with left lateral frontal areas, particularly involving ventrolateral regions, is the ability to set a stimulus response, starting from an a priori association and progressing to a trial and error-based learned association; and (3) **monitoring**, associated with right lateral prefrontal areas, is the process of inspecting the task performance over time, making adjustments to behavior as needed. Interestingly, inhibition (a classic function assigned to frontal lobes) was not identified in their clinical studies as either uniquely affected by frontal brain damage, or perhaps it is subsumed by energization, task setting, and monitoring (Stuss & Alexander, 2007).

From a developmental perspective, some researchers have proposed that executive functioning can be reduced to **working memory** and **inhibition** (e.g., Bell, Wolfe, & Adkins, 2007; Davidson, Amso, Anderson, & Diamond, 2006) or their interactions (Braver & Barch, 2002; Roberts & Pennington, 1996). Current research does show that both, working memory and inhibition, are indeed essential for executive functioning. While some researchers argue that they are not independent from each other (e.g., Munakata, Snyder, & Chatham, 2012; Roberts & Pennington, 1996), others argue that they are independent (Best, Miller, & Jones, 2009) and are extractable as latent factors from sets of tasks performed by children as young as 3–5 years old (Karr et al., 2018). Developmental neuropsychologist, Martha Denckla, proposed to use the term "**central control processes**" when referring to executive functions, and argues that both **inhibition** and **delayed responding** are the core of executive functioning, while maintenance of anticipatory set/preparedness to act and planning of sequences of selected actions are also good candidates for the central control processes denomination. In her approach, working memory is simply a computation that allows "manipulation of representational systems" (Denckla, 1996).

Inspired by Metcalfe and Mischel's (1999) hot–cool systems framework, Zelazo and Müller (2002) proposed a dichotomy involving "**hot**" (affective aspects) and "**cool**" (cognitive aspects) under the umbrella term of executive function. Their approach was supported by evidence from lesion studies demonstrating such dissociation in neural brain systems, as well as developmental research demonstrating that their trajectories differ, with "hot" executive functions lagging behind in their full development (Zelazo & Carlson, 2012). Similarly, Ardila (2008) proposed a simple dichotomous classification, involving metacognitive and emotional executive functions. **Metacognitive** executive functions, such as problem-solving, planning, working memory, are associated with dorsolateral prefrontal cortex and make up the majority of the reasoning-base abilities measured by neuropsychological tests of executive functions. Their core function is the internal representation of actions. The **emotional** or motivational executive functions, accounted by our neuropsychological tests to a lesser amount, are defined as those involved in our "ability to fulfill basic impulses following socially acceptable strategies" (p. 94). They involve inhibitory control, including emotional and behavioral regulation, and coordinate cognition and emotion via the operations of ventral and orbital prefrontal cortex (Ardila, 2008). Despite their similarity with the "hot" and "cool" dichotomy, Ardila proposes that emotional executive functions are observed earlier in development than their metacognitive counterparts (Ardila, 2013a).

Furthermore, in his book titled, *The Myth of Executive Functioning*, Koziol (2014) made every effort to demonstrate that this construct and the current taxonomies are doomed. After a review of the literature, he concluded that there is not enough evidence for the existence of an executive mechanism. He proposed instead an action control framework that includes two stimulus-based, vertically organized, control systems working in tandem: **a cerebro-cerebellar system** (operating based on anticipatory control) and **a cortico-basal ganglia system** (operating under reward-based instrumental learning principles). In his own words:

> The cognitive control system essentially merged anticipatory control with hierarchically organized "rewards" to meet the needs of adaptive behavioral control. This system did not emerge for the purpose of thinking. Instead, cognition evolved from these systems to serve the needs of interactive behavior. (Koziol, 2014, p. 97)

These neuroanatomical and conceptual models are well founded on neurosciences, supported by developmental theories of phylogeny and ontogeny, but they still need to be better bridged with neuropsychological measurement paradigms for executive functioning, as our traditional clinical instruments over-emphasize cognitive and perceptual processing and under-emphasize action control and emotional/affective regulation.

1.5 Developmental Fractionation of the Executive System

1.5.1 Behavioral Fractionation

Cumulative developmental research has demonstrated the fractionation of higher cognitive functions such as intelligence and executive function from childhood to adulthood (Best et al., 2009; Müller & Kerns, 2015; Tsujimoto, 2008). For instance, several behavioral studies have provided evidence of higher inter-task correlations for tasks involving core executive functions such as inhibition and working memory in children as old as 5–6 years of age, than in older children (e.g., Huizinga & van der Molen, 2007; Senn, Espy, & Kaufmann, 2004; Tsujimoto, Kuwajima, & Sawaguchi, 2007). Although research studies have traditionally emphasized instruments that focus on the "cool" cognitive control processes, cumulative evidence from developmental studies using more affective and "hotter" type of tasks (such as adaptations of the adult Iowa Gambling Task for children; e.g., Prencipe et al., 2011) have demonstrated less differentiation between the "cool" and "hot" components in preschoolers than in older children and adolescents (see Peterson & Welsh, 2014, for a review). Indeed, there is cumulative support for the idea of unidimensionality of executive function in preschool children, mostly from latent variable studies (e.g., Fuhs & Day, 2011; Hughes et al., 2010; Karr et al., 2018; Wiebe et al., 2008, 2011; Willoughby, Blair, Wirth, & Greenberg, 2010, 2012; Willoughby, Wirth, & Blair, 2012).

Our re-analysis of latent variable studies also demonstrated that the unitary model converged more frequently (97% mean convergence), was the most frequently accepted (32–36%), and selected (21–53%; Karr et al., 2018). However, the two-factor model with inhibition and working memory followed closely, and overall, these replication success rates remain small. Müller and Kerns (2015) argue that the majority of these studies could have selected acceptable two-factor executive function models consisting of working memory and inhibition, but they were rejected "on grounds of parsimony" (p. 578). There are several examples of studies that selected their two-factor models as they fit their data much better (e.g., Miller, Giesbrecht, Müller, McInerney, & Kerns, 2012; Usai, Viterbori, Traverso, & De Franchis, 2014), including preschoolers with attention-deficit hyperactivity disorders and disruptive behavior disorder (Schoemaker et al., 2012). Although the literature is reporting somewhat inconsistent findings, a common pattern that emerges is the identification of inhibition and working memory factors in preschoolers, with a shifting factor appearing only later in development (e.g., school age and adolescence; Karr et al., 2018).

It is worth noting that most of these latent variable studies have been conducted using performance-based executive function tasks. A few studies have used behavioral rating scales such as the Behavioral Rating Inventory of Executive Function (BRIEF; Gioia, Isquith, Guy, & Kenworthy, 2000), and the executive functioning scale (Garcia-Barrera, Duggan, Karr, & Reynolds, 2014; Garcia-Barrera, Kamphaus, & Bandalos, 2011) from the Behavior Assessment System for Children (BASC; Reynolds & Kamphaus, 1992, 2004), assessing executive functioning as self-rated or observed (by parents and teachers) in everyday life behavior. For instance, Isquith, Gioia, and Espy (2004) used the parent and teacher ratings from the BRIEF on a sample of preschool children aged 2–5 (mean of 3.6) and showed that executive function was less differentiated in younger children than in older children. Using executive behavior-type items from the BASC Teaching Rating Scale for children 6–11 years old (TRS-C), my team has consistently selected an acceptable multi-dimensional model for executive behavior comprised of four factors: problem-solving, attention control (i.e., shifting, sustaining, focusing), behavioral control (i.e., inhibition) and emotional control (i.e., emotional self-regulation; Garcia-Barrera et al., 2011). The original study was completed with teachers' ratings of 2165 children (60% female) from the standardization sample for the BASC (Reynolds & Kamphaus, 1992). Interestingly, we found inter-factor correlations ranging from $r = -0.50$ to -0.87, with the lowest correlations observed between problem-solving and emotional control scales and the highest between problem-solving and attentional control, and between behavioral control and emotional control, suggesting diversity but also a great deal of overlap between the components. An invariance testing analysis did not show any differences on the factorial composition between the younger (6–8 years of age) and older (9–11) children. Similarly, our longitudinal study on at-risk, low-income sample of 1237 (52% female) children aged 6–11 (Garcia-Barrera, Karr, & Kamphaus, 2013), found inter-factor correlations ranging from $r = -0.54$ to -0.86, with the patterns of lowest and highest correlations replicating quite closely those observed in the Garcia-Barrera et al. (2011). In addition, the study demonstrated similar developmental growth trajectories for the components, with emotional control showing a unique pattern not predicted by age, gender, or their interaction.

We were successful at replicating the four-factor model using the BASC-TRS for 6–11 years old on a sample of 1003 6–11-year-old children, comprised of 848 healthy children (47% female, mean age of 8.34 years) and 155 children (24% female, with a mean age of 8.16 years) diagnosed with ADHD, all from Colombia (Garcia-Barrera, Karr, Duran, Direnfeld, & Pineda, 2015). Consistent with all previous studies, the inter-factor correlations ranged from $r = -0.57$ to 0.95, with the highest correlations observed between behavioral control and emotional control, and the lowest between problem-solving and emotional control. We were also successful at replicating these findings when using the second edition of the BASC (BASC-2, Reynolds & Kamphaus, 2004) Teacher Rating Scale (TRS) and Parent Rating Scale (PRS) for children 6–11 years old (Karr & Garcia-Barrera, 2017). For this study, we used the standardization samples, which consisted of 2092 participants normed on the BASC-2-TRS-C and 2556 participants normed on the BASC-2-PRS-C. Participants mean age for both groups approximated 9 years, and gender was roughly equally distributed (TRS-C: 50.14% female; PRS-C: 48.59% female). Our findings demonstrated not only the consistency of the strength of the four-factor model but also similar patterns of inter-factor correlations, ranging from -0.611 to 0.840 on the TRS-C and ranging from -0.657 to -0.876 for the PRS-C. Interestingly, for both forms, the lowest observed correlations were between problem-solving and behavioral control, whereas the highest were between behavioral and emotional control, and between problem-solving and attentional control.

Using the BASC-2, PRS for Adolescents (BASC-2-PRS-A; Reynolds & Kamphaus, 2004), our team examined the four-factor model in a sample of 2722 healthy adolescents (52.6% female, mean age of 14.79 years). Interestingly, inter-factor correlations were slightly lower than those observed in children, and ranged from $r = 0.58$ to 0.76 (Wong, Sakaluk, & Garcia-Barrera, 2018). Furthermore, these inter-factor correlation patterns diminished even more when the four-factor solution was investigated in young adults, using the standardization sample for the BASC-2 Self-Report for College Students (BASC-2-SRP-COL; $N = 765$) and on an independent replication sample ($N = 197$). The correlations ranged from $r = 0.251$ to 0.629, which are considered low to moderate on the derivation sample and from $r = 0.292$ to 0.683 on the replication sample. It is noteworthy that these patterns showed further differentiation of the four behavioral executive functions assessed with this instrument, in such a way that the inter-factor correlation between emotional control and behavioral control is not longer one of the highest correlations (Duggan, Garcia-Barrera, & Müller, 2018).

In summary, examination of the latent factor structure of executive functions, using confirmatory factor analyses using performance-based tasks, as well as with a range of everyday behavior rating instruments (i.e., BRIEF, BASC-TRS-C, BASC-2 TRS-C and PRS-C; BASC-2 PRS-A, and BASC-2 SRP-COL), has consistently demonstrated enough differentiation of executive components in young children and patterns of de-differentiation from adolescence to young adulthood.

While the latent variable approach has facilitated our examination of the fractionation of executive function processes, it is limited in its capacity to facilitate identification of the dynamic changes on executive functioning occurring throughout the lifespan. In addition, models can become idiosyncratic, reflecting the researchers' originated (and likely biased) choices on task selection and study design. Ultimately, factors are derived (emerging from exploratory factor analysis) or proposed and tested for fit (using CFA) from a set of tasks selected by the researchers. Munakata and her colleagues (2012) proposed a developmental framework for cognitive control that eliminates the reliance on latent factors and specific tasks, while emphasizing three key developmental transitions toward flexible and executive-type behavior. Their theory relies on the development of abstract goal representations and task rule generation and maintenance, and the role of the prefrontal cortex in supporting them (Miller & Cohen, 2001). The first transition, from perseverating to overcoming habits, corresponds to children's developing capacity to overcome automatic responses (e.g., perseveration on overlearned behaviors and old rules). The second developmental transition, reactive to proactive control, involves the temporal dynamics of control, that is, when do children activate goal representations. This new stage is observed when children are able to engage proactive rather than reactive control thanks to an increased ability to actively maintain abstract information and monitor goal-relevant cues. The third key transition, from externally driven to self-directed control, occurs when children are able to exert self-control in the presence of internally generated goals rather than when told. Interestingly, Munakata et al. (2012) framework evolved from a unitary perspective (a single function: processing of abstract goal representations) to a dynamic system that incorporates the development of inhibition, endogenous shifting, and monitoring processes within the increasing capacity of the prefrontal cortex to sustain neuronal firing to maintain and monitor goal-relevant information.

1.5.2 Neural Systems Fractionation

Several neuroimaging studies have demonstrated the protracted structural development of the granular frontal cortex, the prefrontal cortex. The prefrontal cortex is a cortical region characterized by its high volume of pyramidal cells, with a larger amount of dendritic arborization than many other cortical areas, a rich pattern of connectivity with other cortical, subcortical, and cerebellar regions, and delimited as the projection zone of the medial dorsal nucleus of the thalamus. Given these characteristics, it has been proposed that the prefrontal cortex has evolved to support higher-order cognition (Elston, 2003; Fuster, 2000; Goldman-Rakic, 1995; Goldman-Rakic, Cools, & Srivastava, 1996; Miller & Cohen, 2001).

Despite the protracted nature of their development, resting-state fMRI studies have demonstrated the existence of fairly established executive control networks in young infants (Doria et al., 2010). The pattern of maturation of gray matter in prefrontal areas follows a developmental gradient such as there is significant volumetric growth between the approximated ages of 4 and 12 years, and then followed by a reduction in gray matter due to pruning (Giedd et al., 1999; Gogtay et al., 2004), which is completed first within the orbitofrontal cortex, followed by ventrolateral and ventromedial areas, and finishing with the gray matter pruning of the dorsolateral prefrontal cortex (Fuster, 2002). At the same time, between childhood and adolescence, higher intrinsic (within the prefrontal cortex) and extrinsic (prefrontal to other areas) connectivity is achieved, with white matter increasing in volume due to myelination of cortico–cortico axons. These connectivity patterns become more coherent with age, and this coherence is reflected in task performance (Müller & Kerns, 2015). Using functional connectivity approaches from functional magnetic resonance imaging (fMRI), researchers have identified a set of functional networks that appear to be associated with executive control, such as the cognitive control network (Cole, Pathak, & Schneider, 2010) and the fronto-parietal and cingulo-opercular networks (Fair, Dosenbach, Church, Cohen, & Brahmbhatt, 2007). Research has demonstrated that these networks are initially anatomically centralized to a local area, and to become more distributed with increasing age (Ezekiel, Bosma, & Morton, 2013; Fair et al., 2009; Müller & Kerns, 2015; Stevens, Kiehl, Pearlson, & Calhoun, 2007).

Some have attributed this gradual and regional maturation patterns to the functional fractionation observed in higher-order functions (Tsujimoto, 2008). Müller and Kerns (2015) summarized these findings in the context of the classic theories that uphold them, by stating:

> Overall, this pattern of findings supports the differentiation hypothesis of the functional organization of cognitive abilities (Garrett, 1946). This hypothesis states that development proceeds from a relatively undifferentiated and global state toward increasing differentiation and articulation (Werner, 1957). It is also consistent with the interactive specialization theory of brain development, according to which neurocognitive development consists of an increasing functional specialization of neural systems that are initially relatively undifferentiated but become more specialized as a result of interactions between individual and environment. (Johnson & Munakata, 2005) (p. 579)

In young adults, neuroimaging studies have suggested that executive functioning relies on both common areas ("unity") and on differentiated networks depending on the type of task demands, such as those associated with inhibition, updating, or shifting ("diversity"; Collette, Hogge, Salmon, & van der Linden, 2006). In a sophisticated study by Collette et al. (2005), using positron emission tomography (PET), unity appears to be represented in the common activation patterns in parietal areas (e.g., left superior parietal gyrus and right intraparietal sulcus) in conjunction with some lower threshold activation of the left middle and inferior frontal gyri. Updating was associated with bilateral fronto-parietal networks and specifically, a higher engagement of the left frontopolar gyrus. Shifting was associated with a network of parietal areas including the right supramarginal gyrus, left precuneus, and left superior parietal areas, in conjunction with a lower threshold activation of right intraparietal gyrus, and left inferior and middle frontal gyri. Inhibition was less differentiated but further analysis showed that the right orbitofrontal gyrus and right middle and superior frontal gyri were more engaged during inhibitory tasks.

These fronto-parietal functional and structural networks supporting executive functioning have been discussed extensively in the literature, and I believe it is a good place to rest this specific theme. Uttal (2001) reminded us of the futility of placing too much emphasis on localization and compartmentalization of the brain, raising the question: "If there is no impending -indeed, no possible- agreement on what mental components are being measured or what a valid taxonomy of mental components should look like, what credence can be given to the quest to localize such phantoms?" (p. 146). In fact, although Uttal's words are somewhat pessimistic, we have actually progressed little from the findings of earlier work (e.g., Teuber, 1972), despite the implementation of sophisticated neuroimaging technologies and statistical analysis, mostly due to the lack of agreement on the structure of the executive function construct. Acknowledgement that prefrontal cortex function does not equal executive function and that there is a gradient of maturation and fractionation of these executive neural systems, are perhaps, our most relevant discoveries.

1.6 Executive Function and Intelligence

One way to approach the question about the conceptualization of executive function is to differentiate it from other similar constructs that are somewhat better understood, such as "intelligence." Several authors have examined the relationships between these two constructs (e.g., Ardila, Pineda, & Rosselli, 2000; Blair, 2006; Demetriou et al., 2018; Duggan & Garcia-Barrera, 2015; Duncan, 2005; Friedman et al., 2006). For instance, Blair (2006) discusses the compelling evidence in support of the differentiation between fluid aspects of cognition (i.e., executive function) and intelligence. Using his dichotomy, Ardila (2018) argues that general intelligence is related to metacognitive executive functions involving reasoning and problem-solving, but not to the affective (i.e., emotional/motivational) executive functions. On a comprehensive meta-analysis, Ackerman, Beier, and Boyle (2005), examined the literature to systematically investigate the relationship between intelligence and working memory. These authors found that while the two constructs are related, they are dissociable and do not represent a unity, their correlations are modest at most. Their meta-analysis included studies conducted in samples between the ages of 13 and 70 years. On a sample of late twin adolescents (16–18 years old), Friedman et al. (2006) used structural equation modeling to demonstrate that among inhibiting, shifting, and updating working memory representations, only updating was significantly associated with both psychometric crystallized and fluid intelligence components. Brydges and his colleagues (2012) applied the Friedman et al.'s (2006) approach on a sample of children 7–9 years old, and demonstrated that while both constructs were dissociable, a single-factor model of executive function integrating updating, shifting, and inhibition, predicted both fluid and crystallized aspects of intelligence. Studies on aging adults have identified correlations between fluid intelligence and updating (e.g., Salthouse, Atkinson, & Berish, 2003), shifting (Salthouse, Fristoe, McGuthry, & Hambrick, 1998), and inhibition (Salthouse et al., 2003).

Other authors have pursued a different approach, exploring the interactions between these two constructs from a developmental perspective. Demetriou et al. (2018) recently introduced an ambitious theory of the architecture of intelligence unifying cognitive developmental theory and psychometric theory. In this valuable effort, the concept of general intelligence or "*g*" was described as the product of the summation of attention control, flexibility, working memory, cognizance of mental processes, and inference ("$g = f$(attention control + flexibility + working memory + cognizance + inference)"; p. 10). However, the term "cognizance" was defined as an attentional supervisory and monitoring system, not unlike Norman and Shallice's SAS (1986); furthermore, inferential processes were defined as being associated with executive control. Thus, on a commentary note (Müller & Garcia-Barrera, 2018), we proposed that, if one accepts that executive function is comprised of processes such as working memory, attention control, and cognitive flexibility, and that cognizance and inference are also associated with executive functioning (Zelazo, 2015, 2018), Demetrious et al.'s formula may be reducible to $g = f$(executive function). Uttal (2001) stated that defining a term using this circular definition approach is a classic problem with psychological constructs: "invoking one mentalist term to denote the meaning of another" (p. 26).

While the construct "intelligence" derived from psychometric traditions ("Intelligence is what intelligence tests measure", Boring, 1923), the construct 'executive function' derived from frontal lesion studies on animal and humans (Pribram, 1973, 1976). Yet, in a review of the literature (Duggan & Garcia-Barrera, 2015), we identified several commonalities between these two constructs, including: (1) the idea that the development of both (i.e., executive function and intelligence) is characterized by an overall inverted U-trajectory, further defined by unique patterns of differentiation across different components, (2) both, executive functioning and intelligence, are observed via behavioral outputs, assumed to be supported by the operations of a fronto-parietal network and the connections of their key nodes (e.g., prefrontal cortex, cingulate cortex, parietal cortex) to the rest of the brain (e.g., cerebellum, basal ganglia, hippocampus, amygdala); and (3) the idea that both may serve as umbrella terms to represent the integration of cognitive states (i.e., *past/crystallized states* generated by processes such as consolidated knowledge, synthesis, and understanding of time, etc.; *current/fluid cognitive states* produced by processes such as flexibility, monitoring, and inhibiting, and *future-oriented states* generated by processes such as planning, decision-making, and forethought, etc.), supported by foundational processes such as attention (for engagement), processing speed (for efficiency) and working memory (for capacity).

Denckla (1996) once stated, "… if one backed off from the tendency to speak of EF [executive function] as "supraordinate" or "higher-order" processes and remained content with designating EF as "central", one might avoid the many occasions on which neuropsychologists are accused of reinventing the *g* of general intelligence" (p. 265). Based on our review, we concluded that the construct of intelligence seems to refer to the "confluence of the abilities to understand complex ideas and use experience and reasoning to solve problems and adapt to the environment" (Duggan & Garcia-Barrera, 2015, p. 437), and we proposed that the key differentiation between the constructs of intelligence and executive function is their unique role in dealing with complexity versus novelty, respectively. Furthermore, we may be closer to understanding the neural networks involved in executive functioning than those involved in intelligent behavior. Ultimately, they seem to share the same neural areas associated with cognitive abilities supporting them; however, clinical studies have shown a pattern of dissociation, characterized by the relative robustness of psychometric crystallized intelligence to the effects of brain lesions, in contrast to the relative vulnerability of fluid intelligence and executive functions to brain lesions (Lezak, Howieson, Bigler, & Tranel, 2012). Given these patterns of commonalities and differentiation between executive function and intelligence, the question remains: Is there enough evidence of a unique dyexecutive syndrome?

1.7 Dysexecutive Syndrome(s)

Uttal (2001) argues that lesion studies could confirm that a brain region is *necessary* for a behavior, but not necessarily that is *sufficient*. Even in modern neuroimaging studies, sufficiency can be often times only assumed. In other words, if we assumed that a collection of interacting brain regions explains a behavior, it could be expected that an observed behavioral change may be the result of damage to any of those regions, however, it could also be that the observed deficit is "the result of an entirely different organizational aspect of the system" (p. 164). Following this logic, one could expect a range of possible manifestations of executive dysfunctions from the lesions studies on cases with damage to prefrontal, parietal, cingulate areas, or their connections. Some of the questions that this book will answer include: Is there a dysexecutive syndrome?, or are there several dysexecutive syndromes?, or perhaps, are there combinations of several clinical manifestations of executive dysfunctions depending on brain pathology and areas affected? And also, how do we assess executive functions and diagnose their dysfunctions?

Stuss and Alexander (2007) explored the question "Is there a dysexecutive syndrome?" on a review of the literature, with a focus on studies examining patients with brain damage circumscribed solely to the frontal lobes. They used their tripartite model including energization, task setting, and monitoring representing the core frontal lobe executive functions, as their framework. They anticipated their findings by quoting their earlier position:

> If we are correct that there is no central executive, neither can there be a dysexecutive syndrome. The frontal lobes (in anatomical terms) or the supervisory system (in cognitive terms) do not function (in physiological terms) as a simple (inexplicable) homunculus. Monitoring, energizing, inhibition, etc. - these are processes that exist at many levels of

> the brain, including those more posterior 'automatic' processes. Owing to their extensive reciprocal connections with virtually all other brain regions, the frontal lobes may be unique in the quality of the processes that have evolved, and perhaps in the level of processing which might be labeled 'executive' or 'supervisory'. (Stuss & Alexander, 2007, p. 902; Stuss et al., 1995)

Indeed, their review yielded a robust conclusion: there is no undifferentiated, unifying, dysexecutive syndrome. Rather, they demonstrated how lesions to specific regions of the frontal lobes produce specific dysexecutive problems. Specifically, damage to bilateral (but mostly right) superior medial areas (and their connection to anterior cingulate cortex and supplementary motor areas) was associated with deficient energization (e.g., apathy, unmotivation, problems with initiation, concentration and task maintenance, verbal fluency, impaired interference control in the Stroop test). Damage to left lateral frontal areas, particularly ventral components, was associated with impaired task setting (e.g., problems with task analysis, setting task criterion toward producing correct responses, set lost in the Wisconsin Card Sorting Test, false-positive responses in memory tests—i.e., identifying non-listed words as correct, false alarms in go/no-go tasks—i.e., incorrect responses to the no-go stimulus, and inability to use verbal task instructions to guide behavior). Finally, damage to the right lateral frontal regions was associated with impaired monitoring (e.g., problems with modulation of expectancy and time estimation in reaction time tasks, monitoring of temporal information in self-timed conditions, poor error checking and monitoring performance overtime, double recalls in memory tasks—i.e., recalling the same word twice). Stuss and Alexander (2007) concluded that this fractionation should not be confused with independence of these functions; according to their view, frontal executive functions interact on an integrated system that assembles itself in different ways depending on task demands.

Using his dichotomous model for executive functions (i.e., metacognition and motivational/emotional), Ardila (2013b) proposed two corresponding dysexecutive syndromes. First, a "metacognitive dysexecutive syndrome", associated with damage to dorsolateral prefrontal cortex, is characterized by the presence of "an inability to organize a behavioral response to novel or complex stimuli" (p. 2); problems addressing complexity are reflected in patients' poor performance in intellectual ability measures. And second, a motivational/emotional syndrome, associated with damage to the orbitofrontal and medial frontal areas, is characterized by the presence of behavioral and emotional dysregulation symptoms including "disinhibition, inappropriate behaviors, personality changes, irritability, mood liability, tactlessness, distractibility, and disregard of important events" (p. 3). A relevant feature of this syndrome is the impaired social cognition, and presence of apathy (and abulia) and problems initiating behaviors overall.

On a review of the literature on executive function impairments on a range of psychopathologies, Snyder, Miyake, and Hankin (2015) identified, as one would have expected, that deficits in executive function task performance are present in many prevalent psychopathologies, including behavioral disorders such as attention-deficit hyperactivity disorder (ADHD), obsessive-compulsive disorder (OCD), and substance use disorders; mood disorders such as major depression

(MDD) and bipolar disorder (BD); and trauma and stressor related disorders such as posttraumatic stress disorder (PTSD). They used the tripartite model from Miyake et al. (2000) as a framework to examine executive functions, in addition to those executive abilities reflected in "complex tasks" for verbal fluency and planning. Although the common feature is poor performance across tasks, within-diagnosis population variations on effect sizes were observed, such as larger deficits for motor response inhibition than interference control (in the Stroop task) for ADHD, and larger deficits for updating working memory than inhibition and shifting for OCD. Overall, an executive impairment (reflecting unity) seems to be more the rule than the exception for several psychopathologies; yet, variability of case-by-case presentation and differences across research studies makes it difficult to generate a classification system for specific dysexecutive syndromes.

Some of the difficulties in examining impairments of executive functioning (e.g., problems with planning, disinhibition) under the goal of creating an integration of symptoms into syndromes (e.g., dysexecutive syndromes) include the lack of a cohesive and consistent approach to define executive function, and the difficulty clinicians experience in drawing the configuration of its components. Packwood et al. (2011) pointed out that having several taxonomies for the concept of executive function generates problems for clinicians when there are so many ways to refer to the components, and for test makers, when there is no agreement in which tasks should be included in an executive assessment battery. As a result, the proposed structures of commercialized test batteries for the assessment of executive functioning become the reigning models of executive function among clinicians.

As a response to this issue, attempts have been made to adjust theory-driven models to typically used tests. For instance, we recently fitted subtests from the Delis–Kaplan Executive Function System (D-KEFS; Delis, Kaplan, & Kramer, 2001) to a latent factor model determined *a priori*, and including components such as shifting, inhibiting, and fluency (Karr, Hofer, Iverson, & Garcia-Barrera, 2018). The D-KEFS is a nine-test battery composed of traditional and more recently developed measures of executive functions, and we selected it among the alternatives because it has shown to be the most commonly administered test battery of executive functioning in clinical practice (Rabin, Paolillo, & Barr, 2016). Past researchers have evaluated the D-KEFS' latent structure using exploratory factor analysis, and identified a set of latent abilities explaining the test performances (Floyd, Bergeron, Hamilton, & Parra, 2010; Latzman & Markon, 2010). However, task impurity, a recognized issue in the measurement of executive functions (Miyake et al., 2000), is not as well controlled in exploratory designs, hence why we used CFA instead. Using as criteria for model fit a comparative fit index (CFI) ≥ 0.90 and a higher-bound cutoff of ≤ 0.07 for the root-mean-square error of approximation (RMSEA), our CFA demonstrated that the three-factor model fit the data well (CFI = 0.938; RMSEA = 0.047), although a two-factor model, with shifting and fluency merged, fit similarly well (CFI = 0.929; RMSEA = 0.048). However, a bi-factor model fit best (CFI = 0.977; RMSEA = 0.032) and explained the most variance in shifting indicators, but rarely converged among 5000 bootstrapped samples (Karr, Hofer, et al., 2018).

If we agree that there are a range of executive functions (e.g., inhibition, monitoring, shifting), and their corresponding dysfunctions (e.g., disinhibition, poor error detection, inflexibility), another problem in diagnosing dysexecutive syndromes relates to the lack of standards or guidelines about how many executive deficits would be needed in order to consider such diagnosis, that is, we have no current established criteria for a diagnosis of dysexecutive syndromes. An important consideration to have in mind is the fact that intra-individual variability in performance across a set of a given executive tasks is more the norm than the exception, beyond having areas of relative strength and weakness. Some of our work examining performance variability on the D-KEFS using multivariate base rates illustrates this issue (Cook et al., 2018; Karr, Garcia-Barrera, Holdnack, & Iverson, 2017, 2018).

Multivariate base rates allow us to quantify the expected prevalence of low scores among healthy individuals, which is particularly useful in clinical assessments when interpreting multiple test scores, as tends to be the case in clinical neuropsychology, and particularly important when assessing executive functioning. We have demonstrated that healthy children, adolescents, and adults commonly obtain low-test scores on the D-KEFS. For example, when considering all 13 D-KEFS scores one or more low scores were obtained by three out of four children and adolescents using a cutoff of $\leq$16th percentile in a sample of 838 children and adolescents between 8 and 19 years old from the D-KEFS normative sample (52% female; Cook et al., 2018).

In adults, our multivariate base rates analyses for the full and four-test (i.e., Trail Making, Color-Word Interference, Verbal Fluency, and Tower Test) D-KEFS batteries also demonstrated the high prevalence of low scores among the D-KEFS normative sample ($N = 1050$; 52.2% female). Among them, 82.6% of participants obtained at least one score $\leq$16th percentile for the full battery (Karr, Garcia-Barrera, et al., 2018) and 62.8% of them had one or more scores $\leq$16th percentile when the multivariate base rates were computed using only seven scores from the four-test battery (Karr et al., 2017). Overall, these results vary but not by much when considering a smaller number of tests. Also, intelligence (as measured by IQ) and education appeared to be inversely related to low score frequency across the lifespan, in that the prevalence of low scores increased with lower intelligence and fewer years of education.

The literature on the diverse range of executive dysfunctions observed across the lifespan, as part of the aftermath of developmental and acquired brain damage, and in personality and neuropsychiatric disorders, is vast. Detailed discussion follows in the next chapters in this book. To conclude, I will end with Denckla's (1996) words, which in my opinion captures quite well the phenomenology of a "dysexecutive syndrome": "This is the picture of a patient with "pure" EF impairment: "a day late and a dollar short" in most of life's undertakings" (p. 264).

References

Ackerman, P. L., Beier, M. E., & Boyle, M. O. (2005). Working memory and intelligence: The same or different constructs? *Psychological Bulletin, 131*(1), 30.

Ardila, A. (2008). On the evolutionary origins of executive functions. *Brain and Cognition, 68*(1), 92–99.

Ardila, A. (2013a). Development of metacognitive and emotional executive functions in children. *Applied Neuropsychology: Child, 2*(2), 82–87.

Ardila, A. (2013b). There are two different dysexecutive syndromes. *Journal of Neurological Disorders, 1*(1), 1–4.

Ardila, A. (2018). Is intelligence equivalent to executive functions? *Psicothema, 30*(2), 159–164.

Ardila, A., Pineda, D., & Rosselli, M. (2000). Correlation between intelligence test scores and executive function measures. *Archives of Clinical Neuropsychology, 15*(1), 31–36.

Baddeley, A. (1996). Exploring the central executive. *The Quarterly Journal of Experimental Psychology Section A, 49*(1), 5–28.

Baddeley, A. D. (2002). Is working memory still working? *European Psychologist, 7*(2), 85–97.

Baggetta, P., & Alexander, P. A. (2016). Conceptualization and operationalization of executive function. *Mind, Brain, and Education, 10*(1), 10–33.

Banich, M. T. (2009). Executive function: The search for an integrated account. *Current Directions in Psychological Science, 18*(2), 89–94.

Beck, A. T., Ward, C. H., Mendelson, M., Mock, J., & Erbaugh, J. (1961). An inventory for measuring depression. *Archives of General Psychiatry, 4*(6), 561–571.

Bell, M. A., Wolfe, C. D., & Adkins, D. R. (2007). Frontal lobe development during infancy and childhood. In D. Coch, G. Dawson, & K. W. Fischer (Eds.), *Human behavior, learning, and the developing brain: Typical development* (pp. 247–276). New York: Guilford.

Best, J. R., Miller, P. H., & Jones, L. L. (2009). Executive functions after age 5: Changes and correlates. *Developmental Review, 29*(3), 180–200.

Blair, C. (2006). How similar are fluid cognition and general intelligence? A developmental neuroscience perspective on fluid cognition as an aspect of human cognitive ability. *Behavioral and Brain Sciences, 29*(2), 109–125.

Boring, E. G. (1923). Intelligence as the tests test it. *New Republic, 36,* 35–37.

Braver, T. S., & Barch, D. M. (2002). A theory of cognitive control, aging cognition, and neuromodulation. *Neuroscience and Biobehavioral Reviews, 26,* 809–817.

Brydges, C. R., Reid, C. L., Fox, A. M., & Anderson, M. (2012). A unitary executive function predicts intelligence in children. *Intelligence, 40,* 458–469.

Burgess, P. W. (1997). Theory and methodology in executive function research. In P. Rabbitt (Ed.), *Methodology of frontal and executive function* (pp. 81–116). Hove, England: Psychology Press.

Cole, M. W., Pathak, S., & Schneider, W. (2010). Identifying the brain's most globally connected regions. *NeuroImage, 49,* 3132–3148.

Collette, F., Hogge, M., Salmon, E., & Van der Linden, M. (2006). Exploration of the neural substrates of executive functioning by functional neuroimaging. *Neuroscience, 139*(1), 209–221.

Collette, F., Van der Linden, M., Laureys, S., Delfiore, G., Degueldre, C., Luxen, A., et al. (2005). Exploring the unity and diversity of the neural substrates of executive functioning. *Human Brain Mapping, 25*(4), 409–423.

Cook, N. E., Karr, J. E., Brooks, B. L., Garcia-Barrera, M. A., Holdnack, J. A., & Iverson, G. L. (2018). Multivariate base rates for the assessment of executive functioning among children and adolescents. Advance Online Publication. *Child Neuropsychology.*

Davidson, M. C., Amso, D., Anderson, L. C., & Diamond, A. (2006). Development of cognitive control and executive functions from 4 to 13 years: Evidence from manipulations of memory, inhibition, and task switching. *Neuropsychologia, 44,* 2037–2078.

de Frias, C. M., Dixon, R. A., & Strauss, E. (2006). Structure of four executive functioning tests in healthy older adults. *Neuropsychology, 20,* 206–214.

Delis, D. C., Kaplan, E., & Kramer, J. (2001). *Delis-Kaplan Executive Function System (D-KEFS)*. San Antonio, TX: Pearson.

Demetriou, A., Makris, N., Spanoudis, G., Kazi, S., Shayer, M., & Kazali, E. (2018). Mapping the dimensions of general intelligence: An integrated differential-developmental theory. *Human Development, 61*(1), 4–42.

Denckla, M. B. (1996). A theory and model of executive function: A neuropsychological perspective. In G. R. Lyons & N. A. Krasnegor (Eds.), *Attention, memory and executive function* (pp. 263–278). Baltimore, MD: Brooks Publishing.

Dennett, D. C. (1991). *Consciousness explained* (p. 511). Boston: Little, Brown and Co.

Doria, V., Beckmann, C. F., Arichi, T., Merchant, N., Groppo, M., Turkheimer, F. E., et al. (2010). Emergence of resting state networks in the preterm human brain. *Proceedings of the National Academy of Sciences, 107*(46), 20015–20020.

Duggan, E. C., & Garcia-Barrera, M. A. (2015). Executive functioning and intelligence. In S. Goldstein, J. A. Naglieri, & D. Princiotta (Eds.), *Handbook of intelligence: Evolutionary theory, historical perspective, and current concepts* (pp. 435–458). New York: Springer Publishing Co.

Duggan, E. C., Garcia-Barrera, M. A., & Müller, U. (2018). Derivation, replication, and validity analyses of a screener for the behavioral assessment of executive functions in young adults. *Assessment, 25*(7), 867–884.

Duncan, J. (2005). Frontal lobe function and general intelligence: Why it matters. *Cortex, 41*(2), 215–217.

Elston, G. N. (2003). Cortex, cognition and the cell: New insights into the pyramidal neuron and prefrontal function. *Cerebral Cortex, 13*(11), 1124–1138.

Epstein, R. (1984). The principle of parsimony and some applications in psychology. *The Journal of Mind and Behavior,* 119–130.

Eslinger, P. J. (1996). Conceptualizing, describing, and measuring components of executive function. In G. R. Lyons & N. A. Krasnegor (Eds.), *Attention, memory and executive function* (pp. 367–395). Baltimore, MD: Brooks Publishing.

Ettenhofer, M. L., Hambrick, D. Z., & Abeles, N. (2006). Reliability and stability of executive functioning in older adults. *Neuropsychology, 20,* 607–613.

Ezekiel, F., Bosma, R., & Morton, J. B. (2013). Dimensional change card sort performance associated with age-related differences in functional connectivity of lateral prefrontal cortex. *Developmental Cognitive Neuroscience, 5,* 40–50.

Fair, D. A., Cohen, A. L., Power, J. D., Dosenbach, N. U. F., Church, J. A., Miezin, F. M., et al. (2009). Functional brain networks develop from a "local to distributed" organization. *PLoS Computational Biology, 5,* 1–14.

Fair, D. A., Dosenbach, N. U. F., Church, J. A., Cohen, A. L., & Brahmbhatt, S. (2007). Development of distinct control networks through segregation and integration. *Proceedings of the National Academy of Sciences, USA, 104,* 13507–13512.

Floyd, R. G., Bergeron, R., Hamilton, G., & Parra, G. R. (2010). How do executive functions fit with the Cattell–Horn–Carroll model? Some evidence from a joint factor analysis of the Delis-Kaplan Executive Function System and the Woodcock-Johnson III tests of cognitive abilities. *Psychology in the Schools, 47,* 721–738.

Fournier-Vicente, S., Larigauderie, P., & Gaonac'h, D. (2008). More dissociations and interactions within central executive functioning: A comprehensive latent-variable analysis. *Acta Psychologica, 129,* 32–48.

Friedman, N. P., Corley, R. P., Hewitt, J. K., & Wright, K. P., Jr. (2009). Individual differences in childhood sleep problems predict later cognitive executive control. *Sleep: Journal of Sleep and Sleep Disorders Research, 32,* 323–333.

Friedman, N. P., & Miyake, A. (2017). Unity and diversity of executive functions: Individual differences as a window on cognitive structure. *Cortex, 86,* 186–204.

Friedman, N. P., Miyake, A., Altamirano, L. J., Corley, R. P., Young, S. E., Rhea, S. A., et al. (2016). Stability and change in executive function abilities from late adolescence to early adulthood: A longitudinal twin study. *Developmental Psychology, 52,* 326–340.

Friedman, N. P., Miyake, A., Corley, R. P., Young, S. E., DeFries, J. C., & Hweitt, J. K. (2006). Not all executive functions are related to intelligence. *Psychological Science, 17,* 172–179.
Friedman, N. P., Miyake, A., Robinson, J. L., & Hewitt, J. K. (2011). Developmental trajectories in toddlers' self-restraint predict individual differences in executive functions 14 years later: A behavioral genetic analysis. *Developmental Psychology, 47,* 1410–1430.
Friedman, N. P., Miyake, A., Young, S. E., DeFries, J. C., Corley, R. P., & Hewitt, J. K. (2008). Individual differences in executive functions are almost entirely genetic in origin. *Journal of Experimental Psychology: General, 137*(2), 201–225.
Fuhs, M. W., & Day, J. D. (2011). Verbal ability and executive functioning development in preschoolers at head start. *Developmental Psychology, 47,* 404–416.
Fuster, J. M. (2000). Executive frontal functions. *Experimental Brain Research, 133*(1), 66–70.
Fuster, J. M. (2002). Frontal lobe and cognitive development. *Journal of Neurocytology, 31*(3–5), 373–385.
Garcia-Barrera, M. A., Duggan, E. C., Karr, J. E., & Reynolds, C. R. (2014). Examining executive functioning using the Behavior Assessment System for Children (BASC). In S. Goldstein & J. A. Naglieri (Eds.), *Handbook of executive functioning* (pp. 283–299). New York, NY: Springer.
Garcia-Barrera, M. A., Kamphaus, R. W., & Bandalos, D. (2011). Theoretical and statistical derivation of a screener for the behavioral assessment of executive functions in children. *Psychological Assessment, 23,* 64–79.
Garcia-Barrera, M. A., Karr, J. E., Duran, V., Direnfeld, E., & Pineda, D. A. (2015). Cross-cultural validation of a behavioral screener for executive functions: Guidelines for clinical use among Colombian children with and without ADHD. *Psychological Assessment, 27*(4), 1349–1363.
Garcia-Barrera, M. A., Karr, J. E., & Kamphaus, R. W. (2013). Longitudinal applications of a behavioral screener of executive functioning: Assessing factorial invariance and exploring latent growth. *Psychological Assessment, 25*(4), 1300–1313.
Garrett, H. E. (1946). A developmental theory of intelligence. *American Psychologist, 1,* 372–378.
Giedd, J. N., Blumenthal, J., Jeffries, N. O., Castellanos, F. X., Liu, H., Zijdenbos, A., et al. (1999). Brain development during childhood and adolescence: A longitudinal MRI study. *Nature Neuroscience, 2*(10), 861.
Gioia, G. A., Isquith, P. K., Guy, S. C., & Kenworthy, L. (2000). *BRIEF: Behavior rating inventory of executive function*. Lutz, FL: Psychological Assessment Resources.
Gogtay, N., Giedd, J. N., Lusk, L., Hayashi, K. M., Greenstein, D., Vaituzis, A. C., et al. (2004). Dynamic mapping of human cortical development during childhood through early adulthood. *Proceedings of the National Academy of Sciences, 101*(21), 8174–8179.
Goldman-Rakic, P. S. (1995). Architecture of the prefrontal cortex and the central executive. *Annals of the New York Academy of Sciences, 769,* 71–84.
Goldman-Rakic, P. S., Cools, A. R., & Srivastava, K. (1996). The prefrontal landscape: Implications of functional architecture for understanding human mentation and the central executive. *Philosophical Transactions: Biological Sciences,* 1445–1453.
Hughes, C., Ensor, R., Wilson, A., & Graham, A. (2010). Tracking executive function across the transition to school: A latent variable approach. *Developmental Neuropsychology, 35,* 20–36.
Huizinga, M., & van der Molen, M. (2007). Age-group differences in set-switching and set-maintenance on the Wisconsin Card Sorting Task. *Developmental Neuropsychology, 31,* 193–215.
Isquith, P. K., Gioia, G. A., & Espy, K. A. (2004). Executive function in preschool children: Examination through everyday behavior. *Developmental Neuropsychology, 26,* 403–422.
Johnson, M. H., & Munakata, Y. (2005). Processes of change in brain and cognitive development. *Trends in Cognitive Science, 9,* 152–158.
Jurado, M. B., & Rosselli, M. (2007). The elusive nature of executive functions: A review of our current understanding. *Neuropsychology Review, 17*(3), 213–233.
Karr, J. E., Areshenkoff, C. N., Rast, P., Hofer, S. M., Iverson, G. L., & Garcia-Barrera, M. A. (2018). The unity and diversity of executive functions: A systematic review and re-analysis of latent variable studies. *Psychological Bulletin, 144*(11), 1147–1185.

Karr, J. E., & Garcia-Barrera, M. A. (2017). The assessment of executive functions using the BASC-2. *Psychological Assessment, 29*(9), 1182–1187.

Karr, J. E., Garcia-Barrera, M. A., Holdnack, J. A., & Iverson, G. L. (2017). Using multivariate base rates to interpret low scores on an abbreviated battery of the Delis-Kaplan Executive Function System. *Archives of Clinical Neuropsychology, 32*(3), 297–305.

Karr, J. E., Garcia-Barrera, M. A., Holdnack, J. A., & Iverson, G. L. (2018). Advanced clinical interpretation of the Delis-Kaplan Executive Function System: Multivariate base rates of low scores. *The Clinical Neuropsychologist, 32*(1), 42–53.

Karr, J. E., Hofer, S. M., Iverson, G. L., & Garcia-Barrera, M. A. (2018). Examining the latent structure of the Delis–Kaplan Executive Function System. Advance Online Publication. *Archives of Clinical Neuropsychology*.

Koziol, L. F. (2014). *The myth of executive functioning: Missing elements in conceptualization, evaluation, and assessment*. Park Ridge, IL: Springer.

Latzman, R. D., & Markon, K. E. (2010). The factor structure and age-related factorial invariance of the Delis-Kaplan Executive Function System (D-KEFS). *Assessment, 17*(2), 172–184.

Lehto, J. E., Juujärvi, P., Kooistra, L., & Pulkkinen, L. (2003). Dimensions of executive functioning: Evidence from children. *British Journal of Developmental Psychology, 21*(1), 59–80.

Lezak, M. D. (1982). The problem of assessing executive functions. *International Journal of Psychology, 17*(1–4), 281–297.

Lezak, M. D., Howieson, D. B., Bigler, E. D., & Tranel, D. (2012). *Neuropsychological assessment* (5th ed.). New York: Oxford University Press.

Luria, A. R. (1973). *The working brain. An introduction to neuropsychology*. New York: Basic Books.

Metcalfe, J., & Mischel, W. (1999). A hot/cool-system analysis of delay of gratification: Dynamics of willpower. *Psychological Review, 106*(1), 3–19.

Miller, E. K., & Cohen, J. D. (2001). An integrative theory of prefrontal cortex function. *Annual Review of Neuroscience, 24*(1), 167–202.

Miller, M. R., Giesbrecht, G., Müller, U., McInerney, R., & Kerns, K. A. (2012). A latent variable approach to determining the structure of executive function in preschool children. *Journal of Cognition and Development, 13*, 395–423.

Miyake, A., Friedman, N. P., Emerson, M. J., Witzki, A. H., Howerter, A., & Wager, T. D. (2000). The unity and diversity of executive functions and their contributions to complex "frontal lobe" tasks: A latent variable analysis. *Cognitive Psychology, 41*(1), 49–100.

Müller, U., & Garcia-Barrera, M. (2018). Developmental *g*: Lost in the construct jungle. *Human Development, 61*(1), 49–53.

Müller, U., & Kerns, K. (2015). The development of executive function. In R. M. Lerner (Ed.), *Handbook of child psychology and developmental science* (7th ed., pp. 571–623). Wiley.

Munakata, Y., Snyder, H. R., & Chatham, C. H. (2012). Developing cognitive control: Three key transitions. *Current Directions in Psychological Science, 21*(2), 71–77.

Nelson, T. O. (1996). Consciousness and metacognition. *American Psychologist, 51*(2), 102–116.

Norman, D. A., & Shallice, T. (1986). Attention to action. In R. J. Davidson, G. E. Schwartz, & D. Shapiro (Eds.), *Consciousness and self-regulation* (pp. 1–18). New York: Plenum Press.

Packwood, S., Hodgetts, H. M., & Tremblay, S. (2011). A multiperspective approach to the conceptualization of executive functions. *Journal of Clinical and Experimental Neuropsychology, 33*, 456–470.

Peterson, E., & Welsh, M. C. (2014). The development of hot and cool executive functions in childhood and adolescence: Are we getting warmer? In *Handbook of executive functioning* (pp. 45–65). New York, NY: Springer.

Prencipe, A., Kesek, A., Cohen, J., Lamm, C., Lewis, M. D., & Zelazo, P. D. (2011). Development of hot and cool executive function during the transition to adolescence. *Journal of Experimental Child Psychology, 108*(3), 621–637.

Pribram, K. H. (1973). The primate frontal cortex: Executive of the brain. In K. H. Pribram & A. R. Luria (Eds.), *Psychophysiology of the frontal lobes* (pp. 293–314). New York, NY: Academic Press.

Pribram, K. H. (1976). Executive functions of the frontal lobes. In T. Desiraju (Ed.), *Mechanisms in transmission of signals for conscious behavior* (pp. 303–322). Amsterdam, The Netherlands: Elsevier.

Rabin, L. A., Paolillo, E., & Barr, W. B. (2016). Stability in test-usage practices of clinical neuropsychologists in the United States and Canada over a 10-year period: A follow-up survey of INS and NAN members. *Archives of Clinical Neuropsychology, 31*(3), 206–230.

Reynolds, C. R., & Kamphaus, R. W. (1992). *Behavior Assessment System for Children (BASC)*. Circle Pines, MN: AGS.

Reynolds, C. R., & Kamphaus, R. W. (2004). *Behavior Assessment System for Children* (2nd ed.). Bloomington, MN: Pearson.

Roberts, R. J., & Pennington, B. F. (1996). An interactive framework for examining prefrontal cognitive processes. *Developmental Neuropsychology, 12,* 105–126.

Salthouse, T. A., Atkinson, T. M., & Berish, D. E. (2003). Executive functioning as a potential mediator of age-related cognitive decline in normal adults. *Journal of Experimental Psychology: General, 132,* 566–594.

Salthouse, T. A., Fristoe, N., McGuthry, K. E., & Hambrick, D. Z. (1998). Relation of task switching to speed, age, and fluid intelligence. *Psychology and Aging, 13,* 445–461.

Schoemaker, K., Bunte, T., Wiebe, S. A., Espy, K. A., Deković, M., & Matthys, W. (2012). Executive function deficits in preschool children with ADHD and DBD. *Journal of Child Psychology and Psychiatry, 53,* 111–119.

Senn, T. E., Espy, K. A., & Kaufmann, P. M. (2004). Using path analysis to understand executive function organization in preschool children. *Developmental Neuropsychology, 26,* 445–464.

Shallice, T. (2002). Fractioning the supervisory attentional system. In D. T. Stuss & R. T. Knight (Eds.), *Principles of frontal lobe functioning* (pp. 261–277). New York: Psychological Press, Oxford University.

Snyder, H. R., Miyake, A., & Hankin, B. L. (2015). Advancing understanding of executive function impairments and psychopathology: Bridging the gap between clinical and cognitive approaches. *Frontiers in Psychology, 6*(328), 1–24.

Stevens, M. C., Kiehl, K. A., Pearlson, G. D., & Calhoun, V. D. (2007). Functional neural networks underlying response inhibition in adolescents and adults. *Behavior & Brain Research, 181,* 12–22.

Stuss, D. T., & Alexander, M. P. (2007). Is there a dysexecutive syndrome? *Philosophical Transactions of the Royal Society B: Biological Sciences, 362*(1481), 901–915.

Stuss, D. T., Shallice, T., Alexander, M. P., & Picton, T. W. (1995). A multidisciplinary approach to anterior attentional functions. *Annals of the New York Academy of Sciences, 769*(1), 191–212.

Teuber, H. L. (1964). The riddle of frontal lobe function in man. In J. M. Warren & K. Akert (Eds.), *The frontal granular cortex and behavior* (pp. 410–477). New York: McGraw-Hill Book Co.

Teuber, H. L. (1972). Unity and diversity of frontal lobe functions. *Acta Neurobiologiae Experimentalis, 32*(2), 615–656.

Tsujimoto, S. (2008). The prefrontal cortex: Functional neural development during early childhood. *The Neuroscientist, 14*(4), 345–358.

Tsujimoto, S., Kuwajima, M., & Sawaguchi, T. (2007). Developmental fractionation of working memory and response inhibition during childhood. *Experimental Psychology, 54,* 30–37.

Usai, M. C., Viterbori, P., Traverso, L., & De Franchis, V. (2014). Latent structure of executive function in five- and six-year-old children: A longitudinal study. *European Journal of Developmental Psychology, 11,* 447–462.

Uttal, W. R. (2001). *The new phrenology: The limits of localizing cognitive processes in the brain.* The MIT Press.

Vaughan, L., & Giovanello, K. (2010). Executive function in daily life: Age-related influences of executive processes on instrumental activities of daily living. *Psychology and Aging, 25,* 343–355.

Warren, J. M., & Akert, K. (1964). *The frontal granular cortex and behavior*. New York: McGraw-Hill Book Co.

Werner, H. (1957). The concept of development from a comparative and organismic point of view. In D. B. Harris (Ed.), *The concept of development: An issue in the study of human behaviour* (pp. 125–148). Minneapolis, MN: Jones Press.

Wiebe, S. A., Espy, K. A., & Charak, D. (2008). Using confirmatory factor analysis to understand executive control in preschool children: I. Latent structure. *Developmental Psychology, 44,* 575–587.

Wiebe, S. A., Sheffield, T., Nelson, J. M., Clark, C. A. C., Chevalier, N., & Espy, K. A. (2011). The structure of executive function in 3-year-olds. *Journal of Experimental Child Psychology, 108,* 436–452.

Willoughby, M. T., Blair, C. B., Wirth, R. J., & Greenberg, M. (2010). The measurement of executive function at age 3 years: Psychometric properties and criterion validity of a new battery of tasks. *Psychological Assessment, 22,* 306–317.

Willoughby, M. T., Blair, C. B., Wirth, R. J., & Greenberg, M. (2012). The measurement of executive function at age 5: Psychometric properties and relationship to academic achievement. *Psychological Assessment, 24,* 226–239.

Willoughby, M. T., Wirth, R. J., & Blair, C. B. (2012). Executive function in early childhood: Longitudinal measurement invariance and developmental change. *Psychological Assessment, 24,* 418–431.

Wong, R. E., Sakaluk, J. K., & Garcia-Barrera, M. A. (2018). Deriving an adolescent executive behaviour screener from the Behavior Assessment System for Children—2. Advance Online Publication. *Archives of Clinical Neuropsychology*.

Zelazo, P. D. (2015). Executive function: Reflection, iterative reprocessing, complexity, and the developing brain. *Developmental Review, 38,* 55–68.

Zelazo, P. D. (2018). Abstracting and aligning essential features of cognitive development. *Human Development, 61*(1), 43–48.

Zelazo, P. D., & Carlson, S. M. (2012). Hot and cool executive function in childhood and adolescence: Development and plasticity. *Child Development Perspectives, 6*(4), 354–360.

Zelazo, P. D., Carter, A., Reznick, J. S., & Frye, D. (1997). Early development of executive function: A problem-solving framework. *Review of General Psychology, 1*(2), 198–226.

Zelazo, P. D., & Müller, U. (2002). Executive function in typical and atypical development. In *Blackwell handbook of childhood cognitive development* (pp. 445–469).

Chapter 2
Executive Functions Brain Functional System

Alfredo Ardila

2.1 Introduction

The term "executive function" (or "executive functions," or "executive functioning") is relatively new in cognitive neurosciences. The observation that the frontal lobes were involved in regulatory behaviors, such as reasoning, problem-solving, planning, inhibiting responses, strategy development and implementation, and working memory, resulted in the comprehensive term "executive function." Although several authors have suggested that the frontal lobes have a regulatory role in behavior, Luria (1976, 1980) can be considered the direct antecessor of the concept of executive functions. He distinguished three functional units in the brain: (1) arousal-motivation (limbic and reticular systems), (2) receiving, processing, and storing information (post-Rolandic cortical areas), and (3) programing, controlling, and verifying activity (frontal lobes). Luria proposed that this third functional unit had an executive role in behavior. It is frequently said that this concept was integrated by Lezak (1983). Later, Baddeley (1986) grouped these behaviors into cognitive domains that, when impaired, include problems in planning, controlling behaviors, perseveration, reduced fluency, and disinhibition, which coined the term "dysexecutive syndrome."

The definition of executive function usually includes a diversity of cognitive and behavioral abilities, such as the ability to control attention, organize goal-directed behaviors, problem-solving, reasoning, temporality of behavior, inhibitory control, and mental flexibility (Denckla, 1996; Stuss & Knight, 2002). The concepts of morality and self-awareness (consciousness) are also usually included in its definition (Jurado & Rosselli, 2007).

Phineas Gage has become the most classical example for prefrontal lobe pathology and impairments in executive functions. Phineas Gage was a responsible and

A. Ardila (✉)
Sechenov University, Moscow, Russia
e-mail: ardilaalfredo@gmail.com

Albizu University, Miami, FL, USA

A. Ardila et al. (eds.), *Dysexecutive Syndromes*,
https://doi.org/10.1007/978-3-030-25077-5_2

hard-working foreman for a railroad company who suffered a tragic accident in which a tampering rod was projected through his skull, significantly damaging his frontal lobes. Surprisingly, he survived, but after this accident, his behavior completely changed. He was described as "profane," "irascible," and "irresponsible." Significant personality changes were observed, and according to Harlow (1868) he began to behave "as an animal." The Phineas Gage case is frequently used as a typical example of executive function disturbances. Phineas Gage's impairments, however, were mostly situated at the behavioral level, not at a purely cognitive level. Overt behavioral changes were documented as frequently found in prefrontal lobe pathology, but purely cognitive impairments were not reported.

During the late nineteenth and early twentieth centuries, clinical investigators analyzed diverse behavioral disturbances in the cases of frontal pathology. The term "frontal lobe syndrome" was usually used to refer to the behavioral and cognitive disturbances associated with prefrontal pathology. "Frontal lobe syndrome" was conceptualized by Feuchtwanger (1923). He correlated frontal pathology to behaviors that were not related to memory, language, sensory, or motor deficits. He emphasized the personality changes in motivation, emotional dysregulation, and the difficulty to regulate and integrate behavior. Later, Goldstein (1944) expanded the capacity of frontal lobes to include the so-called "abstract attitude," behavior initiation, and mental flexibility. Luria (1966, 1969) related prefrontal lobe activity with programming motor behavior, inhibiting immediate responses, abstracting, problem-solving, verbal regulation of behavior, reorienting behavior according to behavioral consequences, temporal integration of behavior, personality integrity, and also consciousness.

During the 1970s, 1980s, and 1990s, several books mainly or exclusively devoted to the analysis of the prefrontal lobes involvement in behavior and cognition were published (e.g., Fuster, 1989; Levin, Eisenberg, & Benton, 1991; Miller & Cummings, 1998; Perecman, 1987; Pribram & Luria, 1973; Roberts, Robbins, & Weiskrantz, 1998; Stuss & Benson, 1986). These works usually assumed that "frontal" ("prefrontal") syndrome was synonymous with executive dysfunction.

Progressively, it became apparent that disturbances in behavior and cognition can be observed in diverse brain pathologies. The idea that "prefrontal syndrome" and "executive dysfunction" are not synonymous was gradually accepted (Tirapu-Ustárroz, García-Molina, Ríos Lago, & Ardila, 2012). The prefrontal cortex plays a key role in monitoring executive functions, but other brain areas are also involved (Elliott, 2003). Intact frontal processes, although not synonymous with intact executive functioning, are an integral part of it.

Research directed to localize executive functions to discrete brain areas has been developed. The emerging view is that executive functions are mediated by a complex brain system involving diverse areas. Neuroimaging results have also implicated posterior, cortical, and subcortical regions involvement in executive functioning.

In summary, "traditionally," it has been assumed that executive functions are dependent on the prefrontal lobe activity. Several recent studies have attempted to pinpoint the specific brain areas supporting executive functions.

2.2 The Traditional Point of View: Executive Functions Are Supported by Prefrontal Lobe Activity

When the concept of executive functioning was introduced, it was assumed that it was simply the functional correlate of the more anatomical concept of "frontal (or prefrontal) syndrome." Executive dysfunction and frontal lobe damage were frequently used as synonymous, considering that frontal lobe pathology usually was associated with executive functioning impairments.

Furthermore, it became accepted that depending on the location of the damage, frontal lobe damage could result in some specific subtypes of syndrome. Generally, three dysexecutive functions syndromes subtypes were distinguished:

(a) **Dorsolateral syndrome**. Cummings (1993) suggested that the dorsolateral circuit is the most important to executive functioning. Dorsolateral damage is associated with an inability to organize a behavioral response to novel or complex stimuli. Symptoms of these types of syndrome are on a continuum and reflect the capacity to shift cognitive sets, use existing strategies, and organize information in order to meet changing environmental demands. Several authors, including Luria (1969), have noted perseveration, stimulus-bound behavior, echopraxia, and echolalia. Lateralization has been noted in executive dysfunction (Goldberg, 2001). According to Fuster (1997a, 1997b, 2002), the most general executive function of the lateral prefrontal cortex is the temporal organization of goal-directed actions in the domains of behavior, cognition, and language.

(b) **Orbitofrontal syndrome**. Orbitofrontal damage has been associated with disinhibition, disturbances in social abilities, inappropriate behaviors, personality changes, impulsivity, tactlessness, and distractibility (Stuss & Knight, 2002). These patients are unable to correctly and appropriately respond to social cues. However, it has been observed that these patients have no difficulty with card-sorting tasks (Laiacona et al., 1989). Eslinger and Damasio (1985) coined the term "acquired sociopathy" to describe dysregulation that couples both a lack of insight and remorse regarding these behaviors. The orbitofrontal cortex is linked predominantly with limbic and basal forebrain areas.

(c) **Medial frontal syndrome**. Medial frontal lobe damage causes apathy or abulia (a severe form of apathy). Acute and extensive bilateral lesions in the medial frontal areas can be associated with so-called akinetic mutism, in which the individual is awake and has self-awareness, but does not initiate behaviors (Ross & Stewart, 1981). Fuster (1997a, 1997b, 2002) has proposed that the ventromedial areas of the prefrontal cortex are involved in expression and control of emotional and instinctual behaviors.

Figure 2.1 illustrates the orbitofrontal and dorsolateral prefrontal areas.

The idea that there are two basic executive functions has been suggested by several authors (e.g., Fuster, 2001; Happaney, Zelazo, & Stuss, 2004; Stuss, 2011). For instance, a distinction between the "cool" cognitive aspects of executive functions has been proposed, which are more associated with dorsolateral regions of the prefrontal

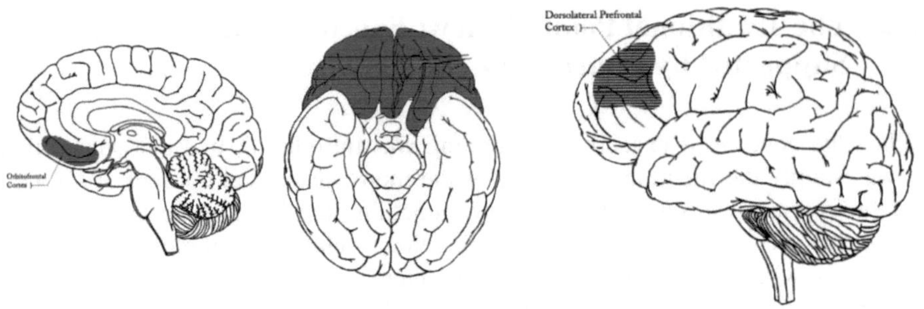

Fig. 2.1 Location of the orbitofrontal and dorsolateral prefrontal areas

cortex, and the "hot" affective aspects, which are more associated with the ventral and medial regions (Zelazo & Muller, 2002). This hot/cool distinction has been applied to the development of executive functions in children (Hongwanishkul, Happaney, Lee, & Zelazo, 2005). Noteworthy, it was observed that whereas cool (metacognitive) executive functions significantly correlate with general intellectual ability ("intelligence") (Ardila, 2018), hot (emotional/motivational) executive functions are not related to general intellectual functioning. As a matter of fact, this basic distinction could be named in diverse ways, for instance, dorsolateral and mesial/orbital executive functions; behavioral and cognitive executive functions; emotion-related and reasoning-related executive functions; intellectual and non-intellectual executive functions, etc.

In a similar vein, Gläscher et al. (2012) applied voxel-based lesion-symptom mapping in 344 individuals with brain focal pathologies, including 165 patients with prefrontal damage. A comprehensive neuropsychological test battery was individually administered. The authors were able to separate two distinct functional–anatomical networks within the prefrontal cortex: (1) the first one associated with cognitive control, involving skills such as response inhibition, conflict monitoring, and switching; this anatomical network included the dorsolateral prefrontal cortex and anterior cingulate cortex. (2) A second functional–anatomical network was associated with value-based decision-making; it included the orbitofrontal, ventromedial, and frontopolar cortex. It was also observed that cognitive control tasks shared a common performance factor related to set shifting; this common factor was linked to the rostral anterior cingulate cortex. By contrast, regions in the ventral prefrontal cortex were required for decision-making.

New findings, both clinical and experimental, progressively suggested that other brain areas in addition to the frontal lobes also participated in executive functions. Although executive function disturbances usually follow focal brain injury of the frontal lobes, not all executive processes are exclusively sustained by the frontal cortex (Andrés & Van der Linden, 2002; Bettcher et al., 2016). Lesions in nearly any part of the brain have been associated with executive dysfunctions (Hausen, Lachmann, & Nagler, 1997).

2.3 A Superordinate Fronto–Cingulo–Parietal Network Supporting Cognitive Control

Departing from an extensive meta-analytic study, Niendam et al. (2012) proposed that there is a superordinate fronto–cingulo–parietal network, supporting cognitive control and may also underlie a range of distinct executive functions.

The authors explain that they performed a search of the BrainMap database (Fox & Lancaster, 2002; Laird et al., 2005) to identify individuals presenting certain specific characteristics: English language, aged 18–60, and using fMRI or PET. One hundred ninety-three functional neuroimaging studies including 2832 healthy individuals were included for their analyses.

The author reports that they selected paradigms that are typically accepted as measures of executive functions or cognitive control. Further filtering and meta-analysis of the experiments was carried out using BrainMap's software applications (Laird et al., 2009).

It was found that across all domains large clusters of significant activation were within certain specific brain areas, including the lateral and medial prefrontal cortex bilaterally, involving the superior, middle, and inferior frontal gyri (Brodmann areas [BAs] 9, 46), as well as the anterior cingulate area (BA32) on the medial aspect of the cerebral hemispheres. In addition to prefrontal activation, large parietal clusters were also found, including the inferior (BA40) and superior (BA7) parietal lobe. Additional activation in frontal regions included the premotor cortex (BA6), frontopolar cortex (BA10), and orbitofrontal cortex (BA11). Activation was also observed in occipital (BA19) and temporal (BAs 22, 37) areas and the insula (BA13). Finally, significant activation was also found in subcortical structures, including the thalamus, caudate, and putamen, as well as some cerebellum regions, such as the posterior declive and anterior culmen. The authors suggest that their findings are consistent with the hypothesis that executive functions are supported by a common set of cortical and subcortical regions including the frontal and parietal areas, as well as the cingulate gyrus and some subcortical structures.

The authors performed an additional analysis to distinguish the activation associated with different executive functions domains: flexibility, inhibition, and working memory. Results revealed similar patterns of common activation in cognitive-control-related frontal and parietal regions, including the dorsolateral prefrontal cortex (BAs 9, 46), anterior cingulate (BA32), inferior (BAs 39, 40) and superior (BA7) parietal lobe, and precuneus (BA19). Domain-specific activation within-group analysis was also found for the three executive function domains:

(1) **Flexibility**. Similar patterns of activation were observed in frontal and parietal regions supporting the cognitive control network, including the dorsolateral prefrontal cortex (BAs 9, 46), cingulate (BAs 32, 24), and both superior (BA7), and inferior (BA40) parietal lobe. Activation was also observed in additional prefrontal (BAs 6, 10, 11), occipital (BA19), and temporal (BAs 37) regions and the insula (BA13).

(2) **Inhibition**. Tasks that require inhibition were associated with activation in frontal and parietal areas, including dorsolateral prefrontal cortex (BAs 9, 46), anterior cingulate gyrus (BA32), and superior (BA7) and inferior (BA40) parietal lobe. Activation was also observed in other prefrontal (BAs 6, 10), occipital (BA19), and temporal (BA13) regions. Subcortical activation included the caudate, thalamus, putamen, and cerebellar declive.
(3) **Working memory**. These tasks elicited the common pattern of frontal–parietal activation associated with the cognitive control network, including the dorsolateral prefrontal cortex (BAs 9, 46), cingulate (BAs 32, 24), and parietal lobe (BAs 7, 40). Activation was also recorded in prefrontal (BAs 6, 10), occipital (BA19), temporal (BAs 37), insular (BA13), and subcortical (thalamus, caudate, putamen, cerebellar declive) regions.

Departing from these results, the authors concluded that executive functions are indeed associated with increased activity in this common cognitive control network, which includes the dorsolateral prefrontal cortex (BAs 9, 46), frontopolar cortex (BA10), orbitofrontal cortex (BA11), and anterior cingulate (BA32). Additional activation is also observed in superior and inferior parietal (BAs 7, 40), occipital (BA19), and temporal (BAs 22, 37), and insular (BA13) cortex, as well as some subcortical areas including the caudate, putamen, thalamus, and cerebellum.

2.4 Cortical-Subcortical Executive Functions Brain System

Ardila, Bernal, and Rosselli (2017) carried out a similar meta-analytic study. The authors also used the same BrainMap database but was accessed on August 2016. Two automatic meta-analyses of peaks of activation across studies/participants were initially conducted (first-level analysis). Two executive functions abilities were selected: reasoning and inhibitory control, considering that they represent the core abilities for the two major subtypes of executive functions (metacognitive and emotional/motivational; see above). The first meta-analysis was intended to assess the brain areas involved in reasoning tasks. The second meta-analysis was intended to assess the specific areas involved in inhibitory control. In the second-level analysis, two between-group contrasts were performed to assess: (a) the areas involved more in reasoning than in inhibitory control (R > I) and (b) the areas involved more in inhibition than in reasoning (I > R).

2.4.1 First-Level Analysis

Query 1: Reasoning. The search conditions were: (1) studies using fMRI; (2) context: normal participants; (3) activations: activation only; (4) handedness: right-handed participants; (5) aged 15–60 years; (6) domain: cognition; and (7) subdomain: reason-

ing. Fifty-four papers with 155 suitable experiments with a total of 2457 participants were found.
Query 2: Inhibition. Search conditions were the same as those used in Study 1, except for subdomain: for this case set to "inhibition." Seventy-seven papers with 191 suitable experiments with a total of 3517 participants were found.

2.4.2 Second Level: Contrast Analysis

Contrast analyses of the two datasets were performed. Two outputs were obtained: (1) inhibition map subtracted from reasoning map (R > I contrast); (2) reasoning map subtracted from inhibition map (I > R contrast). Lateralization indexes (LI) based on the sum of cluster sizes per hemisphere were calculated for each group activation.

2.4.3 Reasoning

It was found that both hemispheres and same brain areas were activated in a relatively symmetrical and similar manner during the performance of reasoning tasks. These areas include: (a) frontal activation area involving some premotor, dorsomedial, and frontopolar zones; (b) parietal area including the superior parietal area and extending toward the inferior parietal (left) and the cingulate gyrus and the occipital (right); (c) the mesial extension of the premotor areas (supplementary motor area). These are the three major areas involved in the "reasoning circuit.". But also—even though in a lesser degree; (d) the insula; and (e) two subcortical areas, located at the level of the basal ganglia and the thalamus. See Fig. 2.2.

2.4.4 Inhibition Control

It was found that (a) very large focus of activation was observed in the right hemisphere, including the insula, the premotor area, and the dorsolateral prefrontal cortex; (b) a second focus of activation, including mesial aspect of the cerebral hemispheres involving the supplementary motor areas and the cingulate gyri; (c) symmetrical clusters of activation in the right and left, including the superior and inferior parietal areas; (d) bilateral activation of the basal ganglia and right thalamus; and (e) a relatively weak activation of the left posterior cingulate gyrus and right posterior inferior temporal gyrus and fusiform gyrus. See Fig. 2.3.

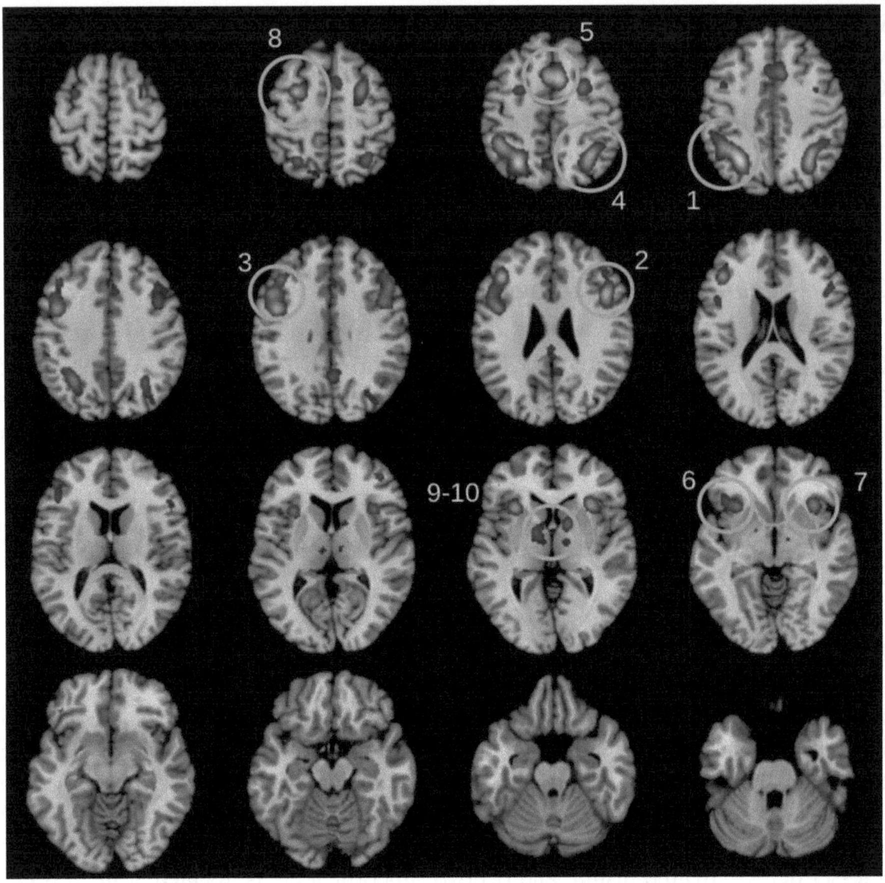

Fig. 2.2 Reasoning: functional connectivity map using meta-analytic connectivity modeling. Sixteen transversal descending cuts have been selected from the brain MRI anatomical volume. Left hemisphere appears on the left side (neurological convention). Clusters are gray-coded for intensity. Main clusters are circled at the most representative level and numbered according to their respective cluster number. *Note* Some areas belonging to the same cluster may appear disconnected due to the discontinuity of the sampling cuts (reproduced with permission)

2.4.5 Contrast Analysis

Areas more involved in reasoning than in inhibitory control. Subtracting the brain areas involved in inhibitory control from the reasoning areas (R > I), it was observed that there are two major and three weaker brain areas involved in reasoning more than in inhibitory control. Both major areas are located in the left hemisphere, and include, on the one hand, a frontal area—BA46, BA9, BA6, and BA8—and on the other, a parietal lobe area—BA39, BA40. In addition, three weaker clusters were found: one bilateral involving the posterior cingulate gyrus; and the other two

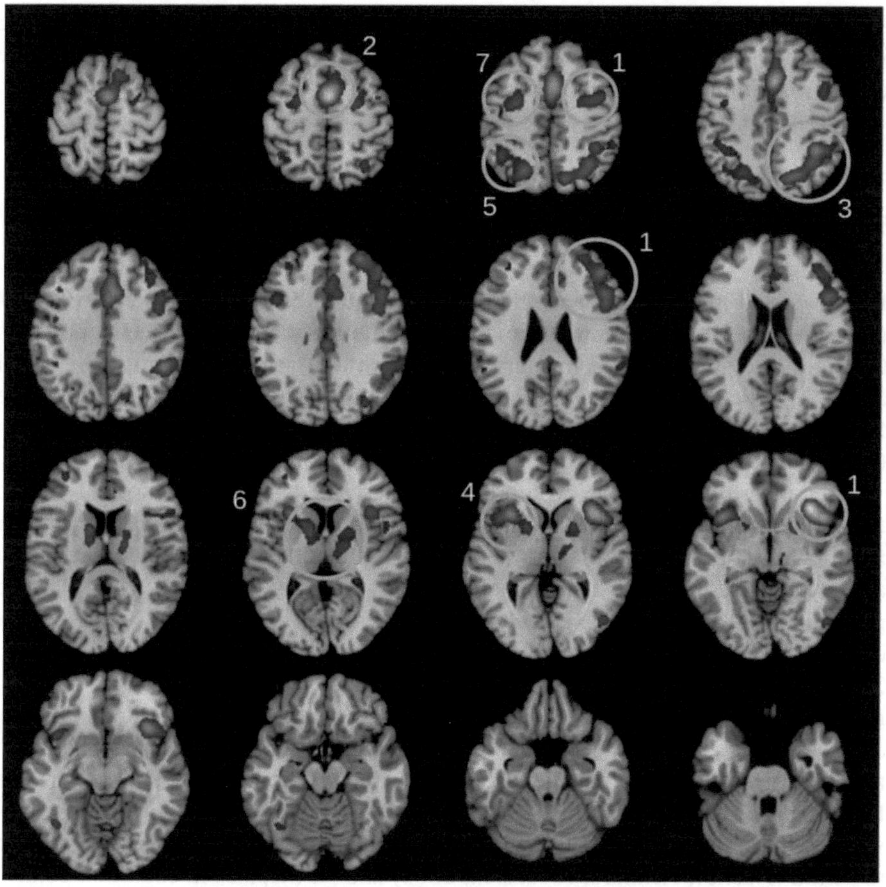

Fig. 2.3 Inhibition: functional connectivity map using meta-analytic connectivity modeling. Image uses the same conventions than the previous one. Main clusters have been circled with their numbers corresponding to cluster numbers. Note that cluster 1 extends from right insula to lateral and dorsal aspects of the frontal lobe (three circles numbered as 1 have been placed in different cuts). Left pre-central and right ganglia-basal clusters mirroring clusters 7 and 4, respectively, have not been circled to avoid cluttering (reproduced with permission)

located in BA6, bilaterally. Strong leftward lateralization was evident. In summary, the major conclusion is that left frontal and parietal areas are more directly involved in reasoning than in inhibition control.

Areas more involved in inhibitory control than in reasoning. Subtracting the brain areas involved in reasoning from the inhibitory control areas, it was deduced those areas participating in the inhibitory control tasks more than in the reasoning tasks (I > R). Results indicated that (a) significant predominant activation of the right hemisphere was observed in inhibition tasks, involving specially the premotor/prefrontal area, and the insula/parietal zones; (b) increased activation was observed bilaterally in some subcortical areas, in particular, the thalamus and the putamen; and (c) in some other cortical areas, an increased activation was observed when performing inhibition tasks; these other areas include the premotor area BA6 and the cingulate area BA32. Summing up, for inhibitory control, leftward lateralization was disclosed.

2.5 Discussion

Results found in both meta-analytic studies are quite coincidental: executive functions are supported by a brain system involving the prefrontal and parietal areas, plus the anterior cingulate/supplementary motor area; it also includes some subcortical areas, in particular, the putamen and the thalamus. If taking two cardinal executive functions, reasoning and inhibitory control, the first one is found to be lateralized to the left and the second one more lateralized to the right hemisphere.

Executive functions have been previously described as localized not only in the frontal lobes but in other lobes (e.g., Andrés & Van der Linden, 2002). Although traditionally it has been supposed that executive functions depend on the prefrontal activity, diverse previous studies, including fMRI studies, have also found that the parietal lobe is directly involved in executive functions (Diamond, 2013; Fassbender et al., 2004; Niendam et al., 2012; Sauseng, Klimesch, Schabus, & Doppelmayr, 2005; Sylvester et al., 2003). Similarly, diverse studies have illustrated the involvement of the supplementary motor area in executive functions. As an example, Bonini and colleagues (2014), using intracerebral recording, observed that the leading role in the neural network underlying the capacity to evaluate the outcomes of our actions—a fundamental executive function—is played by the supplementary motor area. Noteworthy, it has been suggested that the supplementary motor area links cognition to action (Nachev, Kennard, & Husain, 2008) and participates in cognition control (Ridderinkhof, Ullsperger, Crone, & Nieuwenhuis, 2004). Sylvester and colleagues (2003), using fMRI, found the medial "frontal cortex" (BA6/32) participates both in the switching of attention between tasks, and the resolution of interference between competing task responses.

Functional neuroimaging studies have also shown the involvement of the basal ganglia and particularly the putamen in executive functions (Lewis, Dove, Robbins, Barker, & Owen, 2004; Monchi, Petrides, Strafella, Worsley, & Doyon, 2006; Owen, 2004; Rogers, Andrews, Grasby, Brooks, & Robbins, 2000; Sylvester et al., 2003). There is also evidence that the thalamus participates in an executive functions brain system (Alexander, DeLong, & Strick, 1986). Furthermore, there is clear evidence that in the cases of basal ganglia diseases, such as Parkinson and Huntington diseases, impairments in executive functions are found (e.g., Lawrence et al., 1996; Robbins et al., 1994; Owen et al., 1992; Taylor, Saint-Cyr, & Lang, 1986).

Current description of the executive functions' brain system seems to be the best available explanation of the neurological correlates of so-called "executive functions."

References

Alexander, G. E., DeLong, M. R., & Strick, P. L. (1986). Parallel organization of functionally segregated circuits linking basal ganglia and cortex. *Annual Review of Neuroscience, 9,* 357–381.

Andrés, P., & Van der Linden, M. (2002). Are central executive functions working in patients with focal frontal lesions? *Neuropsychologia, 40*(7), 835–845.

Ardila, A. (2018). Is intelligence equivalent to executive functions? *Psicothema, 30*(2), 159–164.

Ardila, A., Bernal, B., & Rosselli, M. (2017). Executive functions brain system: An activation likelihood estimation meta-analytic study. *Archives of Clinical Neuropsychology, 33*(4), 379–405.

Baddeley, A. (1986). *Working memory*. Oxford: Oxford University Press.

Bettcher, B. M., Mungas, D., Patel, N., Elofson, J., Dutt, S., Wynn, M., et al. (2016). Neuroanatomical substrates of executive functions: Beyond prefrontal structures. *Neuropsychologia, 85,* 100–109.

Bonini, F., Burle, B., Liégeois-Chauvel, C., Régis, J., Chauvel, P., & Vidal, F. (2014). Action monitoring and medial frontal cortex: Leading role of supplementary motor area. *Science, 343*(6173), 888–891.

Cummings, J. L. (1993). Frontal-subcortical circuits and human behavior. *Archives of Neurology, 50,* 873–880.

Denckla, M. B. (1996). A theory and model of executive function: A neuropsychological perspective. In G. R. Lyon & N. A. Krasnegor (Eds.), *Attention, memory and executive function* (pp. 263–277). Baltimore: Paul H Brooks.

Diamond, A. (2013). Executive functions. *Annual Review of Psychology, 64,* 135–168.

Elliott, R. (2003). Executive functions and their disorders. *British Medical Bulletin, 65,* 49–59.

Eslinger, P. J., & Damasio, A. R. (1985). Severe disturbance of higher cognition after bilateral frontal lobe ablation: Patient EVR. *Neurology, 35,* 1731–1741.

Fassbender, C., Murphy, K., Foxe, J. J., Wylie, G. R., Javitt, D. C., Robertson, I. H., et al. (2004). A topography of executive functions and their interactions revealed by functional magnetic resonance imaging. *Cognitive Brain Research, 20,* 132–143.

Feuchtwanger, E. (1923). *Die Funktionen des Stirnhirns*. Berlin: Springer.

Fox, P. T., & Lancaster, J. L. (2002). Mapping context and content: The BrainMap model. *Nature Reviews Neuroscience, 3,* 319–321.

Fuster, J. M. (1989). *The prefrontal cortex*. New York: Raven Press.

Fuster, J. M. (1997a). *The prefrontal cortex—Anatomy physiology, and neuropsychology of the frontal lobe*. Philadelphia: Lippincott-Raven.

Fuster, J. M. (1997b). *The prefrontal cortex: Anatomy, physiology, and neuropsychology of the frontal lobe* (3rd ed.). New York: Lippincott, Williams & Wilkins.

Fuster, J. M. (2001). The prefrontal cortex—An update: Time is of the essence. *Neuron, 30,* 319–333.

Fuster, J. M. (2002). Frontal lobe and cognitive development. *Journal of Neurocytology, 31,* 373–385.

Gläscher, J., Adolphs, R., Damasio, H., Bechara, A., Rudrauf, D., Calamia, M., et al. (2012). Lesion mapping of cognitive control and value-based decision making in the prefrontal cortex. *Proceedings of the National Academy of Sciences of the United States, 109*(36), 14681–14686.

Goldberg, E. (2001). *The executive brain*. New York: Oxford University Press.

Goldstein, K. (1944). The mental changes due to frontal lobe damage. *Journal of Psychology, 17,* 187–208.

Happaney, K., Zelazo, P. D., & Stuss, D. T. (2004). Development of orbitofrontal function: Current themes and future directions. *Brain and Cognition, 55,* 1–10.

Harlow, J. M. (1868). Recovery from the passage of an iron bar through the head. *Massachusetts Medical Society Publications, 2,* 327–346.

Hausen, H. S., Lachmann, E. A., & Nagler, W. (1997). Cerebral diaschisis following cerebellar hemorrhage. *Archives of Physical Medicine and Rehabilitation, 78,* 546–549.

Hongwanishkul, D., Happaney, K. R., Lee, W. S., & Zelazo, P. D. (2005). Assessment of hot and cool executive function in young children: Age-related changes and individual differences. *Developmental Neuropsychology, 28*(2), 617–644.

Jurado, M. B., & Rosselli, M. (2007). The elusive nature of executive functions: A review of our current understanding. *Neuropsychology Review, 17,* 213–233.

Laiacona, M., De Santis, A., Barbarotto, R., Basso, A., Spagnoli, D., & Capitani, E. (1989). Neuropsychological follow-up of patients operated for aneurysms of anterior communicating artery. *Cortex, 25,* 261–273.

Laird, A. R., Fox, P. M., Price, C. J., Glahn, D. C., Uecker, A. M., Lancaster, J. L., et al. (2005). ALE meta-analysis: Controlling the false discovery rate and performing statistical contrasts. *Human Brain Mapping, 25,* 155–164.

Laird, A. R., Eickhoff, S. B., Kurth, F., Fox, P. M., Uecker, A. M., Turner, J. A., et al. (2009). ALE meta-analysis workflows via the BrainMap database: Progress towards a probabilistic functional brain atlas. *Frontiers in Neuroinformatics, 3,* 23.

Lawrence, A. D., Sahakian, B. J., Hodges, J. R., Rosser, A. E., Lange, K. W., & Robbins, T. W. (1996). Executive and mnemonic functions in early Huntington's disease. *Brain, 119,* 1633–1645.

Levin, H. S., Eisenberg, H. M., & Benton, A. L. (1991). *Frontal lobe function and dysfunction.* New York: Oxford University Press.

Lewis, S. J., Dove, A., Robbins, T. W., Barker, R. A., & Owen, A. M. (2004). Striatal contributions to working memory: A functional magnetic resonance imaging study in humans. *European Journal of Neuroscience, 19,* 755–760.

Lezak, M. D. (1983). *Neuropsychological assessment.* New York: Oxford University Press.

Luria, A. R. (1966). *Human brain and psychological processes.* New York: Harper & Row.

Luria, A. R. (1969). Frontal lobe syndromes. In P. J. Vinken & G. W. Bruyn (Eds.), *Handbook of clinical neurology* (Vol. 2, pp. 725–757). Amsterdam: North Holland.

Luria, A. R. (1976). *Basic problems of neurolinguistics.* Berlin: Walter de Gruyter.

Luria, A. R. (1980). *Higher cortical functions in man.* New York: Consultants Bureau.

Miller, B. L., & Cummings, J. L. (1998). *The human frontal lobes: Functions and disorders.* New York: The Guilford Press.

Monchi, O., Petrides, M., Strafella, A. P., Worsley, K. J., & Doyon, J. (2006). Functional role of the basal ganglia in the planning and execution of actions. *Annals of Neurology, 59,* 257–264.

Nachev, P., Kennard, C., & Husain, M. (2008). Functional role of the supplementary and pre-supplementary motor areas. *Nature Reviews Neuroscience, 9,* 856–869.

Niendam, T. A., Laird, A. R., Ray, K. L., Dean, Y. M., Glahn, D. C., & Carter, C. S. (2012). Meta-analytic evidence for a superordinate cognitive control network subserving diverse executive functions. *Cognitive, Affective & Behavioral Neuroscience, 12,* 241–268.

Owen, A. M. (2004). Cognitive dysfunction in Parkinson's disease: The role of frontostriatal circuitry. *The Neuroscientist, 10,* 525–537.

Owen, A. M., James, M., Leigh, P. N., Summers, B. A., Marsden, C. D., Quinn, N. A., et al. (1992). Fronto-striatal cognitive deficits at different stages of Parkinson's disease. *Brain, 115,* 1727–1751.

Perecman, E. (Ed.). (1987). *The frontal lobes revisited.* New York: The IRBN Press.

Pribram, K. H., & Luria, A. R. (Eds.). (1973). *Psychophysiology of the frontal lobes.* New York: Academic Press.

Ridderinkhof, K. R., Ullsperger, M., Crone, E. A., & Nieuwenhuis, S. (2004). The role of the medial frontal cortex in cognitive control. *Science, 306,* 443–447.

Robbins, T. W., James, M., Owen, A. M., Lange, K. W., Lees, A. J., Leigh, P. N., et al. (1994). Cognitive deficits in progressive supranuclear palsy, Parkinson's disease, and multiple system atrophy in tests sensitive to frontal lobe dysfunction. *Journal of Neurology, Neurosurgery and Psychiatry, 57,* 79–88.

Roberts, A. C., Robbins, T. W., & Weiskrantz, L. (1998). *The prefrontal cortex: Executive and cognitive functions.* Oxford: Oxford University Press.

Rogers, R. D., Andrews, T. C., Grasby, P. M., Brooks, D. J., & Robbins, T. W. (2000). Contrasting cortical and subcortical activations produced by attentional-set shifting and reversal learning in humans. *Journal of Cognitive Neuroscience, 12,* 142–162.

Ross, E. D., & Stewart, R. M. (1981). Akinetic mutism from hypothalamic damage: Successful treatment with dopamine agonists. *Neurology, 31,* 1435–1439.

Sauseng, P., Klimesch, W., Schabus, M., & Doppelmayr, M. (2005). Fronto-parietal EEG coherence in theta and upper alpha reflect central executive functions of working memory. *International Journal of Psychophysiology, 57,* 97–103.

Stuss, D. T. (2011). Functions of the frontal lobes: Relation to executive functions. *Journal of the International Neuropsychological Society, 17,* 759–765.

Stuss, D. T., & Benson, D. F. (1986). *The frontal lobes.* New York: Raven Press.

Stuss, D. T., & Knight, R. T. (2002). *Principles of frontal lobe function.* Oxford: Oxford University Press.

Sylvester, C. Y. C., Wager, T. D., Lacey, S. C., Hernandez, L., Nichols, T. E., Smith, E. E., et al. (2003). Switching attention and resolving interference: fMRI measures of executive functions. *Neuropsychologia, 41,* 357–370.

Taylor, A. E., Saint-Cyr, J. A., & Lang, A. E. (1986). Frontal lobe dysfunction in Parkinson's disease. *Brain, 109,* 845–883.

Tirapu Ustárroz, J., García-Molina, A., Ríos Lago, M., & Ardila, A. (2012). *Neuropsicología de la corteza prefrontal y las funciones ejecutivas [Neuropsychology of prefrontal cortex and executive functions].* Barcelona: Editorial Viguera.

Zelazo, P. D., & Muller, U. (2002). Executive function in typical and atypical development. In U. Goswami (Ed.), *Handbook of childhood cognitive development.* Oxford, UK: Blackwell.

Part II
Developmental Executive Dysfunction

Chapter 3
Executive Dysfunctions in Attention-Deficit Hyperactivity Disorder

Shameem Fatima

Executive functions (EFs) are the mental control processes that are primarily subserved by the prefrontal area. These functions include processes such as working memory, prioritization, initiation, inhibition allowing to break out maladaptive habits, planning for future goals, decision making and risk evaluation, sequential processing of actions, and flexible adaptation. These processes allow self-regulation by controlling lower cognitive processes such as attention, perception, and motor processes and enable self-directed behaviors for successful routine functioning across the life span. The EFs are, especially, vital in children because these processes allow successful social interaction.

Accordingly, executive dysfunctions represent impaired higher-order cognitive and communicative functions. Executive dysfunctions have been frequently observed in neuro-developmental disorders of autism spectrum disorder, attention-deficit/hyperactivity disorder, phenylketonuria, fetal alcohol syndrome, schizophrenia, obsessive compulsive disorder, and Tourette syndrome. The chapter focuses on attention-deficit/hyperactivity disorder.

Attention-deficit/hyperactivity disorder (ADHD) is a neuro-developmental disorder that is described by a persistent pattern of inattention and/or hyperactivity in an individual which is not seen in healthy individuals at comparable developmental levels. The disorder has been defined in the Diagnostic and Statistical Manual of Mental Disorders-5th edition (DSM-5) as a persistent pattern of inattentive and hyperactive behavior that interferes significantly with functioning of the individual in a variety of contexts including home, school, workplace, social context, etc. (American Psychiatric Association [APA], 2013). It is further explained that the symptoms are classified into two main categories: (i) inattention and (ii) hyperactivity and/or impulsivity. Functional manifestations of inattention are commonly observed in various forms such as disorganization, lack of persistence/perseverance, and problems with maintaining attention which cannot be attributed to a lack of understanding

S. Fatima (✉)
COMSATS University Islamabad, Lahore, Pakistan
e-mail: shameemfatima@cuilahore.edu.pk

A. Ardila et al. (eds.), *Dysexecutive Syndromes*,
https://doi.org/10.1007/978-3-030-25077-5_3

or a challenge. The behavioral manifestations of hyperactivity symptoms are seen in form of unnecessary motor actions, and impulsivity is expressed in quick actions without considering consequences which is mainly derived from a failure in delaying gratification or from a desire for immediate reward.

The problem develops during the neuro-developmental period of childhood but likely to persist for many years or may be for the whole life. The problem is described to be prevalent in approximately 5% children and 2.5% adults around the world (APA, 2013). Other studies have estimated that even two-third (67%) of ADHD children grow up to adulthood period with these symptoms (Ranby et al., 2012). With a particular reference to the symptoms, Sobanski and colleagues have proposed that hyperactivity symptoms incline to decrease, while inattention symptoms tend to increase when an ADHD child grows toward adulthood (Sobanski et al., 2010). In adulthood, individuals with ADHD show symptoms of impulsivity, inattention, and executive deregulation which are manifested in behavioral problems such as impulsive decision-making, trouble in following instructions, high distractibility, difficulty in managing time, working memory impairment, and trouble with quietly involving in leisure activities (Barkley, Murphy, & Fischer, 2008).

The American Psychiatric Association (APA, 2013) contends that during early childhood years, symptoms appear in the form of excessive motor behavior in an ADHD child but due to variability in symptoms, it becomes very difficult to differentiate the symptoms of excessive motor activity from a normal behavior. Arnett, MacDonald, and Pennington (2013) explain that the available screeners are not developmentally sensitive enough to detect any behavioral and cognitive markers of ADHD in preschool years. Therefore, ADHD is quite commonly diagnosed at school when inattention symptoms become apparent and influence school performance. These symptoms tend to stabilize during the early adolescent years. The hyperactivity symptoms in most ADHD individuals become less evident during adolescent or adulthood years but problems of impatience, impulsivity, inattention, and planning difficulty may continue throughout adulthood. This abnormality is relatively stable but some individuals may develop antisocial behavior during adolescence. Prevalence of ADHD is more common in males compared to females with a ratio of 2:1 in children. Females with ADHD commonly show inattention symptoms of ADHD as primary features (APA, 2013).

3.1 Executive Dysfunctions Associated with ADHD

Broadly, the literature describes general cognitive deficits such as deficits in attention, memory, perception, and executive functions in individuals with ADHD (Arnett et al., 2013). More specifically, impairment in executive functions has been considered to be clearly associated with ADHD symptoms. Several theories spotlight the role of executive function deficits in individuals with ADHD (Barkley, 1997; Berger & Posner, 2000; Pennington & Ozonoff, 1996). As executive functions encompass a range of higher regulatory abilities including attention and planning, flexible thinking, ability to use feedback, ability to generate and implement strategies which are critical for goal achievement and successful adaptation in social and academic context, so executive dysfunctions in these regulatory mechanisms can lead to poor adaptation and behavioral and emotional problems (Anderson, Anderson, Northam, Jacobs, & Catroppa, 2001).

Earlier studies have described that these individuals show deficits on several EF measures (Barkley, 1997; Doyle, 2006; Rapport, Chung, Shore, & Isaacs, 2001); however, deficits on inhibitory control measures and inability to inhibit distractions are among the most consistent findings (see for a review Willcutt, Doyle, Nigg, Faraone, & Pennington, 2005; Wodka et al., 2007). Accordingly, based on Barkley's theory of executive dysfunctions in ADHD, it was found that ADHD combined type was clearly associated with executive dysfunctions but no evidence for executive dysfunctions could be found for ADHD inattentive type (Barkley, 1997). Contrarily, a review of differences in executive dysfunctions in ADHD types proposed that ADHD combined type was strongly associated with inhibition difficulties, while the inattentive type was associated with disorganized and lazy behavior (Milich, Balentine, & Lynam, 2001). Similarly, Willcutt et al. (2005) argued that symptoms of ADHD were connected to executive control disorder manifested mainly in inhibitory difficulties in working memory and planning.

Particularly, the research highlights the role of impaired inhibitory control and working memory processes in ADHD symptomology (Doyle, 2006; Martinussen, Hayden, Hogg-Johnson, & Tannock, 2005; Nigg, 2000). Two competing views describe the primacy of inhibition or working memory in ADHD. One view proposed by Barkley (1997) describes that deficit in inhibitory control mechanisms including inhibiting an automatic/well-learned response, discontinuing an ongoing response, and interference control are the primary cognitive impairments central to ADHD symptoms. These primary deficits in inhibitory processes explain secondary deficiencies in working memory system and associated functions. The second view proposes working memory impairment as a "core" deficit in ADHD (Kofler, Rapport, Bolden, & Altro, 2008; Rapport et al., 2001) and inhibition deficits as the downstream products of this core deficit. They explain that a stimulus must reach the working memory system before a response can be inhibited. However, Nigg (2001) contends that although executive inhibitory responses are clearly impaired in ADHD individuals, the concept of inhibition in ADHD should be refined to differentiate between inhibition of executive control and inhibition of motivational control. To Nigg, ADHD symptoms are more likely to be the effect of executive inhibitory control deficits, particularly, of executive motor inhibition deficits in the case of combined type ADHD.

Critically, Gargaro, Rinehart, Bradshaw, Tonge, and Sheppard (2011) have argued that inhibition difficulties are not the only cognitive deficiencies in individuals with ADHD. Johnson and colleagues have compared an ADHD group, a high functioning autism group, and a control group on Sustained Attention to Response Task on fixed and random order presentations. The individuals with ADHD compared to high functioning autism group and normal controls have shown clear deficits of sustained attention as assessed by commission and omission errors as well as greater response time variability. The researchers also explain that impaired arousal and top-down control processes are indicative of involvement of sub-cortical arousal systems and attentional networks in the ADHD pathology (Johnson et al., 2007). Barkley (2006) extends that less activation of behavioral inhibition mechanisms, particularly related to poor interference control may cause problems with sustaining attention.

Furthermore, in a meta-analysis review, Willcutt and colleagues have reported that ADHD individuals compared to controls show deficits on EF measures of planning, working memory (spatial and verbal), vigilance, and inhibition (Willcutt et al., 2005). Moreover, Arnett et al. (2013) have contended that these individuals show marked difficulty in abstracting ideas and anticipating consequences of their actions which may explain their increased impulsivity levels. Additionally, the ADHD group has been reported to display weaker iconic memory compared to normal controls at 50 and 100 ms presentation of visual symbols (Ahmadi et al., 2013).

3.2 Executive Dysfunctions and Functioning of Individual with ADHD

It is suggested that deficits in executive functions, emotional regulation, and inhibitory control mechanisms may explain emotional, behavioral, and academic problems in ADHD individuals (Schoemaker et al., 2012; Sobanski et al., 2010). Executive functions are top-down control mechanisms which regulate cognitions, emotions, and behaviors. Impairment in these regulatory abilities has important cognitive, behavioral, emotional, and social consequences for individuals with ADHD. These individuals are at a higher risk of failure in schools, prone to developing emotional and behavioral problems, and face difficulties in forming and maintaining social relationships. Evidence shows that ADHD children show compromised academic performance in forms of poor grades and lower scores on achievement tests compared to their healthy counterparts (Frazier, Youngstrom, Glutting, & Watkins, 2007). Additionally, other school problems such as higher use of counseling services at schools, a higher dropout rate, and grade retention are also reported frequently in these children (DuPaul et al., 2004; Loe & Feldman, 2007; Molina et al., 2009). It is proposed that inattention symptoms compared to hyperactivity symptoms are more strongly associated with academic problems. Evidence also supports attention problems to be the predictors of poor academic performance in ADHD children (Galera, Melchior, Chastang, Bouvard, & Fombonne, 2009; Merrell & Tymms, 2001) and in children who are below the diagnostic threshold (Breslau et al., 2009; Currie & Stabile, 2006). With particular reference to specific EF deficits, previous researchers have reported working memory to be a correlate of poor school performance and learning problems in children with and without ADHD (Alloway & Alloway, 2010; Alloway, Elliott, & Place, 2010). The role of working memory seems important in classroom assignments, remembering rules and instructions, complex task management, etc. (Alloway, Gathercole, & Elliott, 2010). In the school context, academic difficulties are generally associated with symptoms of inattention while problems in peer interaction are associated with impulsivity and hyperactivity.

In addition to cognitive and academic difficulties, individuals with ADHD face problems in modulating affective conditions and understanding emotional stimuli. Barkley (2006) defines emotional self-regulation as a set of mechanisms that activates appropriate modular emotional reactions to stimuli. Emotional problems of ADHD individuals can be attributed to dysfunctions in the inhibitory control mechanisms. Poor emotional regulation can result in either excessive emotional reactions to certain stimuli, in poor emotional empathy, or in a decreased ability to regulate emotional states. This, in turn, may lead to increased levels of irritability, frustration, or aggressiveness. These individuals show emotional symptoms of emotional instability, emotional liability, extreme emotional reactivity, and low frustration tolerance (Martel & Nigg, 2006; Sobanski et al., 2010). Their family and peer relationships are characterized by frequent discords and negative interactions in the form of peer rejection and neglect. The deficits in emotional regulation are said to be the product of impaired executive control processes (Sobanski et al., 2010). To Barkley (2006), although problems with emotional regulation are not included in the diagnostic criteria of ADHD, yet, these are fundamental features of the disorder.

Evidence from several studies indicates that children with ADHD demonstrate difficulties with self-regulation and behavioral problems due to alterations in sustained attention and inhibitory control (Puentes-Rozo, Barceló-Martínez, & Pineda, 2008). As children with ADHD are unable to put adequate efforts on tasks requiring sustained attention, so they are perceived as lazy, irresponsible, and non-cooperative individuals. In adults with ADHD, the symptoms predict poor occupational success in terms of output, attendance, achievements, and promotions as well as a higher likelihood of unemployment and interpersonal problems (APA, 2013). Other behavioral problems associated with EF deficiencies in individuals with ADHD are problems with financial decisions and deadlines, motivational instability, losing enthusiasm, a lack of self-monitoring, not completing tasks, etc. Additionally, they face problems with taking initiative, inhibiting automatic responses, planning, setting priorities and goals, and time management (Wasserstein & Lynn, 2001). Overall, these individuals complete less schooling and achieve lower grades and poor vocational success. In case of severe symptoms, the individual's academic, occupational, familial, and social adaptability is significantly impaired.

3.3 Neurobiology of Attention-Deficit/Hyperactivity Disorder

Previous literature suggests ADHD symptoms to be correlated with impaired performance on inhibition measures as well as on associated neuropsychological measures assessing sustained attention, delayed gratification, insight, organization and planning, time management, and response time (e.g., Johnson et al., 2007; Willcutt et al.,

2005). To Barkley (2006), these findings suggest the contribution of multioperational location systems of brain which are likely to be mediated by specific neurotransmitter. Currently, researchers have started neurophysiological and neuroimaging assessments of individuals with ADHD alongside the neuropsychological assessment and cognitive testing. Although the related research is still in its infancy, the neural correlates of executive dysfunctions in ADHD have been started to be discovered by structural and functional neuroimaging studies.

A growing body of neuroimaging studies link abnormalities in brain regions related to prefrontal cortex with compromised performance on tasks assessing executive functions (Moore, Schettler, Killiany, Rosene, & Moss, 2012; Petrides, 2000; Ravizza & Ciranni, 2002; Stern et al., 2000). More specifically, neuroimaging studies provide evidence for the link of inhibitory deficits with deficient neural activity within the fronto-striatal and fronto-parietal circuits in ADHD individuals (Arnsten, 2009; De La Fuente, Xia, Branch, & Li, 2013; Dickstein, Bannon, Castellanos, & Milham, 2006; Hart, Radua, Nakao, Mataix-Cols, & Rubia, 2013; Seidman, Valera, & Makris, 2005). Due to PFC changes, these individuals suffer from executive control disorders generally expressed in inhibitory difficulties (Willcutt et al., 2005). Also, evidence from meta-analysis studies describes a consistent pattern of hypoactivation in frontal areas of the brain in ADHD compared with controls individuals (Cortese et al., 2012; Dickstein et al., 2006). Due to PFC changes, these individuals suffer from executive control disorders generally expressing in inhibitory difficulties (Willcutt et al., 2005).

Neuroimaging studies have tried to recognize the pathophysiology of ADHD by assessing the abnormal structural and functional patterns in brain areas that are typically involved in attention, executive functions, response inhibition, working memory, motor control, and emotional regulations. Accordingly, several studies describe the involvement of brain structures in the frontal cortex including prefrontal cortex, basal ganglia, and posterior cortex in ADHD symptoms (Arnsten & Li, 2005). Additionally, a review study by Cortese and colleagues, based on 55 MRI studies, has shown bilaterally reduced size of putamen, reduced volumes of right anterior frontal cortex and left caudate nucleus in individuals with ADHD (Cortese et al., 2012). Also, the review has reported that children with ADHD show lower measurements on cerebellum activity throughout their childhood and adolescent years. In addition, they reported a slightly reduced right PFC and a more symmetrical left PFC in individuals with ADHD that may likely affect higher regulatory cognitive abilities of inhibition, planning, sustained focus, and organization of information (Cortese et al., 2012; Doyle, 2006).

The findings from studies conducted on samples of children with ADHD compared to controls have revealed a consistent pattern of hypoactivation in frontal brain areas involved in executive functioning and attention including fronto-parietal areas and ventral attentional network. Further studies with children samples have shown hypoactivation in somatomotor networks (Cortese et al., 2012). Furthermore, findings from electroencephalogram studies indicate the link of ADHD symptoms with brain activity, supporting the increased activity level in the EEG (Boutros, Fraenkel, & Feingold, 2005). A different activity pattern in electrophysiological measurements have been shown in children with ADHD compared to controls on exposure to emotional stimuli (Singhal et al., 2012), on inhibitory tasks (Bruckmann et al., 2012), and in reaction time in cognitive testing (McLoughlin, Palmer, Rijsdijk, & Makeig, 2014).

3.4 Biochemical Correlates of ADHD

Research on the neurobiological basis of ADHD shows dysfunctional biochemical processes particularly related to dopamine, noradrenaline, and serotonin which may cause impairments in cognitive processes (Volkow et al., 2011). Accordingly, dopamine transmission theory of ADHD proposes dysfunctional dopaminergic activation in two brain regions: first, hypoactivation in anterior cingulate cortical regions causing cognitive deficits, and second, hyper-activation in sub-cortical regions particularly in caudate nucleus leading to excessive motor activation (Castellanos, 1997). Additionally, Arnsten, Steere, and Hunt (1996) propose abnormal activation of noradrenaline in two brain regions: (i) underactivation in cortical dorsolateral prefrontal region which relates to core working memory deficits; and (ii) overactivation of the subcortical region of locus coeruleus relating to over-alertness in ADHD.

3.5 Treatment

Treatment for ADHD symptoms can help reduce the symptoms and improve attention and concentration.

3.5.1 Multimodal Treatment of ADHD

Although pharmacotherapy has been proven helpful and successful for treating ADHD symptoms, it should be combined with psychotherapy for more effectiveness and better results. Therefore, a multimodal treatment plan is better recommended for ADHD treatment. Medical treatment may include medications that may help the patient to concentrate better, remain calm, and be less impulsive. The stimulant drugs such as methylphenidate may work by activating brain areas relation to attention. Other drugs such as Atomoxetine, a noredrenaline reuptake inhibitor may increase noradrenaline in brain areas which in turn can also help concentrate and reduce impulsive behavior.

Alongside medical treatment, different psychological therapies can be useful for relieving the ADHD symptoms. Among these are included: psycho-education, cognitive behavior treatment, social skills training, and parent education and training. Many of these psychotherapies have been implemented previously with effective outcomes in ADHD patients. For example, implementing cognitive behavior therapy, coaching, and behavior therapy including parent training in clinical setting or at home and in school setting have been shown to be effective (e.g., Knight, Rooney, & Chronis-Tuscano, 2008; Pelham & Fabiano, 2008). Furthermore, interventions aimed at promoting attention skills such as "the Pay Attention! Program" has also shown positive improvement in attention (Tamm et al., 2010). Empirical evidence suggests that interventions aiming at alleviating not only the ADHD symptoms but also the patient's day to day functioning using multimodal treatments including medical and psychosocial, prove more effective than the medical treatment alone (Reeves & Anthony, 2009).

Psycho-education may aid in educating the individual with ADHD about the symptoms of the disease and its effects on daily life. It can also educate the individual to become an active part of the treatment agency for effective results. *Behavior therapy* commonly targets behavior problems. By using reward system, it controls disorganized and impulsive behavior. For improvement, first list down the behavior problems and identify good behaviors needed to be introduced, set rewards, implement step by step, but consistently. The therapy can include teachers and parents in the treatment plan to make them learn how to plan and structure behaviors and activities and to motivate and admire the child on improvements. *Cognitive behavior therapy* may help the patients identify, analyze, and change maladaptive thinking patterns with more rational and adaptive thinking pattern which may, in turn, result in adaptive behavior. *Social skills training* should be used in combination with other psychological and pharmacological treatment plans. It involves teaching the child how to behave in different social contexts using adaptive social skills. It may involve role-playing and modeling techniques. *Parent education and training* should be an integral part of the psychosocial intervention. It involves educating parents about the disease and its effect on daily functioning. It also includes tailoring parents to learn specific ways of talking to and playing, involving, and working with the child with ADHD. This may help the child in focusing attention and reducing impulsive and disorganized behavior.

Other possible treatments may include healthy diet and use of food supplements. Individuals with ADHD are recommended to use a healthy and a balanced diet. Deficiencies in certain nutritious dietary elements can worsen ADHD symptoms. Protein-rich and healthy food helps in making neurotransmitters and is important for brain health, so it is a protective factor against ADHD symptoms. Also, these individual are recommended to avoid processed and junk food as well as fizzy drinks. Some studies have suggested that certain food supplements such as omega 3 and omega 6 fatty acids as well as zinc, iron, and magnesium can supplement nutrient deficiencies and help in making neurotransmitter involved in attention and concentration (Konofal, Lecendreux, Arnulf, & Mouren, 2004; Johnson, Ostlund, Fransson, Kadesjö, & Gillberg, 2009).

3.5.2 Executive Functioning Interventions

A new line of research suggests that interventions aiming at specific executive dysfunctions may also help in relieving ADHD symptoms. Recently, empirical evidence proposes that executive functions can be promoted in children and adolescents through specific activities as well as by using EF training. Researchers recommend that EF improvement in children with ADHD can help reduce impulsive behaviors and improve attention and memory which may, in turn, promote better self and emotional regulation (Diamond, Barnett, Thomas, & Munro, 2007). Menezes and colleagues contend that instead of cognitive training, ecological EF intervention should be focused for more generalization and improvement in EF-related daily functioning in these individuals (Menezes, Dias, Trevisan, Carreiro, & Seabra, 2015).

3.6 Comorbid Disorders with ADHD

Clinical research and related discussion in DSM-5 describes the presence of several comorbid disorders in individuals with ADHD (APA, 2013). The ADHD is described to be extremely comorbid disorder with more than 60–70% of individual with ADHD showing symptoms of other psychiatric disorders (Cherkasova, Sulla, Dalena, Pondé, & Hechtman, 2013; Spencer, 2006).

3.6.1 Comorbid Disorders in Childhood

Behavioral problems are the most frequent comorbidities in children with ADHD. Among these are oppositional defiant disorders (ODD) and conduct disorder (CD). Other comorbid conditions include autism spectrum disorder and specific learning disabilities.

3.6.1.1 Oppositional Defiant Disorder

The comorbidity of the ODD is described to be in about 50% of the combined type and in about 25% of the inattentive type ADHD children (APA, 2013). In such comorbid cases, children are psychologically and emotionally more impaired. During early school years, comorbidity of ADHD and oppositional defiant behavioral problems likely predispose children in bullying involvement. However, effective treatments are likely to decrease the risk of further psychological problems in adulthood years such as anxiety, depression, or substance abuse. For the optimal treatment of individuals with comorbid ADHD and ODD, it is better recommended to combine pharmacotherapy with psychosocial treatment particularly behavior therapy. Behavior therapy should incorporate treatment plans targeting time management, response inhibition training, setting rules, and establishing goals. For ODD, the treatment usually involves the introduction of rules and aims to re-establish generational limits.

3.6.1.2 Conduct Disorder

The occurrence of conduct disorder is reported in about a quarter of combined-type ADHD children and adolescents (APA, 2013). Prevalence of conduct disorder has been reported to be in about 2–9% of the population, and its prevalence is particularly higher in individuals from low socioeconomic status (Baker, 2013). Comorbidity of CD with ADHD also adds to the severity of the cognitive and behavioral problems. Children with comorbidity of ADHD and CD symptoms are reported to have a poor prognosis and are vulnerable to develop disorders including substance abuse and antisocial personality disorder in adulthood (Barkley, Fischer, Smallish, & Fletcher, 2004). The comorbidity of both can be explained by the shared risk factor hypothesis which states that each of the two disorders is a risk as well as the precursor of developing the other disorder (Shachar & Tannock, 1995). With comorbid symptoms of the two disorders, medications for ADHD symptoms in combination with drugs for aggressive symptoms are recommended. However, it is strongly recommended to use psychosocial intervention along with pharmacotherapy in a multimodal approach for more effective outcomes.

3.6.1.3 Autism Spectrum Disorder

Estimates suggest that two-third of individuals with ADHD manifest symptoms of autism (Davis & Kollins, 2012). Therefore, neurological studies seek to identify common neurological substrates that may link with similarities in neuropsychological profiles in individuals with both disorders or with comorbid conditions. Empirical evidence shows that patients with autism as well ADHD patients are impaired on working memory and cognitive flexibility, while impairment on inhibitory control differentiates between two with ADHD combined-type patients showing inhibition deficiencies compared to autistic patients (Paloscia et al., 2013).

3.6.1.4 Learning Disorder

Specific learning disorders are also reported to be a comorbid diagnosis in ADHD children. It is estimated that nearly one-fourth of ADHD children (20–25%) also meet the diagnostic criteria for any learning disorder (Pliszka, 2000). However, the adverse effects of ADHD symptoms on academic output persist even after controlling the effects of learning disorders (Currie & Stabile, 2006) and behavior problems (Giannopulu, Escolano, Cusin, Citeau, & Dellatolas, 2008).

3.6.2 Comorbidities with ADHD in Adulthood

Comorbidities of psychiatric disorders with ADHD also differ depending on the life stage. For example, as discussed above, children with ADHD are more likely to share symptoms of ODD, CD, autism, and learning disorder. However, adults with ADHD are more likely to develop any anxiety disorder, substance abuse, antisocial or any other personality disorder, or social phobia, but children are more likely to have comorbid oppositional disorder and separation anxiety (Biederman et al., 1993).

It has been reported that adults with ADHD have co-occurring diagnosis of anxiety in 47%, any mood disorder in 38%, impulse control in 20%, and substance use disorders in 15% of patients (Kessler et al., 2006). However, sometimes symptoms of ADHD are obscured due to more robust symptoms of the comorbid disorder or the vice versa. Few of these comorbid symptoms may be the outcome of the impact of ADHD symptoms. For example, anxiety may be the aftereffect of poor academic outcome due to ADHD. On the other side, depression may share the common environmental risk factor with ADHD (Faraone & Biederman, 1997).

References

Ahmadi, N., Goodarzi, M. A., Hadianfard, H., Mohamadi, N., Farid, D., et al. (2013). Comparing iconic memory in children with and without attention deficit hyperactivity disorder. *Iranian Journal of Psychiatry, 8*(3), 131–137.

Alloway, T. P., & Alloway, R. G. (2010). Investigating the predictive roles of working memory and IQ in academic attainment. *Journal of Experimental Child Psychology, 106*(1), 20–29.

Alloway, T. P., Elliott, J., & Place, M. (2010). Investigating the relationship between attention and working memory in clinical and community samples. *Child Neuropsychology, 16*(3), 242–254.

Alloway, T. P., Gathercole, S. E., & Elliott, J. (2010). Examining the link between working memory behavior and academic attainment in children with ADHD. *Developmental Medicine & Child Neurology, 52*(7), 632–636.

American Psychiatric Association. (2013). *Diagnostic and statistical manual of mental disorders* (5th ed.). Washington, DC, USA: American Psychiatric Association.

Anderson, V. A., Anderson, P., Northam, E., Jacobs, R., & Catroppa, C. (2001). Development of executive functions through late childhood and adolescence in an Australian sample. *Developmental Neuropsychology, 20*(1), 385–406.

Arnett, A. B., MacDonald, B., & Pennington, B. F. (2013). Cognitive and behavioral indicators of ADHD symptoms prior to school age. *Journal of Child Psychology and Psychiatry and Allied Disciplines, 54,* 1284–1294.

Arnsten, A. F. (2009). Toward a new understanding of attention-deficit hyperactivity disorder pathophysiology: An important role for prefrontal cortex dysfunction. *CNS Drugs, 23,* 33–41.

Arnsten, A. F., & Li, B. M. (2005). Neurobiology of executive functions: Catecholamine influences on prefrontal cortical functions. *Biological Psychiatry, 57*(11), 1377–1384.

Arnsten, A. F., Steere, J. C., & Hunt, R. D. (1996). The contribution of alpha 2-noradrenergic mechanisms of prefrontal cortical cognitive function. Potential significance for attention deficit hyperactivity disorder. *Archives of General Psychiatry, 53,* 448–455.

Baker, K. (2013). Conduct disorders in children and adolescents. *Paediatrics and Child Health, 23,* 24–29.

Barkley, R. A. (1997). Behavioral inhibition, sustained attention, and executive functions: Constructing a unifying theory of ADHD. *Psychological Bulletin, 121*(1), 65–94.
Barkley, R. A. (2006). A theory of ADHD. In R. A. Barkley (Ed.), *Attention-deficit hyperactivity disorder. A handbook for diagnosis and treatment* (pp. 297–334). New York, NY: Guilford Press.
Barkley, R. A., Fischer, M., Smallish, L., & Fletcher, K. (2004). Young adult follow-up of hyperactive children: Antisocial activities and drug use. *Journal of Child Psychology and Psychiatry, 45,* 24–36.
Barkley, R. A., Murphy, K. R., & Fischer, M. (2008). *ADHD in adults: What the science says.* New York, NY: Guilford Press.
Berger, A., & Posner, M. (2000). Pathologies of brain attentional networks. *Neuroscience & Biobehavioral Reviews, 24*(1), 3–5.
Biederman, J., Faraone, S. V., Spencer, T., Wilens, T., Norman, D., Lapey, K. A., et al. (1993). Patterns of psychiatric comorbidity, cognition, and psychosocial functioning in adults with attention deficit hyperactivity disorder. *American Journal of Psychiatry, 150*(12), 1792–1798.
Boutros, N., Fraenkel, L., & Feingold, A. (2005). A four-step approach for developing diagnostic tests in psychiatry: EEG in ADHD as a test case. *Journal of Neuropsychiatry and Clinical Neuroscience, 17,* 455–464.
Breslau, J., Miller, E., Breslau, N., Bohnert, K., Lucia, V., & Schweitzer, J. (2009). The impact of early behavior disturbances on academic achievement in high school. *Pediatrics, 123*(6), 1472–1476.
Bruckmann, S., Hauk, D., Roessner, V., Resch, F., Freitag, C. M., Kammer, T., et al. (2012). Cortical inhibition in attention deficit hyperactivity disorder: New insights from the electroencephalographic response to transcranial magnetic stimulation. *Brain, 135,* 2215–2230.
Castellanos, F. X. (1997). Toward a pathophysiology of attention-deficit/hyperactivity disorder. *Clinical Pediatrics, 36,* 381–393.
Cherkasova, M., Sulla, E. M., Dalena, K. L., Pondé, M. P., & Hechtman, L. (2013). Developmental course of attention deficit hyperactivity disorder and its predictors. *Journal of Canadian Academy of Child and Adolescent Psychiatry, 22*(1), 47–54.
Cortese, S., Kelly, C., Chabernaud, C., Proal, E., Di Martino, A., Milham, M. P., et al. (2012). Toward systems neuroscience of ADHD: A meta-analysis of 55 fMRI studies. *American Journal of Psychiatry, 169,* 1038–1055.
Currie, J., & Stabile, M. (2006). Child mental health and human capital accumulation: The case of ADHD. *Journal Health Economics, 25*(6), 1094–1118.
Davis, N. O., & Kollins, S. H. (2012). Treatment for co-occurring attention deficit/hyperactivity disorder and autism spectrum disorder. *Neurotherapeutics, 9*(3), 518–530.
De La Fuente, A., Xia, S., Branch, C., & Li, X. (2013). A review of attention-deficit/hyperactivity disorder from the perspective of brain networks. *Frontiers in Human Neuroscience, 7.*
Diamond, A., Barnett, W. S., Thomas, J., & Munro, S. (2007). Preschool program improves cognitive control. *Science, 318*(5855), 1387–1388.
Dickstein, S. G., Bannon, K., Castellanos, F. X., & Milham, M. P. (2006). The neural correlates of attention deficit hyperactivity disorder: An ALE meta-analysis. *Journal of Child Psychology and Psychiatry, 47*(10), 1051–1062.
Doyle, A. E. (2006). Executive functions in attention-deficit/hyperactivity disorder. *Journal of Clinical Psychiatry, 67,* 21–26.
DuPaul, G. J., Volpe, R. J., Jitendra, A. K., Lutz, J. G., Lorah, K. S., et al. (2004). Elementary school students with AD/HD: Predictors of academic achievement. *Journal of School Psychology, 42,* 285–301.
Faraone, S. V., & Biederman, J. (1997). Do attention deficit hyperactivity disorder and major depression share familial risk factors? *Journal of Nervous and Mental Disorder, 185*(9), 533–541.
Frazier, T. W., Youngstrom, E. A., Glutting, J. J., & Watkins, M. W. (2007). ADHD and achievement: Meta-analysis of the child, adolescent, and adult literatures and a concomitant study with college students. *Journal of Learning Disabilities, 40*(1), 49–65.

Galera, C., Melchior, M., Chastang, J. F., Bouvard, M. P., & Fombonne, E. (2009). Childhood and adolescent hyperactivity-inattention symptoms and academic achievement 8 years later: The GAZEL Youth study. *Psychological Medicine, 39*(11), 1895–1906.

Gargaro, B. A., Rinehart, N. J., Bradshaw, J. L., Tonge, B. J., & Sheppard, D. M. (2011). Autism and ADHD: How far have we come in the comorbidity debate? *Neuroscience and Biobehavioral Reviews, 35*(5), 1081–1088.

Giannopulu, I., Escolano, S., Cusin, F., Citeau, H., & Dellatolas, G. (2008). Teachers' reporting of behavioural problems and cognitive-academic performances in children aged 5–7 years. *British Journal of Educational Psychology, 78,* 127–147.

Hart, H., Radua, J., Nakao, T., Mataix-Cols, D., & Rubia, K. (2013). Meta-analysis of functional magnetic resonance imaging studies of inhibition and attention in attention-deficit/hyperactivity disorder: Exploring task-specific, stimulant medication, and age effects. *JAMA Psychiatry, 70,* 185–198.

Johnson, K. A., Robertson, I. H., Kelly, S. P., et al. (2007). Dissociation in performance of children with ADHD and high-functioning autism on a task of sustained attention. *Neuropsychologia, 45*(10), 2234–2245.

Johnson, M., Ostlund, S., Fransson, G., Kadesjö, B., & Gillberg, C. (2009). Omega-3/omega-6 fatty acids for attention deficit hyperactivity disorder: A randomized placebo-controlled trial in children and adolescents. *Journal of Attention Disorders, 12*(5), 394–401.

Kessler, R. C., Adler, L., Barkley, R., Biederman, J., Conners, C. K., Demler, O., et al. (2006). The prevalence and correlates of adult ADHD in the United States: Results from the National Comorbidity Survey Replication. *American Journal of Psychiatry, 163*(4), 716–723.

Knight, L. A., Rooney, M., & Chronis-Tuscano, A. (2008). Psychosocial treatments for attention deficit/hyperactivity disorder. *Current Psychiatry Reports, 10*(5), 412–418.

Kofler, M. J., Rapport, M. D., Bolden, J., & Altro, T. A. (2008). Working memory as a core deficit in ADHD: Preliminary findings and implications. *The ADHD Report, 16,* 8–14.

Konofal, E., Lecendreux, M., Arnulf, I., & Mouren, M. C. (2004). Iron deficiency in children with attention-deficit/hyperactivity disorder. *Archives of Pediatrics & Adolescent Medicine, 158*(12), 1113–1115.

Loe, I. M., & Feldman, H. M. (2007). Academic and educational outcomes of children with ADHD. *Journal of Pediatric Psychology, 32*(6), 643–654.

Martel, M. M., & Nigg, J. T. (2006). Child ADHD and personality/temperament traits of reactive and effortful control, resiliency, and emotionality. *Journal of Child Psychology and Psychiatry and Allied Disciplines, 47,* 1175–1183.

Martinussen, R., Hayden, J., Hogg-Johnson, S., & Tannock, R. (2005). A meta-analysis of working memory impairments in children with attention-deficit/hyperactivity disorder. *Journal of the American Academy of Child and Adolescent Psychiatry, 44*(4), 377–384.

McLoughlin, G., Palmer, J. A., Rijsdijk, F., & Makeig, S. (2014). Genetic overlap between evoked frontocentral theta-band phase variability, reaction time variability, and attention-deficit/hyperactivity disorder symptoms in a twin study. *Biological Psychiatry, 75,* 238–247.

Menezes, A., Dias, N. M., Trevisan, B. T., Carreiro, L. R., & Seabra, A. G. (2015). Intervention for executive functions in attention deficit and hyperactivity disorder. *Arqquivos di Neuro-Psiquiatria, 73*(3), 227–236.

Merrell, C., & Tymms, P. B. (2001). Inattention, hyperactivity and impulsiveness: Their impact on academic achievement and progress. *British Journal of Educational Psychology, 71*(1), 43–56.

Milich, R. B., Balentine, A. C., & Lynam, D. R. (2001). ADHD combined type and ADHD predominantly inattentive type are distinct and unrelated disorders. *Clinical Psychology: Science and Practice, 8,* 463–488.

Molina, B. S., Hinshaw, S. P., Swanson, J. M., Arnold, L. E., Vitiello, B., et al. (2009). The MTA at 8 years: Prospective follow-up of children treated for combined-type ADHD in a multisite study. *Journal of the American Academy of Child and Adolescent Psychiatry, 48*(5), 484–500.

Moore, T. L., Schettler, S. P., Killiany, R. J., Rosene, D. L., & Moss, M. B. (2012). Impairment in delayed nonmatching to sample following lesions of dorsal prefrontal cortex. *Behavioral Neuroscience, 126*(6), 772–780.

Nigg, J. T. (2000). On inhibition/disinhibition in developmental psychopathology: Views from cognitive and personality psychology and a working inhibition taxonomy. *Psychological Bulletin, 126*(2), 220–246.

Nigg, J. T. (2001). Is ADHD a disinhibitory disorder? *Psychological Bulletin, 127*(5), 571–598.

Paloscia, C., Baglioni, V., Alessandrelli, R., Rosa, C., Guerini, R., Aceti, F., et al. (2013). Executive function deficits in ADHD and Asperger syndrome. *Rivista di Psichiatria, 48*(6), 441–447.

Pelham, W. E., Jr., & Fabiano, G. A. (2008). Evidence-based psychosocial treatments for attention-deficit/hyperactivity disorder. *Journal of Clinical Child and Adolescent Psychology, 37*(1), 184–214.

Pennington, B. F., & Ozonoff, S. (1996). Executive functions and developmental psychopathology. *Journal of Child Psychology and Psychiatry, 37*(1), 51–87.

Petrides, M. (2000). The role of the mid-dorsolateral prefrontal cortex in working memory. *Experimental Brain Research, 133*(1), 44–54.

Pliszka, S. R. (2000). Patterns of psychiatric comorbidity with attention-deficit/hyperactivity disorder. *Child & Adolescent Psychiatric Clinics of North America, 9*(3), 525–540.

Puentes-Rozo, P. J., Barceló-Martínez, E., & Pineda, D. A. (2008). Behavioral and neuropsychological characteristics of children of both sexes, between 6 and 11 years of age, with attention deficit hyperactivity disorder. *Revista de Neurologia, 47,* 175–184.

Ranby, K. W., Boynton, M. H., Kollins, S. H., McClernon, F. J., Yang, C., & Fuemmeler, B. F. (2012). Understanding the phenotypic structure of adult retrospective ADHD symptoms during childhood in the United States. *Journal of Clinical Child and Adolescence Psychology, 41,* 261–274.

Rapport, M. D., Chung, K. M., Shore, G., & Isaacs, P. (2001). A conceptual model of child psychopathology: Implications for understanding attention deficit hyperactivity disorder and treatment efficacy. *Journal of Clinical Child Psychology, 30*(1), 48–58.

Ravizza, S. M., & Ciranni, M. A. (2002). Contributions of the prefrontal cortex and basal ganglia to set shifting. *Journal of Cognitive Neuroscience, 14*(3), 472–483.

Reeves, G., & Anthony, B. (2009). Multimodal treatments versus pharmacotherapy alone in children with psychiatric disorders: Implications of access, effectiveness, and contextual treatment. *Pediatric Drugs, 11*(3), 165–169.

Schoemaker, K., Bunte, T., Wiebe, S. A., Andrews, K., Deković, M., & Matthys, W. (2012). Executive function deficits in preschool children with ADHD and DBD. *Journal of Child Psychology and Psychiatry and Allied Disciplines, 53,* 111–119.

Seidman, L. J., Valera, E. M., & Makris, N. (2005). Structural brain imaging of attention-deficit/hyperactivity disorder. *Biological Psychiatry, 57*(11), 1263–1272.

Shachar, R., & Tannock, R. (1995). Test of four hypotheses for the comorbidity of attention-deficit hyperactivity disorder and conduct disorder. *Journal of American Academy of Child and Adolescent Psychiatry, 34,* 639–648.

Singhal, A., Shafer, A. T., Russell, M., Gibson, B., Wang, L., Vohra, S., et al. (2012). Electrophysiological correlates of fearful and sad distraction on target processing in adolescents with attention deficit-hyperactivity symptoms and affective disorders. *Frontiers in Integral Neuroscience, 6,* 119.

Sobanski, E., Banaschewski, T., Asherson, P., Buitelaar, J., Chen, W., Franke, B., et al. (2010). Emotional liability in children and adolescents with attention deficit/hyperactivity disorder (ADHD): Clinical correlates and familial prevalence. *Journal of Child Psychology and Psychiatry and Allied Disciplines, 51,* 915–923.

Spencer, T. J. (2006). ADHD and comorbidity in childhood. *Journal of Clinical Psychiatry, 67*(Suppl 8), 27–31.

Stern, C. E., Owen, A. M., Tracey, I., Look, R. B., Rosen, B. R., & Petrides, M. (2000). Activity in ventrolateral and mid-dorsolateral prefrontal cortex during nonspatial visual working memory processing: Evidence from functional magnetic resonance imaging. *Neuroimage, 11*(1), 392–399.

Tamm, L., Hughes, C., Ames, L., Pickering, J., Silver, C. H., Stavinoha, P., et al. (2010). Attention training for school-aged children with ADHD: Results of an open trial. *Journal of Attention Disorders, 14*(1), 86–94.

Volkow, N. D., Wang, G. J., Newcorn, J. H., Kollins, S. H., Wigal, T. L., Telang, F., et al. (2011). Motivation deficit in ADHD is associated with dysfunction of the dopamine reward pathway. *Molecular Psychiatry, 16,* 1147–1154.

Wasserstein, J., & Lynn, A. (2001). Metacognitive remediation in adult ADHD: Treating executive function deficits via executive functions. *Annals of the New York Academy of Sciences, 931*(1), 376–384.

Willcutt, E. G., Doyle, A. E., Nigg, J. T., Faraone, S. V., & Pennington, B. F. (2005). Validity of the executive function theory of attention-deficit/hyperactivity disorder: A meta-analytic review. *Biological Psychiatry, 57*(11), 1336–1346.

Wodka, E. L., Mahone, E. M., Blankner, J. G., Larson, J. C., Fotedar, S., et al. (2007). Evidence that response inhibition is a primary deficit in ADHD. *Journal of Clinical and Experimental Neuropsychology, 29*(4), 345–356.

Chapter 4
Executive Dysfunctions in Autism Spectrum Disorders

Shameem Fatima

Autism spectrum disorder (ASD), a neurodevelopmental disorder, is characterized by socio-communicative problems. Autistic individuals are impaired on social interaction and communication as well as they show repetitive behaviors and restricted interests (American Psychological Association, 2013). However, presentation of ASD symptoms varies depending on the range of functioning and severity of symptoms. Although, the level of impairment varies in autistic individuals, however, the functional consequences are universally life altering for both the individual and the family (Newschaffer et al., 2007). So, individuals with ASD at each end of the spectrum are labeled differently, i.e., low functioning individuals with ASD are known to be autistic, while high functioning individuals are diagnosed to have an Asperger syndrome. But autistic term has been used in this chapter to refer to whole spectrum of the disorder.

In 2002, the disorder has been described to be prevalent in 6 or 7 out of 1000 persons with a ratio of 3:1 for males versus females (Fombonne, 2009). Recently, APA (2013) reports that prevalence of ASD has been increased to 1 in 100 individuals with similar prevalence rates in children and adults. However, it is unclear whether the increased ratio reveals a true increase in frequency or is an artifact of expanded diagnostic criteria for the disorder or of increased awareness. Of note, the diagnostic criteria in DSM 5 have been expanded to include individuals diagnosed with DSM-IV diagnosis of (a) autistic disorders including early infantile autism, childhood autism, Kanner's autism, and atypical autism, (b) Asperger's disorder, (c) pervasive developmental disorder not otherwise specified, and (d) childhood disintegrative disorder. Among clinically referred cases, male to female diagnostic ratio is 4:1. Interestingly, clinically referred diagnosed female patients commonly show symptoms of co-occurring intellectual or learning disabilities. Therefore, it may be the case that females with subtle socio-communication symptoms may remain undiagnosed, if they do not show intellectual disabilities (APA, 2013).

S. Fatima (✉)
COMSATS University Islamabad, Lahore, Pakistan
e-mail: shameemfatima@cuilahore.edu.pk

A. Ardila et al. (eds.), *Dysexecutive Syndromes*,
https://doi.org/10.1007/978-3-030-25077-5_4

4.1 Diagnostic Symptoms of ASD

American Psychiatric Association (2013) classifies ASD symptoms into two major categories: criteria A—social impairment and communication difficulties, and criteria B—repetitive and restricted behaviors. More generally, the symptoms of the disorder are classified into three core deficits: (i) impairment in social interaction, (ii) communication difficulties, (iii) repetitive and stereotyped behavior (Newschaffer et al., 2007).

4.1.1 Impairment in Social Interaction

Early signs of social impairment in autistic children can be seen in the first or second year of life in the form of lack of joint attention. These early children are unable to point, show, or bring any object to an adult to share enjoyment and interest. They are described to be unable to show spontaneous but functional and contextual gestures in communication. Children and adolescents with autism show clear deficits of social and emotional reciprocity. They are unable to successfully share their thoughts and feelings with others. They show little interest in initiating social interaction. Their language is usually one-sided and lacking social reciprocity because the language is usually used to request or label rather than to exchange conversation and share thoughts and emotions. Even the adults with ASD who have learned strategies to compensate their social skill deficits face difficulties in novel and unusual social situations. They may also have to struggle very hard to recognize differential appropriateness of same behavior in multiple contexts because the behavior suitable in one context is not necessarily suitable in other contexts. Usually, they prefer solitary activities or prefer to interact with much younger or much older participants (APA, 2013).

4.1.2 Communication Difficulties

Individuals with ASD experience varying levels of language difficulties from no speech at all to poor expression and comprehension of speech, language delays, and stiff or literal language. They are unable to successfully reciprocate language and exchange conversation. However, language impairment profile changes with age and developmental maturation level. Communication difficulties become evident since early years of life from problems in joint attention and deficient vocal outputs. Normal language developmental processes are absent in children with ASD. Oral motor impairment in addition to a lack of motivation for social communication may cause language difficulties (Mody & Belliveau, 2013); therefore, social impairment and communication difficulties go side by side in autism, and thus kept in one category

(category A) in APA (2013). Even the high functioning adults with good language may feel problem in coordinating verbal language with nonverbal communication or may show exaggerated body language.

4.1.3 Repetitive and Stereotyped Behaviors

Individuals with ASD also manifest some repetitive and restricted behaviors and activities. These behaviors may include simple repetitive behaviors (e.g., fingers taping, toy flipping, etc.), repetitive speech, and stereotypical use of words or phrases. They show high resistance to novelty or change and prefer to stick to routine and restricted activities. They even show distress and resistance on packing of out of season wears. Some of their routine activities may relate to their excessive or lesser sensitivity to external sensory stimuli that may be expressed in heightened responses to specific sounds, smells, or textures. However, many autistic adults without co-occurring language or intellectual impairment are able to suppress their repetitive or stereotyped behaviors in social situations.

4.2 Functional Consequences of Autism Spectrum Disorder

Symptoms of ASD can have many functional consequences. Social symptoms and communication disabilities of autism may slow down learning processes, particularly the learning which is based on social or peer interaction. Adaptive and intellectual skills in more than 70% of these individuals are below average. Due to severe problems with planning, organization, and their inability to cope with novelty and change, academic achievement of students with ADHD, even those having above average IQ, is hampered.

In the context of home, their sensory sensitivities and resistance to change may pose difficulties in daily activities of eating, sleeping, and routine care—for example, nail and haircuts, dental care, and self-care. High co-occurrence with below average intellectual abilities may make their adaptation and adjustment very difficult. Daily activities such as meal preparation, personal hygiene, money handling, and time management are important life skills to live independently. Due to planning and organization difficulties, they feel severely deficient in such daily activities. Also, language skills in childhood years correlate with daily life skills in children with autism (Szatmari et al., 2009). Gray et al. (2014) have reported that autistic children and adolescents with poor daily life skills are less likely to achieve post-secondary education and employment. High functioning autistics children and adolescents can manage routine activities in close supervision. However, as adults, they cannot live independently. Even autistic adults without intellectual disabilities experience poor psychosocial functioning in terms of independent living and useful employment.

Functional consequences of autism in older age are not clear, but social and communication problems may likely to have challenging health consequences (APA, 2013).

4.3 Cognitive Theories in Relation to ASD

Many theories have tried to explain the autistic symptomology in relation to executive dysfunctions. Among these, three main cognitive theories have tried to explain the brain and behavior link in autism. These theories are: the Theory of Mind Deficit Hypothesis (Frith, 2003a; Kimhi, 2014), Weak Central Coherence (Noens & van Berckelaer-Onnes, 2008), and Executive Dysfunction Theory (see Hill, 2004, for a review).

The former two hypotheses together can account many of the symptoms, deficits, and assets of ASD. The third one, the theory of executive dysfunctions, may best explain repetitive behaviors and restricted interests.

4.3.1 Theory of Mind

The theory of mind, also known as mentalising is described as the cognitive ability to recognize, attribute, and manipulate mental states such as beliefs and desires. Mentalising ability rapidly develops in typically developing young children but develops at a very slow rate in children with autism (Frith, 2003a). For example, Joseph and Tager-Flusbergs (2004) predicted autism symptoms from theory of mind and executive functions on a sample of 31 school-aged autistics children. It was reported that theory of mind and executive control explained a significant amount of variance in communication symptoms of ASD beyond the effects of language but no such evidence could be found for social interaction or repetitive behaviors symptoms. Neuroimaging studies have identified a neural network that centers on the para-cingulate cortex, the superior temporal cortex, and the bilateral temporal poles, which is active during mentalising. It has been found that high functioning individuals with ASD show insignificant activation in the neural network and related brain areas involved in mentalising (Castelli, Frith, Happé, & Frith, 2002; Happé et al., 1996).

4.3.2 Weak Central Coherence

Some of the features of autistic individuals can be explained by the account of weak central coherence (Noens & van Berckelaer-Onnes, 2008). The central coherence account illustrates a processing style rather than a deficit. The account describes the tendency of the individual to process information in its relevant context. In the case of strong coherence, the contextual information is processed at the cost of details of the event. While, on the other hand, piecemeal and detailed information is attended and memorized at the expense of contextual information in the case of weak central coherence. For example, when a typically developing individual is asked to retell a story, he would describe the general picture of the story in its context, but would not be able to describe the details of chunks. On the other hand, individuals with autism would find it easier to describe the detail of the subparts rather than the general gist of the story.

The individuals with autism possess some strengths which become weaknesses on certain occasions. These individuals express enhanced local processing but weak integrated processing. These individuals show highest scores on tests taping factual knowledge as well as on tasks requiring focused attention on details. On the other hand, they score very poorly on tasks assessing common sense comprehension and on tasks taping overall/contextual explanation of the event. The theory of weak central coherence explains this deficit of common sense comprehension and/or deviance from the theme. Studies also support the role of enhanced local processing in auditory modalities in individuals with ASD (Mottron, Peretz, & Menard, 2000). However, later extensions of this account suggest that weak central coherence account emphasizes on enhanced focus on individual elements but does not propose poor gestalt integration.

Neurological bases for this account have not yet been studied sufficiently. However, a beginning postulation proposes that bottom up information processing stages, where sensory information is processed, are mature enough in these individuals to pay full attention to sensory details of the event. However, top-down information processing stages where information is related with the reserved cognitive resources are not fully functional in these individuals (Frith, 2003b).

4.3.3 Executive Dysfunction Theory

Third and well-documented account is the Executive Dysfunction Theory (see Hill, 2004, for a review), which proposes that executive dysfunctions are responsible for behavioral manifestations of autistic symptoms, particularly, the repetitive and restricted behaviors. Executive functions as an umbrella term for several higher order mental regulatory operations allow an individual to disengage from the immediate context to plan, organize, coordinate, and execute actions to achieve their goals. Interest in executive dysfunctions in autistic individuals has been increased over the last 2–3 decades. Prior studies have investigated EFs in high- and low-functioning individuals with ASD, and in almost all situations, both children and adolescents with autism have shown clear behavioral problems associated with impairments of several executive functions, including planning, cognitive flexibility, shifting attention, selective or sustained attention, verbal fluency, visual working memory, and inhibition (e.g., Courchesne et al., 1994; see O'Hearn, Asato, Ordaz, & Luna, 2008 for review; Ozonoff, 1995a). These executive dysfunctions are proposed to be a likely explanation of the rigid and repetitive behaviors as well as non-core cognitive symptoms of ASD. Although, a little consensus has developed regarding the specificity of executive dysfunctions related to autistic symptoms, most of the studies have concluded a developmental delay in executive functions in ASD. A review based on functional MRI studies also provides evidence for these delays in high functioning autism which are likely to be related to less adapted use of executive functions in adulthood (O'Hearn et al., 2008).

4.3.3.1 Early Signs of Executive Dysfunctions in ASD

Given the fact that frontal lobe starts developing in young children, the researchers have assessed samples of preschool-aged children using less complex tasks of executive functions developed for young children or for non-human primates. Many studies have reported problems in joint attention as an early sign of ASD (Leekam, López, & Moore, 2000; Osterling & Dawson, 1994).The joint attention is a phenomenon of sharing attention between infant, mother, and an object (e.g., pointing to a toy while looking at the mother to share enjoinment) that develops from 6 to 12 months. Other studies have found deficient performance of older children on tasks taping mental flexibility (McEvoy, Rogers, & Pennington, 1993). Additionally, in another longitudinal study, joint attention was found to be the significant predictor of cognitive flexibility in ASD group compared with typically developing group after one year at time 2 assessment. In the same study, around four years of age, deficits in cognitive flexibility were evident in children with ASD compared with typically developing controls. However, online manipulation of information was found to be intact in both groups (Griffith, Pennington, Wehner, & Rogers, 1999). Further evidence comes from Dawson and colleagues who have compared autistic children with two groups: a group of normal young children and a group of children with Down syndrome. Three- to four-year-old autistic children have shown impaired performance on behavioral tasks associated with ventromedial PFC and dorsolateral PFC. Furthermore, joint attention have predicted performance on tasks associated with only ventromedial prefrontal areas but not the dorsolateral prefrontal areas at 4 years as well as at 5 years (assessed from delayed response and delayed non-matching task, while co-varying nonverbal mental ability). The findings suggest the important role of ventromedial areas in core autism symptoms (Dawson, Meltzoff, Osterling, & Rinaldi, 1998).

Indeed, each of the three accounts including theory of mind deficits, weak central coherence, and executive dysfunctions describe some of the autistic symptoms, but cannot explain the broader spectrum of ASD. In this regard, another hypothesis has been proposed by Happé, Ronald, and Plomin (2006), who suggest that none of these single accounts can explain all the symptoms of ASD, including social and non-social symptoms. They propose a fraction able triad approach by explaining that in the triad, the variations in the three main component symptoms of ASD including social impairment, communication problems, and repetitive behaviors are independent of each other both phenotypically as well as biologically.

4.4 Specificity of Executive Dysfunctions in Autism

Although primacy of executive dysfunctions is widely reported in ASD, yet, the pre-eminence of specific executive dysfunctions in ASD is a topic of debate and needs further attention of future researchers. During the last two decades, researchers have examined several executive functions in autism, particularly planning, cognitive flexibility, inhibition, and working memory. Although the previous researchers are not yet able to develop a complete consensus on the specific domains of executive dysfunctions in ASD, however, the individuals with autism have been shown to manifest consistent impairment on measures of planning, cognitive flexibility, and working memory. Still the findings for inhibition are inconsistent. The specific executive dysfunctions have been discussed in detail below.

4.4.1 Planning

Planning is defined as a sequential and dynamic mental process which involves in monitoring, prioritizing, reducing/clustering information, rearranging, and updating of a sequence of planned actions. Individuals with ASD are consistently reported to be impaired on planning tests. Several studies have found that autistic children, adolescents, and adults show poor performance on planning tests, such as the Tower of London compared to age-matched clinical control groups including dyslexia, ADHD, and Tourette syndrome, and age-matched normally developing individuals (Ozonoff & Jensen, 1999; Sergeant, Geurts, & Oosterlaan, 2002). Importantly, poor performance of autistic individuals on neuropsychological tests tapping planning is maintained over time (Ozonoff & McEvoy, 1994).

Among these studies, another study compared children and adolescents with ASD with two control groups. One group was matched to the autistic group on age and learning disability, and the second group, a younger and typically developing group, matched to the autistic group on verbal and non-verbal mental ages. They used a computerized test of planning, the Stockings of Cambridge, a variant of the Tower of London test. The researchers reported two interesting findings in addition to a general finding of poor performance of autistic group compared to both groups. First, autistic group showed planning deficits, particularly on puzzles requiring a longer sequence of moves; second, planning success was directly associated with non-verbal mental age. Their finding suggested that autism and intellectual disability lead to an additive deficit in planning (Hughes, Russell, & Robbins, 1994).

4.4.2 Cognitive Flexibility

Mental flexibility is a neuropsychological skill that is defined as a flexible adaptation of attention to focus on different aspects of the goal and to think about different and alternative perspectives. Deficits in cognitive flexibility are represented in the form of an inability to shift to a different thought or action according to situational requirements. In behavioral form, good mental flexibility is represented in adaptive variations in behavior, generating variety of solutions in a problem situation, revising plans, and transition of attention between tasks. Behavioral manifestation of poor cognitive flexibility is represented in perseverative and stereotyped behaviors as well as in difficulties regulating and modulating motor acts. Several studies have reported that individuals with ASD show poor mental flexibility. The literature shows that poor cognitive flexibility is observed in autistic individuals in the form of perseverative errors (Hughes et al., 1994). Additionally, these individuals show deficits in shifting or sustaining attention or in selective attention (Courchesne et al., 1994; Noterdaeme, Mildenberger, Minow, & Amorosa, 2002).

Previous studies using samples of autistic individuals have quite commonly used Wisconsin card sorting test to assess mental flexibility. Review studies (e.g., Hill, 2004) also highlight that individuals with ASD compared with normally developing controls show consistent impairment on at least two key components of executive functions: planning and mental flexibility assessed by Wisconsin Card Sorting Test.

4.4.3 Working Memory

Working memory is defined as an ability to hold, select, and use relevant information in mind for completing the task or achieving the goal. Despite the presence of clear theoretical and empirical evidence for the association between working memory and social cognition, limited research on working memory is available on samples of ASD. Among available studies, though few studies could not find working memory impairment in high functioning autistic individuals, many studies clearly demonstrate working memory impairment, particularly related to spatial domain in adolescents with ASD symptoms (e.g., Steele, Minshew, Luna, & Sweeney, 2007; Williams, Goldstein, Carpenter, & Minshew, 2005). Additionally, McGonigle-Chalmers and colleagues compared autistics group with a control group on a size-sequencing executive functioning task. Autistic group showed higher scores on errors and reaction time measures suggesting the impairment in the prospective component of working memory that might have caused problems in context dependent information updating and task relevant biased cognitions and behaviors (McGonigle-Chalmers, Bodner, Fox-Pitt, & Nicholson, 2008). A review report also supports the role of working memory impairment in autistic symptomology (O'Hearn et al., 2008).

Of note, working memory problems in autistics individuals become more prominent when cognitive task imposes heavy load on working memory related to more complex social information in some severe social situations (McGonigle-Chalmers et al., 2008; Landa & Goldberg, 2005; Williams, Goldstein, & Minshew, 2006). The differential cognitive load on working memory may likely explain why some studies could not find working memory impairment in high functioning autistic individuals. However, Neuroimaging studies show deficiencies of more universal working memory processes instead of focused impairments in the prefrontal cortex (Barendse et al., 2013).

4.4.4 Inhibition

Inhibition is considered an ability to control one's mode of attention and thought to change an automatic response with a novel response and. Self-inhibiting behavior is represented in appropriate behavior according to situations, impulse control, following rules or criteria, managing extraneous distractions, or interference, and in delaying response. The findings regarding inhibition deficits in individuals with ASD are inconsistent. Some studies are able to find deficits on inhibition ability in autistic individuals (Brian, Tipper, Weaver, & Bryson, 2003), but majority of the studies have shown that autistic children and adolescents are unimpaired (Ozonoff & Jensen, 1999) on a classic test, the Stroop color word task, taping this ability. The findings are in clear contrast to findings based on samples of individuals with other neuro-developmental disorders such as ADHD and phenylketonuria which show clear inhibition dysfunction (Diamond, Prevor, Callender, & Druin, 1997; Ozonoff & Jensen, 1999; Wodka et al., 2007).

4.5 Specificity of Executive Dysfunctions in Specific Symptomology of ASD

Although executive dysfunctions have been extensively reported in ASD, yet, the role of specific executive dysfunctions in specific autistic symptoms is a much debated topic which needs serious attention of future researchers. Accordingly, it has been proposed that specific executive dysfunctions may explain some of the autistic symptoms. Executive dysfunctions have been described to be associated with the social and communicative as well as with repetitive and restricted behaviors in ASD individuals.

Generally, available studies have reported executive dysfunctions to be related to restricted and repetitive symptoms of ASD (Kenworthy, Black, Harrison, Della Rosa, & Wallace, 2009; Lopez, Lincoln, Ozonoff, & Lai, 2005; South, Ozonoff, & McMahon, 2007). More specifically, it has been suggested that deficits in set shifting and mental flexibility may explain repetitive and restricted behaviors of individuals with ASD (Hill, 2004; Lopez et al., 2005). Moreover, alongside the theory of mind, empirical, though limited number of studies have reported that executive dysfunctions are correlated with socio-communicative symptoms in ASD individuals (Gilotty, Kenworthy, Sirian, Black, & Wagncer, 2002; Joseph & Tager-Flusberg, 2004; Kenworthy et al., 2009; McEvoy et al., 1993). For example, social impairments that are the defining characteristics of ASD may be attributed to problems in specific aspects of executive functions such as inhibition, mental and behavioral flexibility, and the ability to select, monitor, and reorganize/adjust socially appropriate responses (Channon, Charman, Heap, Crawford, & Rios, 2001; Dennis, Agostino, Roncadin, & Levin, 2009; Joseph & Tager-Flusberg, 2004). However, the findings are limited in that majority of the existing studies have used either archival clinical data without control groups or relied on laboratory tasks for the assessment of specific executive dysfunctions. The use of behavioral observation in conjunction with neuroimaging studies is needed to rule out specificity of executive dysfunctions in relation to specific autistic symptoms.

Other studies have assessed two broader executive functioning categories: behavioral regulation and metacognition, in relation to autistic symptomology. One of these studies has found clear association of behavioral regulation processes (inhibition, emotional control, and set shifting) with social functioning in both groups of ASD and typically developing children. However, metacognitive executive processes have been differentially associated with social functioning with significant association in autistic group but no such association in typically developing group. The researchers have proposed that autistic children may require more widespread use of executive processes in order to adapt in social situations in contrast to typically developing children who require only a focused and refined use of behavioral regulation executive processes for efficient and successful social interaction. Evidence from functional neuroimaging studies also support different neural activation patterns in individuals with autism and typically developing children underlying social and non-social processing and executive functioning (see Di Martino et al., 2009 for a review; Just, Cherkassky, Keller, Kana, & Minshew, 2007). The proposed association of metacognitive processes with social interaction can also be supported by linking both processes with theory of mind. Consistent associations between metacognitive executive processes and theory of mind have been reported on the one hand and impaired theory of mind has been reported to explain socio-communicative deficits of ASD individuals on the other hand (see review by Hughes & Leekam, 2004). Furthermore, interventions targeting metacognitive abilities have also shown improvement in social processes in autistic adolescents (Kenworthy et al., 2014).

4.6 Neuroanatomical Considerations in ASD

Executive functions are higher regulatory cognitive mechanisms that are thought to be regulated by frontal areas of brain. Different propositions have tried to explain the brain-behavior link in ASD by focusing on executive dysfunctions. Among these, one proposition suggests that irregularities in medial temporal lobe may likely to result in executive dysfunctions, and variable severity of medial temporal lobe impairment co-vary with variation in executive dysfunctions (Dawson et al., 2002). One of the two explanations of this proposition describes executive dysfunctions to be the correlate instead of cause of the core symptoms of autism. According to this view, functional irregularities in prefrontal areas which appear in adult samples may likely be the secondary outcomes of an early medial temporal lobe dysfunction (Dawson et al., 2002). The second explanation proposes a more direct association of frontal lobe abnormalities with the executive dysfunctions in ASD. Accordingly, it has been suggested that: (i) executive dysfunctions in autistic individuals may be correlated with dysfunctional integration of the frontal areas with other brain areas, (ii) abnormal myelination process, or (iii) abnormal neuronal maturation process (Chugani, 1998; Luna et al., 2002). This proposition is supported by the findings of reduced functional connectivity of frontal lobe with other cortical and subcortical areas (Luna et al., 2002), and transient delayed postnatal maturation of the frontal areas in individuals with autism (Ohnishi et al., 2000; Zilbovicius et al., 1995).

Although neuroanatomical studies of the frontal lobes in relation to executive dysfunctions in autism are limited, nevertheless, several structural abnormalities in cortical and subcortical areas have been identified (Kemper & Bauman, 1998). Among these include delayed postnatal maturation of the frontal areas (Zilbovicius et al., 1995), serotonergic irregularities in prefrontal areas (Chugani et al., 1997), and structural abnormalities in amygdale and orbitofrontal cortical areas (Salmond, de Haan, Friston, Gadian, & Vargha-Khadem, 2003). Also, reduced activation in dorsolateral PFC has been described in a spatial working memory task (Luna et al., 2002). Importantly, more detailed structural studies of autistic brain as well as functional imaging studies during executive function task performance are vital to rule out the biological basis of executive dysfunctions and their functional consequences in autism. Particularly, considering the neurodevelopmental nature of the disorder, longitudinal studies are recommended for tracking participants over their lifespan.

4.7 Further Concerns and Recommendations

Clearly, detailed functional brain imaging studies of autistic individuals as well as longitudinal studies over their lifespan are needed to delineate brain and behavior connection and lifelong development of the abnormality.

Many other concerns related to executive dysfunction studies in autism needed to be addressed in the future studies. First, **task complexity and task presentation** should be considered while interpreting results. For example, many executive function tasks such as Wisconsin card sorting test and Stroop tests are multi-component tasks requiring mental flexibility, inhibition, working memory, monitoring, and reorganization. Future studies are recommended to assess detailed investigation of all cognitive processes involved in a single test. Also, computerizing versus face-to-face presentation of the executive function tasks to the autistic individuals will help to identify how much independent or related are executive and social problems in autism, given the finding that computerized presentation gives different results than that of face to face administration (Ozonoff, 1995b).

The second concern is whether **specific executive dysfunction can be defined as a diagnostic marker** for autism? One problem is that many neurodevelopmental disorders such as ADHD, Tourette syndrome, and conduct disorder share executive dysfunctions. However, recent developments have provided initial evidence for different executive dysfunction profiles in individuals with autism (show poor profiles of planning and mental flexibility) versus ADHD (clear deficits in inhibition). However, given the task complexity and task presentation, continued, and detailed investigation of specific executive dysfunctions in different neurodevelopmental disorders are recommended to delineate if we can make specific executive dysfunction as a diagnostic marker for autistic diagnosis.

A related concern is that **executive dysfunctions must be a universal feature of all autistic individuals**, if we want to make it a diagnostic marker. It is explained that executive dysfunctions must have been the characteristic feature of every individual with ASD to include these in the primary symptoms. To date, although majority of the studies have reported specific executive dysfunctions such as deficits in cognitive flexibility, planning, and working memory in autistic individuals, so far, many of the studies could not find consistent evidence for executive dysfunctions, particularly related to inhibition, in these individuals (e.g., Ozonoff & Jensen, 1999; Diamond et al., 1997). This lack of consistent evidence may simply be an artifact of methodological issues such as measures selected, however, based on inconsistent findings, universality of executive dysfunctions in ASD cannot be ruled out. Future researchers are recommended to assess wide range of executive functions using ecologically valid executive functioning measures along with naturalistic observations of behaviors relying on executive functions, and parent's and teacher's reports of behaviors. This multi-measure technique will not only enable to rule out specificity of executive dysfunctions but also the universality of these dysfunctions to make it diagnostic criteria. Assessment of wide range of executive functions would also be beneficial to delineate the pattern of correlation and differentiation between different EF constructs and to identify whether this pattern coincides with the pattern found in normal individuals.

4.8 Comorbidities of ASD with Other Disorders

Many of the individuals with ASD also develop other neurodevelopmental or psychiatric disorders. Nearly 70% of these individuals have one comorbid mental disorder, and around 40% of have two or more co-occurring mental disorders (APA, 2013). Such comorbid conditions can occur at any stage in life, and some autistic individuals do not develop any such comorbid disorder until their adulthood. As the comorbid conditions can affect the functional consequences as well as response of the individual to therapeutic treatment, therefore, it is very important to identify such comorbidities in individuals with autism. Several comorbidities in autistic individuals have been described in APA (2013) including intellectual impairment, language disorders, learning disorders, attention deficit hyperactivity disorder, developmental coordination disorders, anxiety, or depression.

4.8.1 *Intellectual Impairment and Language Difficulties*

Children with ASD are frequently reported to have intellectual disability and structural language disorder. Intellectual disability is diagnosed when a child of six years or older age has a below 70 IQ and shows difficulties in daily tasks. The structural language disorder is described as an inability to format sentences using proper grammar and inability to comprehend language. The co-occurrence of intellectual disability was previously reported to be in 70% of ASD individuals; however, later studies have reported reduced comorbidity of intellectual disability, which is 40–50% (Matson & Shoemaker, 2009). Early intervention and awareness trainings, betterment in addressing learning needs of the individual, and better assessment of IQ may have caused this drop rate.

4.8.2 *Specific Learning Difficulties*

Occurrence of learning disabilities in children with ASD is also commonly reported; however, estimates of learning disability in children with ASD vary. As each of the two disorders is associated with neurocognitive weaknesses, so presence of learning disabilities along with autism may have cognitive and behavioral consequences. McGuinness et al., (2017) found that youth having ASD and learning disability were at more risk of impairment in working memory, planning, and processing speed compared to their counterparts having ASD alone.

4.8.3 *Attention Deficit/Hyperactivity Disorder*

During the past decade, research on ASD has shown increased prevalence of co-occurring attention deficit/hyperactivity disorder (ADHD) and autism spectrum disorders (Reiersen & Todd, 2008). Such a high prevalence of the reported co-occurring disorder may suggest that some common gene may likely cause the onset of both abnormalities. The identification of co-occurring symptoms of ASD and ADHD is very important as these individuals usually respond poorly to standard ASD treatments or may have exaggerated side effects of medications. Such individuals may benefit from pharmacological treatment in addition to the behavior therapy, social skills therapy as well as individual and family psychotherapy (Reiersen & Todd,

2008). The APA (2013) has stated that if the individual meets criteria for both ASD and ADHD, he/she will be given both diagnoses.

4.8.4 Anxiety

Individuals with ASD are more vulnerable to experience some co-occurring mental health problem, as compared to the general population. Among mental health problems, co-occurrence of anxiety symptoms has been reported to be in nearly 50% of the children and adolescents with ASD (van Steensel, Bögels, & Perrin, 2011). Most importantly, as discussed above, many of the 50% ASD cases who develop co-occurring intellectual disability also develop symptoms of mental health problems, particularly anxiety (Matson & Shoemaker, 2009). Co-occurring anxiety with ASD is often a very complex condition because commonly multiple anxiety disorders occur concurrently with varying levels of additive and interactive effects. This in turn may pose many challenges to the individuals and their families as well as to the clinician in selecting the focused treatment for both anxiety and autistic symptoms. It is recommended that tailored assessment methods and adapting cognitive behavioral treatments to address anxiety symptoms in autistic individuals would be more effective for improvement in functional consequences of the disorder (Kerns, Roux, Connell, & Shattuck, 2016).

4.8.5 Depression

Among co-occurring mental health problems, depressive symptoms are also common. However, in children with ASD, the identification of depressive syndrome becomes very difficult because the presentation of these symptoms is usually atypical or overlaps with social and communicative difficulties. Traditional self-report measures of depressive symptoms are difficult to use with many children with ASD. Additionally, no evidence is available for reliability or validity of these measures for assessment of children and adolescents with ASD. Prevalence rate estimation for depression in autistic individuals vary because of overlapping symptoms of both disorders. Insight of one's disability may also predispose autistic individuals to depressive symptoms. Manifestation of depressive symptoms may also vary according to the age and maturation level of the individual.

Further, APA (2013) also describes developmental coordination disorder as a co-occurring disorder in individuals with autism. It is recommended that concurrent diagnosis of both disorders should be given for co-occurring disorders of developmental coordination disorder, anxiety disorders, depressive disorders, and other comorbid diagnoses.

4.9 Conclusion

In short, symptoms of ASD fall in three major categories including: (i) social impairment, (ii) communication difficulties, and iii) repetitive and restricted behaviors. Three different cognitive theories including theory of mind, weak central coherence, and executive dysfunctions have tried to explain the symptoms of ASD. Theory of mind deficits in ADHD may explain some social and communicative symptoms. Weak central coherence account explains that individuals with ASD process piecemeal information at the expense of contextual detail. Executive dysfunctions account describes that socio-communicative deficits and repetitive behavior of autistic individuals may be the consequence of executive dysfunctions such as deficits of planning, cognitive flexibility, working memory, and inhibition. However, it is argued that these three cognitive accounts, though tried to explain specific ASD symptoms, cannot explain the broader spectrum of ASD. In this regard, a more recent hypothesis proposed by Happé et al. (2006) suggests that none of these single accounts can explain all the symptoms, including social and non-social symptoms of ASD. Despite all this, our understanding regarding specific executive dysfunctions in ASD has been improved since the last decade. Overall, the studies during the past two decades have shown that almost all individuals with ASD including children, adolescents, and adults present consistent impairment on tasks tapping planning and cognitive flexibility. Furthermore, these individuals show impairment on working memory tasks, particularly related to spatial working memory capacity. Also, preschools autistic children show deficits of joint attention, which is a predictor of cognitive flexibility in late childhood or early adolescence. However, findings are inconsistent regarding inhibition as some studies have found impaired performance of autistic individuals on tasks tapping inhibition, while others have been failed to find such impairment. While this can simply be the result of selection of measures (complex versus simple measures) or presentation of the task (face to face versus computerized presentation), still much research is needed to delineate whether executive dysfunctions can be included in the core autistics symptoms and whether these can be the diagnostic marker of autism. Therefore, it is concluded that more detailed assessment of executive functions, using a wide range of executive functioning tasks along with ecologically valid executive functioning measures, is needed. Furthermore, natural observation of behavioral components relying on executive cognitive abilities and parents and teachers reports of day-to-day behavior should be used in complement with executive functioning measures for a clearer understanding. Additionally, longitudinal studies are recommended to identify the executive dysfunction trajectory in autistic individuals. A clearer understanding of executive dysfunctions in autistic individuals will help in improving clinical techniques and trainings to ameliorate the undesirable consequences of executive dysfunctions on daily activities of these individuals.

References

American Psychiatric Association. (2013). *Diagnostic and statistical manual of mental disorders* (5th ed.). Washington, DC: USA.

Barendse, E. M., Hendriks, M. P., Jansen, J. F., Backes, W. H., Hofman, P. A., Thoonen, G., … Aldenkamp, A. P. (2013). Working memory deficits in high-functioning adolescents with autism spectrum disorders: Neuropsychological and neuroimaging correlates. *Journal of Neurodevelopmental Disorders, 5*(1), 14. https://doi.org/10.1186/1866-1955-5-14.

Brian, J. A., Tipper, S. P., Weaver, B., & Bryson, S. E. (2003). Inhibitory mechanisms in autism spectrum disorders: Typical selective inhibition of location versus facilitated perceptual processing. *Journal of Child Psychology and Psychiatry and Allied Disciplines, 44*(4), 552–560.

Castelli, F., Frith, C., Happé, F., & Frith, U. (2002). Autism, Asperger syndrome and brain mechanisms for the attribution of mental states to animated shapes. *Brain, 125,* 1839–1849.

Channon, S., Charman, T., Heap, J., Crawford, S., & Rios, P. (2001). Real-life-type problem-solving in Asperger's syndrome. *Journal of Autism and Developmental Disorders, 31*(5), 461–469.

Chugani, D. C. (1998). A critical period of brain development: Studies of cerebral glucose utilization with PET. *Preventative Medicine, 27,* 184–188.

Chugani, D. C., Muzik, O., Rothermel, R., Behen, M., Chakraborty, P., Mangner, T., … Chugani, H. T. (1997). Altered serotonin synthesis in the dentatothalamocortical pathway in autistic boys. *Annals of Neurology, 42*(4), 666–669.

Courchesne, E., Townsend, J., Akshoomoff, N. A., Saitoh, O., Yeung-Courchesne R., Lincoln, A. J., … Lau, L. (1994). Impairment in shifting attention in autistic and cerebellar patients. *Behavioral Neuroscience, 108*(5), 848–65.

Dawson, G., Meltzoff, A. N., Osterling, J., & Rinaldi, J. (1998). Neuropsychological correlates of early symptoms of autism. *Child Development, 69,* 1276–1285.

Dawson, G., Webb, S., Schellenberg, G. D., Dager, S., Friedman, S., Aylward, E., et al. (2002). Defining the broader phenotype of autism: Genetic, brain, and behavioral perspectives. *Development and Psychopathology, 14,* 581–611.

Dennis, M., Agostino, A., Roncadin, C., & Levin, H. (2009). Theory of mind depends on domain-general executive functions of working memory and cognitive inhibition in children with traumatic brain injury. *Journal of Clinical and Experimental Neuropsychology, 31*(7), 835–847. https://doi.org/10.1080/13803390802572419.

Diamond, A., Prevor, M. B., Callender, G., & Druin, D. P. (1997). Prefrontal cortex cognitive deficits in children treated early and continuously for PKU. *Monographs of the Society for Research in Child Development, 62,* 1–208.

Di Martino, A., Ross, K., Uddin, L. Q., Sklar, A. B., Castellanos, F. X., & Milham, M. P. (2009). Functional brain correlates of social and nonsocial processes in autism spectrum disorders: An activation likelihood estimation meta-analysis. *Biological Psychiatry, 65*(1), 63–74. https://doi.org/10.1016/j.biopsych.2008.09.022.

Fombonne, E. (2009). Epidemiology of pervasive developmental disorders. *Pediatric Research, 65*(6), 591–598.

Frith, U. (2003a). *Autism: Explaining the Enigma* (2nd ed.). Blackwell.

Frith, C. D. (2003b). What do imaging studies tell us about the neural basis of autism? In M. Rutter (Ed.), *Autism: Neural basis and treatment possibilities*. London: Wiley.

Gilotty, L., Kenworthy, L., Sirian, L., Black, D. O., & Wagncer, A. E. (2002). Adaptive skills and executive function in autism spectrum disorders. *Child Neuropsychology, 8*(4), 241–248.

Gray, K. M., Keating, C. M., Taffe, J. R., Brereton, A. V., Einfeld, S. L., Reardon, T. C., et al. (2014). Adult outcomes in autism: Community inclusion and living skills. *Journal of Autism and Developmental Disorders, 44,* 3006–3015.

Griffith, E. M., Pennington, B. F., Wehner, E. A., & Rogers, S. J. (1999). Executive functions in young children with autism. *Child Development, 70,* 817–832. https://www.jstor.org/stable/1132244.

Happé, F., Ehlers, S., Fletcher, P., Frith, U., Johansson, M., Gillberg, C., … Frith, C. (1996). 'Theory of mind' in the brain. Evidence from a PET scan study of Asperger syndrome. *Neuroreport, 8*, 197–201.

Happé, F., Ronald, A., & Plomin, R. (2006). Time to give up on a single explanation for autism. *Nature Neuroscience, 9*(10), 1218–1220. https://doi.org/10.1038/nn1770.

Hill, E. L. (2004). Executive dysfunction in autism. *Trends in Cognitive Sciences, 8*(1), 26–32.

Hughes, C., & Leekam, S. (2004). What are the links between theory of mind and social relations? Review, reflections and new directions for studies of typical and atypical development. *Social Development, 13,* 590–619. https://doi.org/10.1111/j.1467-9507.2004.00285.x.

Hughes, C., Russell, J., & Robbins, T. W. (1994). Evidence for executive dysfunction in autism. *Neuropsychologia, 32,* 477–492.

Joseph, R. M., & Tager–Flusberg, H. (2004).The relationship of theory of mind and executive functions to symptom type and severity in children with autism. *Development and Psychopathology, 16*(1), 137–155. https://doi.org/10.1017/s095457940404444x.

Just, M. A., Cherkassky, V. L., Keller, T. A., Kana, R. K., & Minshew, N. J. (2007). Functional and anatomical cortical underconnectivity in autism: Evidence from an FMRI study of an executive function task and corpus callosum morphometry. *Cereberal Cortex, 17*(4), 951–961.

Kemper, K. L., & Bauman, M. L. (1998). Neuropathology of infantile autism. *Journal of Neuropathology and Experimental Neurology, 57*(7), 645–652. https://doi.org/10.1097/00005072-199807000-00001.

Kenworthy, L., Anthony, L. G., Naiman, D. Q., Cannon, L., Wills, M. C., Luong-Tran, C., … Wallace, G. L. (2014). Randomized controlled effectiveness trial of executive function invention for children on the autism spectrum. *Journal of Child Psychology and Psychiatry and Allied Sciences, 55*(4), 374–383. https://doi.org/10.1111/jcpp.12161.

Kenworthy, L., Black, D. O., Harrison, B., Della Rosa, A., & Wallace, G. L. (2009). Are executive control functions related to autism symptoms in high-functioning children? *Child Neuropsychology, 15*(5), 425–440. https://doi.org/10.1080/09297040802646983.

Kerns, C. M., Roux, A. M., Connell, J. E., & Shattuck, P. T. (2016). Adapting cognitive behavioral techniques to address anxiety and depression in cognitively able emerging adults on the autism spectrum. *Cognitive Behavior Practices, 23*(3), 329–340. https://doi.org/10.1016/j.cbpra.2016.06.002.

Kimhi, Y. (2014). Theory of mind abilities and deficits in autism spectrum disorders. *Top Language Disorders, 34*(4), 329–343.

Landa, R. J., & Goldberg, M. C. (2005). Language, social, and executive functions in high functioning autism: A continuum of performance. *Journal of Autism and Developmental Disorders, 35*(5), 557–573. https://doi.org/10.1007/s10803-005-0001-1.

Leekam, S. R., Lόpez, B., & Moore, C. (2000). Attention and joint attention in preschool children with autism. *Developmental Psychology, 36*(2), 261–273.

Lopez, B. R., Lincoln, A. J., Ozonoff, S., & Lai, Z. (2005). Examining the relationship between executive functions and restricted, repetitive symptoms of autistic disorder. *Journal of Autism and Developmental Disorders, 35*(4), 445–460.

Luna, B., Minshew, N. J., Garver, K. E., Lazar, N. A., Thulborn, K. R., Eddy, W. F., et al. (2002). Neocortical system abnormalities in autism. An fMRI study of spatial working memory. *Neurology, 59,* 834–840.

Matson, J. L., & Shoemaker, M. (2009). Intellectual disability and its relationship to autism spectrum disorders. *Research in Developmental Disabilities, 30*(6), 1107–1114.

McEvoy, R. E., Rogers, S. J., & Pennington, B. F. (1993). Executive function and social communication deficits in young autistic children. *Journal of Child Psychology and Psychiatry and Allied Disciplines, 34,* 563–578.

McGonigle-Chalmers, M., Bodner, K., Fox-Pitt, A., & Nicholson, L. (2008). Size sequencing as a window on executive control in children with autism and Asperger's syndrome. *Journal of Autism and Developmental Disorders, 38,* 1382–1390. https://doi.org/10.1007/s10803-007-0396-y.

McGuinness, P. S., Cook, B. E., Bush, H., Lind, H., Vuijk, P. J., Doyle, A. E., & Braaten, E. B. (2017). Children with autism spectrum disorder and comorbid specific learning disorder demonstrate cognitive weakness compared to autism spectrum disorder alone. *Journal of the American Academy of Child & Adolescent Psychiatry, 56*(10suppl.), S231.

Mody, M., & Belliveau, J. W. (2013). Speech and language impairments in autism: Insights from behavior and neuroimaging. *New American Journal of Medical Sciences (Boston), 5*(3), 157–161.

Mottron, L., Peretz, I., & Ménard, E. (2000). Local and global processing of music in high-functioning persons with autism: Beyond central coherence? *Journal of Child Psychology and Psychiatry and Allied Disciplines, 41*(8), 1057–1065.

Noens, I. L. J., & van Berckelaer-Onnes, I. A. (2008). The central coherence account of autism revisited: Evidence from the ComFor study. *Research in Autism Spectrum Disorder, 2*(2), 209–222. https://doi.org/10.1016/j.rasd.2007.05.004.

Newschaffer, C. G., Croen, L. A., Daniels, J., Giarelli, E., Grether, J. K., Levy, S. E., … Windham, G. C. (2007). The epidemiology of autism spectrum disorders. *Annual Review of Public Health, 28*, 235–258. https://doi.org/10.1146/annurev.publhealth.28.021406.144007.

Noterdaeme, M., Mildenberger, K., Minow, F., & Amorosa, H. (2002). Evaluation of neuromotor deficits in children with autism and children with a specific speech and language disorder. *European Child and Adolescent Psychiatry, 11*(5), 219–225.

O'Hearn, K., Asato, M., Ordaz, S., & Luna, B. (2008). Neurodevelopment and executive function in autism. *Development and Psychopathology, 20*(4), 1103–1132. https://doi.org/10.1017/s0954579408000527.

Ohnishi, T., Matsuda, H., Hashimoto, T., Kunihiro, T., Nishikawa, M., Uema, T., et al. (2000). Abnormal regional cerebral blood flow in childhood autism. *Brain, 123*, 1838–1844.

Osterling, J., & Dawson, G. (1994). Early recognition of children with autism: A study of first birthday home videotapes. *Journal of Autism and Developmental Disorders, 24*, 247–257.

Ozonoff, S. (1995a). Executive functions in autism. In E. Schopler & G. Mesibov (Eds.), *Learning and cognition in autism* (pp. 199–219). New York: Plenum Press.

Ozonoff, S. (1995b). Reliability and validity of the Wisconsin card sorting test in studies of autism. *Neuropsychology, 9*, 491–500.

Ozonoff, S., & Jensen, J. (1999). Brief report: Specific executive function profiles in three neurodevelopmental disorders. *Journals of Autism and Developmental Disorders., 29*, 171–177.

Ozonoff, S., & McEvoy, R. E. (1994). A longitudinal study of executive function and theory of mind development in autism. *Development and Psychopathology, 6*, 415–431.

Reiersen, A. M., & Todd, R. D. (2008). Co-occurrence of ADHD and autism spectrum disorders: Phenomenology and treatment. *Expert Review Neurotherapy, 8*(4), 657–669.

Salmond, C. H., de Haan, M., Friston, K. J., Gadian, D. G., & Vargha-Khadem, F. (2003). Investigating individual differences in brain abnormalities in autism. *Philosophical Transactions of the Royal Society of London. Series B: Biological Sciences, 358*(1430), 405–413. https://doi.org/10.1098/rstb.2002.1210.

Sergeant, J. A., Geurts, H., & Oosterlaan, J. (2002). How specific is a deficit of executive functioning for attention-deficit/hyperactivity disorder? *Behavioral Brain Research, 130*, 3–28.

South, M., Ozonoff, S., & McMahon, W. M. (2007). The relationship between executive functioning, central coherence, and repetitive behaviors in the high-functioning autism spectrum. *Autism, 11*, 437–451.

Steele, S. D., Minshew, N. J., Luna, B., & Sweeney, J. A. (2007). Spatial working memory deficits in autism. *Journal of Autism and Developmental Disorder, 37*(4), 605–612. https://doi.org/10.1007/s10803-006-0202-2.

Szatmari, P., Bryson, S., Duku, E., Vaccarella, L., Zwaigenbaum, L., Bennett, T., et al. (2009). Similar developmental trajectories in autism and Asperger syndrome: From early childhood to adolescence. *Journal of Child Psychology and Psychiatry and Allied Disciplines, 50*(12), 1459–1467.

Van Steensel, F. J., Bögels, S. M., & Perrin, S. (2011). Anxiety disorders in children and adolescents with autistic spectrum disorders: A meta-analysis. *Clinical Child and Family Psychological Review, 14*(3), 302–317.
Williams, D. L., Goldstein, G., Carpenter, P. A., & Minshew, N. J. (2005). Verbal and spatial working memory in autism. *Journal of Autism and Developmental Disorder, 35*(6), 747–756. https://doi.org/10.1007/s10803-005-0021-x.
Williams, D. L., Goldstein, G., & Minshew, N. J. (2006). The profile of memory function in children with autism. *Neuropsychology, 20,* 21–29.
Wodka, E. L., Mahone, E. M., Blankner, J. G., Larson, J. C., Fotedar, S., Denckla, M. B., et al. (2007). Evidence that response inhibition is a primary deficit in ADHD. *Journal of Clinical and Experimental Neuropsychology, 29*(4), 345–356. https://doi.org/10.1080/13803390600678046.
Zilbovicius, M., Garreau, B., Samson, Y., Remy, P., Barthélémy, C., Syrota, A., et al. (1995). Delayed maturation of the frontal cortex in childhood autism. *The American Journal of Psychiatry, 152*(2), 248–252. https://doi.org/10.1176/ajp.152.2.248.

Part III
Acquired Executive Dysfunction

Chapter 5
Executive Dysfunction After Traumatic Brain Injury

Mauricio A. Garcia-Barrera, F. Taylor Agate, Ryan E. Wong, Colette M. Smart and Justin E. Karr

5.1 Introduction

Sam is a 19-year-old female varsity soccer player, at the center forward position, who sustained a sports-related concussion during her last game. This was a high-stakes game, as her team was competing for a championship. Earlier in the game, Sam experienced a head-to-elbow collision against another player; she collapsed to the ground without losing consciousness or incurring an open head wound, recovered within 30 s, and continued playing. Later, she recalled having felt dizzy and experiencing some acute-onset nausea. Her head was pounding in anticipation of a headache. She ignored these symptoms as the game continued. During the second half, within the same game, Sam found herself in position to receive a long ball pass from their team's goalkeeper, a pass they have rehearsed several times during practice. With a quick head rotation, her heading of the ball was astute, precise, and she achieved a goal. Her team jumped in celebration, while she collapsed to the ground and could not stand up. She was carried off of the field on a stretcher, and the sports physician on site ordered an ambulance for admission to the local hospital's emergency department (ED). Another player reported she might have lost consciousness for a few seconds while lying in the grass. Video examination confirmed that she remained in the grass immobile for about 6 s before being awakened by other players. Although Sam recalled most of the game, she did not recall details of the incident, or having scored a goal. Her Glasgow Coma Scale (GCS) score was 13 out of 15. Sam was diagnosed with mild Traumatic Brain Injury (mTBI) and was hospitalized for 3 days for preventive monitoring as her computerized tomography

M. A. Garcia-Barrera (✉) · F. T. Agate · R. E. Wong · C. M. Smart
Department of Psychology, University of Victoria, Victoria, BC, Canada
e-mail: mgarcia@uvic.ca

J. E. Karr
Department of Physical Medicine and Rehabilitation, Harvard Medical School, Spaulding Rehabilitation Hospital, Home Base, A Red Sox Foundation and Massachusetts General Hospital Program, Boston, MA, USA

A. Ardila et al. (eds.), *Dysexecutive Syndromes*,
https://doi.org/10.1007/978-3-030-25077-5_5

(CT) scan revealed a small intracranial hematoma in her frontal lobes. Surgery was not required, and anti-inflammatory medication was administered to diminish risk of brain swelling.

Sam was evaluated by a clinical neuropsychologist 2 months later. The clinical interview revealed a past history of two unreported concussions, both sports-related and without loss of consciousness. She had clinically recovered from the recent mTBI, presenting no neurological signs during examination, but reported difficulty with problem-solving and making decisions, as she felt quickly overwhelmed and emotionally dysregulated; she also reported feeling defensive when others pointed out she was not herself. With guidance from coaches and her family doctor, she had progressively returned to soccer practice, and was regaining fitness, but reported to have withdrawn from social interactions with team members outside of practice. She was feeling isolated but unmotivated to initiate engagement. Her fear about experiencing another concussion had arisen and was a major concern for her, producing a heightened anxiety. On testing, Sam's overall performance was within normal limits for most areas assessed, and her performance level was consistent with estimated levels of premorbid functioning based on word reading and pre-injury school performance. There was no baseline testing available. Sam is majoring in business and was considered a B+ student. However, there were reports of diminished performance in school post-concussion, mostly due to difficulty concentrating during midterm exams despite extended time allowance and having missed a few deadlines due to disorganization with her calendar. Sam's self-ratings on the Behavior Rating Inventory of Executive Function (BRIEF) demonstrated self-awareness of her everyday difficulties, which were also confirmed by parents' report. Given the risk of more concussive events, Sam was recommended psycho-education, to gain knowledge about sport-related concussion symptoms and expected recovery trajectory, informing any future return-to-play decisions. She was also recommended individual psychotherapy to work on her social withdrawal and anxiety, in addition to cognitive rehabilitation of executive functions with a problem-solving focus to work on her difficulties with planning, problem-solving, emotional regulation, and disorganization. Given her CT scan, she was recommended to continue soccer practice but to withdraw from playing competitive soccer for 12 months. Follow-up CT scan and neuropsychological assessment 13 months later revealed a full recovery, and Sam reported that she discussed with coaches a gradual return to competitive play, but she stopped heading practice and changed field positions; now she is playing on a right-midfield position in which she has been able to reduce her ball heading during games down to zero.

5.2 Traumatic Brain Injury

5.2.1 Definition

Sam suffered an mTBI. Although the term "Traumatic Brain Injury" (TBI) seems self-explanatory, there is no one sole definition available in the literature. Researchers have moved from the vague "head injury" terminology, to terms that emphasize damage to the brain structure and function. Looking for parsimony, a consensus position statement from The Demographics and Clinical Assessment Working Group of the International and Interagency Initiative toward Common Data Elements for Research on Traumatic Brain Injury and Psychological Health, refers to TBI as "an alteration in brain function, or other evidence of brain pathology, caused by an external force" (Menon Schwab, Wright, & Maas, 2010; p. 1638). With this definition, it is further proposed that an *alteration in brain function* may present as (1) loss of or decreased consciousness (LOC), (2) loss of memory of the event and the periods before or after it, (3) the presence of neurological deficits such as muscle weakness, loss of balance, change in vision, or (4) alteration in mental state, such as confusion, disorientation, etc. Only one of these clinical signs is required. Also, *evidence of damage* to the brain may include neuroradiological, visual, or other laboratory tests, and the *external force* may include the head being struck or penetrated by an object, sharp acceleration and deceleration movement, forces generated by an explosion or blast, etc. (Menon et al., 2010).

TBI severity is classified on a continuum, ranging from mild to moderate to severe. About 80% of traumatic brain injuries are mild (Bruns & Hauser, 2003). Most of the debate has arisen from the diagnosis of mild TBI, and in establishing proper guidelines to differentiate injury severities. The most frequently used index of TBI severity is the Glasgow Coma Scale (GCS, Teasdale & Jennett, 1974). This scale produces a score from 3 to 15, including examination of responsiveness in eye opening, and level of verbal and motor response. The higher the score, the better the response. It has been proposed that a score between 3 and 5 corresponds to a very severe brain injury, a score between 6 and 8 is associated with a severe brain injury, 9–12 corresponds to moderate, and a score between 13 and 15 is associated with mild brain injury. Some authors proposed that the presence of positive CT scan findings (as in Sam's case) would be considered as a complicated mTBI (Roebuck-Spencer & Sherer, 2008). The now-classic scale is free and can be downloaded from this Web site: https://www.glasgowcomascale.org/.

The scores obtained with the GCS offer robust indicators of prognosis, but they can be affected by several factors, including patient's intoxication at admission, facial injuries, and aphasia that can compromise verbal response, visual or auditory processing, and early management such as intubation and medications (e.g., sedatives and other anesthetic drugs). The Glasgow Outcome Scale (GOS, Jennett & Bond, 1975) has been used to measure recovery outcome after TBI. The best outcome is "good recovery" for a full functional recovery with some residual emotional or cognitive lingering deficits; "moderate disability" for some recovery of function, reflective of some independent living but presenting with inability to return to work or function socially; "severe disability" when the patient is conscious but requires full support to meet their physical and cognitive needs; and "vegetative state" when the patient is unable to communicate and follow commands, and there is no other discernable cognitive functioning (Lezak, Howieson, Bigler, & Tranel, 2012; Roebuck-Spencer & Sherer, 2008). Other diagnostic and predictive factors that have been proposed include duration of coma (≤20 min = mild, ≤6 h = moderate, and >6 h = severe injury; Lezak, Howieson, Loring, Hannay, & Fischer, 2004), and duration of post-traumatic amnesia (PTA; <5 min = very mild, 5–60 min = mild, 1–24 h = moderate, 1–7 seven days = severe, 1–4 weeks = very severe, and >4 weeks = extremely severe; Lezak et al., 2012; p. 185). Although length of PTA is a better predictor of global outcomes than coma duration and than the GOS (Lezak et al., 2012), it is recognized that these variables have poor predictive power when in isolation (Roebuck-Spencer & Sherer, 2008).

In Sam's case, she meets criteria for a diagnosis of complicated mTBI, and she experienced a short LOC (estimated at 6 s) and had a PTA of less than 5 min, and her GOS would classify her in the "good recovery" category. Even though we would expect positive neuropsychological findings (e.g., poor performance in a few areas), her overall performance was "within normal limits," but in the absence of prior testing, some acute cognitive capacity loss could have been masked. Her recovery was remarkable, and somewhat unpredicted by the presence of PTA and LOC. Researchers have discussed potential confounders that muddle the precision of the diagnosis of mTBI (Menon et al., 2010; Ruff et al., 2009). For instance, accounts of PTA can be confounded by the LOC; accounting for the LOC period can be problematic, as a delayed LOC could be a consequence of other secondary issues, not necessarily the original TBI (e.g., intracranial pressure due to extradural hematoma, or seizure activity); some of the information obtained by the clinician may be the outcome of self-experience, whereas some may be the outcome of information relayed to the patients by others. For instance, in Sam's case, she could not report LOC with confidence due the PTA. Another issue is that the PTA may be associated with stress (as in psychogenic amnesia observed in cases of posttraumatic stress disorder -PTSD), not necessarily the brain injury. Similarly, the LOC and PTA could be the outcome of substance use before the accident, or drugs administered to the patient while in transport to the ED. Finally, some of the symptoms that are relevant to diagnosis are less specific to TBI (e.g., fatigue, headache, sleep disorders), and could be best accounted for by stress, depression, PTSD, or anxiety).

The definition of mTBI is an area of continuing debate. A review of mTBI by the World Health Organization (WHO) identified 38 definitions of mTBI with varying degrees of overlap. Based on these findings, the WHO proposed the following operational definition:

> mTBI is an acute brain injury resulting from mechanical energy to the head from external physical forces. Operational criteria for clinical identification include: (1) One or more of the following: confusion or disorientation, loss of consciousness for 30 min or less, post-traumatic amnesia for less than 24 h, and/or other transient neurological abnormalities such as focal signs, seizure, and intracranial lesion not requiring surgery; (2) Glasgow Coma Scale

> score of 13–15 after 30 min post-injury or later upon presentation for health care; (3) these manifestations of mTBI must not be due to drugs, alcohol, medications, caused by other injuries or treatment for other injuries (e.g., systemic injuries, facial injuries, or intubation), caused by other problems (e.g., psychological trauma, language barrier, or coexisting medical conditions), or caused by penetrating craniocerebral injury. (Kristman et al., 2014, p. S266)

5.2.2 Neuroimaging Techniques as Useful Instruments in Examining the Outcomes of MTBI

Given the difficulty in properly identifying and diagnosing instances of mTBI, and the reliance on self-report, alternative methodologies have been developed. Early studies on concussion noted that neuropsychological testing had limited utility at detecting mTBI (Binder, Rohling, & Larrabee, 1997); however, meta-analytic evidence suggests that clinical neuropsychological assessment can reliably detect mTBI symptoms (or lack thereof) in the acute phase of the injury, but appears to fail to detect and/or predict long-term cognitive deficits in mTBI patients (Martin, 2003). Neuropsychological assessment has in fact become a common method for evaluating the sequelae of mTBI, particularly in cases classified as complicated (such as Sam's). Neuropsychological assessment was included in the recent recommendations for the assessment of long-term effects of sports-related concussions (McCrory et al., 2017). Past researchers have applied several tests to evaluate post-mTBI cognitive outcomes among working adults (Sherer et al., 2002); however, no gold-standard instrument exists for the neuropsychological assessment of workers following occupational mTBI. Although past studies have historically used validated paper-and-pencil assessment tests to evaluate the cognitive outcomes of mTBI, recent advances in computerized neuropsychological assessment have emphasized the added sensitivity of response time (RT) data at detecting impairment following mTBI (Collie, McCrory, & Makdissi, 2006; Iverson, Brooks, Lovell, & Collins, 2006; Sosnoff, Broglio, Hillman, & Ferrara, 2007). Further, specific cognitive abilities appear vulnerable to the effects of mTBI based on past meta-analytic findings, including memory, processing speed, and executive functions (Belanger, Curtiss, Demery, Lebowitz, & Vanderploeg, 2005; Belanger, Spiegel, & Vanderploeg, 2010; Frencham, Fox, & Maybery, 2005; Zakzanis, Leach, & Kaplan, 1999).

Based on these considerations, the best instrument for a cognitive evaluation of mTBI would assess these cognitive domains through reliable and valid computerized tests with accurate RT measurement. Recently, the National Institute of Health (NIH) has developed a Cognition Battery known as the **NIH-Toolbox**, which provides a computerized toolkit of neuropsychological tests evaluating cognitive domains such as crystallized knowledge, memory, processing speed, and executive functions. Notably, although crystallized knowledge should not decrease as a result of concussion, these tasks measure a level of premorbid ability and provide guidance on the level of a participant's functioning prior to head injury. As a validated tool for the cognitive assessment of adults (Weintraub et al., 2014), the NIH-Toolbox has established psychometric qualities, including convergent validity with gold standard measures currently used for neuropsychological assessment (Mungas et al., 2014). The composite scores for the toolbox (i.e., crystallized, fluid and total cognition) present high test–retest reliability ($r = 0.92$, 0.86, and 0.90, respectively) and only small to medium practice effects (Heaton et al., 2014), making the variables largely appropriate for a longitudinal design so long as the analytical methods take the impact of repeated measurement into consideration (Cysique et al., 2011). The NIH-Toolbox includes tests for the assessment of *Executive functions such as:* (1) Flanker Inhibitory Control and Attention: The participant views an arrow central to the screen and other arrows on either side in the same or opposite direction. The participant must identify the direction of the central arrow and ignore the directions of the other arrows; and (2) Dimensional Change Card Sort: The participant observes two pictures that vary based on shape and color. The participant must match these shapes to a target shape based on shape and color, but the correct dimension by which to sort will change during a switch task, which requires the individual to shift back and forth with changing task rules.

From a clinical perspective, neuroimaging techniques are widely used to diagnose moderate and severe brain injuries, although traditional techniques (e.g., CT, T1-weighted MRI) are not sensitive to the microstructural damage and small tears associated with mTBI, and it is only in some complicated cases, such as Sam's, when the CT scan may show positive findings. Although not yet used for diagnostic purposes, two of the most common neuroimaging techniques for detecting and studying mTBI in research settings are Electroencephalograms (EEG), and advanced magnetic resonance imaging (MRI, both structural approaches and functional—*f*MRI) (Eierud et al., 2014). These techniques have demonstrated that a main outcome of the brain injury sustained after a concussion is mostly circumscribed to axons and the bundles they form; structures that comprise white matter tissue in the brain (Shenton et al., 2012). Specifically, mTBI often involves twisting and shearing of axons. Such axonal injuries can cause changes in brain function, but are not typically visualized with traditional brain imaging techniques, such as CT or high-resolution T1-weighted MRI scans. An alternative method is diffusion tensor imaging (DTI), an MRI-based technique that can be used to measure the diffusion of water in the brain. Given that diffusion occurs parallel to axon bundles, rather than perpendicular, DTI is particularly useful in the study of white matter tissue. In fact, DTI imaging is emerging as a strong candidate for detecting long-term white matter structural brain anomalies associated with chronic cognitive deficits of mTBI, which traditional clinical neuropsychological assessments may fail to detect (Eierud et al., 2014; Shenton et al., 2012). Specifically, DTI results reveal decreased integrity in white matter regions (as evidenced by increased mean diffusivity and decreased fractional anisotropy) following mTBI (Cubon, Putukian, Boyer, & Dettwiler, 2011; Kinnunen et al. 2010; Messé et al., 2011). The mild injuries visualized with DTI can be diffuse, but are often seen in large white matter tracts, such as the corpus callosum and internal capsule (Sharp & Ham, 2011). Importantly, DTI results have been shown to positively correlate with cognitive impairment following mTBI (Kinnunen et al., 2010; Lipton et al., 2009), and to relate to post-concussion symptoms (Inglese et al., 2005). More recently, DTI has been used longitudinally, at 2 weeks and 2 months post-injury, to examine changes in white matter tracts after sports-related mTBI. The results showed changes in DTI-based metrics (e.g., radial diffusivity) over time, providing evidence that DTI is a sensitive measure of neurological recovery following concussive injury (Murugavel et al., 2014).

Along with structural injury come changes in brain function. Such changes can be reliably captured with techniques such as *f*MRI and EEG. Functional MRI is a technique that allows for the visualization of the brain in action. Essentially, structural MRI collects high-resolution images of the brain that can be combined with blood-oxygen level-dependent (BOLD) *f*MRI to track blood flow in the brain during a cognitive task or at rest. Since the conception of *f*MRI in the early 1990s (Ogawa et al., 1992), significant advances in research have broadened our understanding of how the brain functions under both healthy and diseased conditions (e.g., Dolan, 2008; Haller & Bartsch, 2009; Rosen, Buckner, & Dale, 1998). Using functional connectivity approaches from *f*MRI, researchers have identified a set of functional networks that appear to be associated with executive control, such as the cognitive control network (Cole, Pathak, & Schneider, 2010) and the fronto-parietal and cingulo-opercular networks (Fair, Dosenbach, Church, Cohen, & Brahmbhatt, 2007). However, relatively few studies have used *f*MRI to assess concussion. According to a review, approximately 20 studies have used *f*MRI to examine mTBI (McDonald, Saykin, & McAllister, 2012). In spite of this, functional imaging has been identified as a novel technological platform that has clinical potential for concussion evaluation (McCrory et al., 2017). To date, studies have revealed differences in brain activation in mTBI groups compared to healthy controls, even when behavioral performance is equivalent (McDonald et al., 2012). One of the few studies in concussions using resting-state *f*MRI revealed differences in functional connectivity between mTBI and controls (Mayer, Mannell, Ling, Gsparovic, & Yeo, 2011).

Mathematical models derived from graph theory have been recently used to analyze brain network organization (Bullmore & Sporns, 2009). Graph theory characterizes the brain as a set of networks. Each network is made up of distinct brain regions called nodes. The graph theory approach allows for the quantitative analysis of network properties such as organization and efficiency, and characterizes the network according to both global (whole brain) and local (specific brain regions) attributes. The healthy human brain generally functions as an efficient "small-world" network, characterized by connections between nodes that allow for both local specialization and global integration (Watts & Strogatz, 1998). In contrast, a "random" network is characterized by connections that promote global integration but not local specialization, and an "organized" network promotes local specialization but not global integration. Investigation with graph theory analysis of adult concussion/mTBI demonstrates a shift toward suboptimal network organization (Caeyenberghs et al., 2014; Nakamura, Hillary, & Biswal, 2009; Pandit et al., 2013). Resting-state EEG is a useful technique to capture differences in the global and/or local connectivity measures of network organization. These analytical approaches have been applied in adolescents who have experienced concussion (Virji-Babul et al., 2014).

5.2.3 *How Prevalent Is TBI?*

Sam's mTBI is one on millions of the yearly diagnosed TBIs in the world. There is variability in the accounts of prevalence and incidence of TBI both in the world and within nations, due to differences in the parameters used for the diagnosis of TBI in a given population (e.g., no LOC is required to diagnose a mTBI in cases such as sports-related concussion, but it is often used for other mTBI cases). Most published work report prevalence data from developed nations that have invested in epidemiological record keeping. Worldwide reports estimate that at least 10 million TBIs resulting in either hospitalization or death occur annually; as a result, an estimated 57 million people have been hospitalized due to having experienced a TBI (Langlois, Rutland-Brown, & Wald, 2006). A meta-analysis including 25,134 individuals from a selected pool of 15 papers (out of 1261 articles yielded by the search) examined the prevalence of TBI in adults in the USA, Australia, New Zealand, and Canada, finding a general prevalence rate of 12.1% when the diagnosis of TBI is specifically delimited by the presence of LOC (Frost, Farrer, Primosch, & Hedges, 2013). In the USA alone, there were close to 2.8 million TBI-related ED visits, hospitalizations, and deaths in 2013 (Taylor, Bell, Breiding, & Xu, 2017a). Over 5 million Americans that survived their TBI are dealing with the long-term outcomes (including lifelong disability) associated with injuries severe enough to have required hospitalization (Langlois et al., 2006). In Europe, TBI is listed as one of the top three causes of highest injury-related medical costs (Maas, Stocchetti, & Bullock, 2008). According to data from the Center for Disease Prevention and Control, the leading causes of TBI in adults (when known and when visits to the ER, hospitalizations and death rates are considered) are falls, motor vehicle traffic accidents, struck by or against events, and assaults, in that order (Frost et al., 2013; Langlois et al., 2006). Of those, traffic accidents are also the leading cause of TBI-related death (Faul, Xu, Wald, & Coronado, 2010), and the World Health Organization (WHO) projected that by 2020 it will be among the top causes of global burden of disease and injury (Maas et al., 2008).

There were a few risk factors detected by epidemiological research. Consistent with other epidemiological studies (e.g., Faul et al., 2010; Langlois et al., 2006), Frost and colleagues' meta-analysis found an odds ratio of 2.22 ($p \leq 0.0001$) for **gender** indicating that men are at twofold higher risk of suffering a TBI than women. This gender difference may be associated with a higher rate of men engaging in risky behaviors, contact sports and substance use (e.g., alcohol) (Frost et al., 2013). However, an area of growing concern is the increasing amount of woman experiencing intimate partner violence (IPV)-related TBIs, which are particularly unreported, unaccounted, and under-investigated mild TBIs. Valera, Campbell, Gill, and Iverson (2019) reported that "Approximately one-third of women globally have experienced physical or sexual IPV (Devries et al., 2013) and in a group of community and shelter women who had experienced IPV, it was shown that approximately 75% sustained at least one IPV-related TBI […]" (p. 2). In the USA alone, that number is estimated to be approximately 31,500,000 (Valera et al., 2019), a staggering and worrisome proportion, considering the aftermath effects of mTBI. Overall, violence is the cause of closed head injury in 7–10% of cases based on studies in the USA and China (Maas et al., 2008). In Canada, results from the Canadian Community Health Survey demonstrated a significant 10-year trend in increased self-reported traumatic brain injury among Canadians seeking care in EDs within the first 48 h post-injury, with 30,879 patients admitted in 2005, 45,452 in 2009, and 79,037 in 2014 (Rao, McFaull, Thompson, & Jayaraman, 2018).

Age emerged as another risk factor, with children 0–4, older adolescents 15–19, and older adults (≥65 years old) presenting as the groups at higher risk for TBI (Faul et al., 2010; Langlois et al., 2006). Adults over 75 years of age present the highest prevalence of hospitalization and death after TBI (Faul et al., 2010). In a report by Coronado et al. (2015), an estimated 329,290 children (age 19 or younger) were treated in US EDs in 2012 for sports and recreation-related injuries that included a diagnosis of concussion or TBI, showing a twofold increase from 2001 to 2012. Consistent with the literature identifying gender and age as risk factors for TBI, a systematic review we conducted synthesizing the data from 11 meta-analyses meeting inclusion criteria, identified that females and high school adolescents presented with the highest deficits on cognitive outcomes, including executive functioning, which was the most sensitive to the effects of multiple mTBI (Karr, Areshenkoff, & Garcia-Barrera, 2014b).

The following sections focus on a review of the effects of TBI on executive functioning across the lifespan, with an emphasis on four vulnerable groups: children and adolescents (**pediatric TBI**), and in adults (**occupational TBI**, **sports-related concussions**, and **military TBI**). Chapter 8 in this book includes discussion of executive dysfunctions observed in older adults.

5.3 Pediatric TBI and Executive Functioning

Pediatric brain injuries are a significant and growing concern, especially mTBI. Epidemiology studies in the USA reported that just from 2005 to 2009, children made over 5 million visits to either outpatient clinics (2 million) or the ED (3 million) seeking care for mTBI (Mannix, O'Brien, & Meehan III, 2013). According to the electronic database of the Canadian Hospitals Injury Reporting and Prevention Program, approximately 46,000 concussion s were reported in children and adolescents between the ages 5–19 years from 2016 to 2017 (Government of Canada, 2018). Overall, preventable injuries lead to nearly 3.5 million ED visits with a total economic cost of 26.8 billion dollars each year in Canada (Parachute Canada, 2015). Among those adolescents entering EDs with sports-related head injuries, the vast majority suffers from concussions with over 15,000 individuals visiting EDs in Alberta and Ontario in 2015 alone (Canadian Institute for Health Information, 2016). Epidemiological studies in Canada identified that over 30% of individuals who played sports as children or adolescents reported suffering concussions or suspected concussions, with half of these individuals never being formally diagnosed (Angus Reid Institute, 2015). This finding supports the idea that epidemiological data for concussion rates are generally considered to be far lower than the actual incidence rate as many people do not seek medical attention when they receive concussions (McCrea, Hammeke, Olsen, Leo, & Guskiewicz, 2004).

5.3.1 Developmental Sensitivity of Executive Systems to Damage

Executive functions are broadly understood to be an integrated system of complex cognitive processes that govern flexible, goal-directed behavior and are reliant on subordinate processes like inhibitory control, updating working memory, and shifting attention (Diamond, 2013). Akin to a machine with many moving parts, executive functioning relies upon an interconnected system of frontal-parietal regions and subcortical pathways. Like a complex piece of machinery, there are simply more pieces or places where something could go wrong and this leads to an increased vulnerability to damage in the executive system as it predominantly relies upon whole-brain integrity. Indeed, executive functions and associated brain regions are disproportionately impacted by neurological insults.

Relative to adults, children, and adolescents are considered to have weaker executive function; however, if taken from a neurodevelopmental lens, this difference should be considered normative as opposed to pathological. The beginnings of executive control can be observed as early as 12 months and as children age, they progressively show improvements on measures of executive function, beginning to perform at approximately adult levels by adolescence (Crone, 2009; Jurado & Rosselli, 2007). Unlike in adults, where the executive system is assumed to be fully formed and therefore more robust in the face of neurological damage, there is an even greater vulnerability for developing executive deficits in children and adolescents as maturational brain processes (e.g., synaptic pruning) are underway and are easily altered or disrupted by environmental factors like traumatic brain injury.

Due to the extended developmental trajectory of executive functions, deficits may not be observed until later ages when certain abilities that are expected to develop, fail to emerge (Ashton, 2010; Chapman & McKinnon, 2000; Gil, 2003; Li & Liu, 2013). In a study following 433 children with mild-to-severe TBI or orthopedic injury controls, the proportion of children aged 5–15 with observed executive dysfunction doubled for mild TBI and tripled for moderate-to-severe TBI 3 months after baseline. Indeed, in that same study, observable deficits in executive functioning were seen via parental reports on the BRIEF in up to 40% of pediatric TBI cases within a year of injury, despite relatively few differences with non-TBI controls at baseline (Sesma, Slomine, Ding, & McCarthy, 2008). The neurocognitive foundations for executive functioning are laid in early childhood but not fully realized until adulthood; and in recognition of this increased vulnerability even for the mildest of neurological insults, contemporary injury management protocols for mild traumatic brain injuries like concussion tend to be more conservative for youth than for adults and err on the side of caution (Lumba-Brown et al., 2018; McCrory et al., 2017). Any damage or disruption to the development of executive functioning is a matter of great concern as executive deficits observed in childhood are predictive of a variety of outcomes ranging from reduced individual quality of life to increases in community-level public safety concerns (Diamond, 2013; Moffitt et al., 2011).

5.3.2 *Pediatric TBI: In a Nutshell*

When examining the current literature on TBI and executive functioning in pediatric populations, there appear to be two general rules governing the relationship between the two:

(1) Any neurological insult impacting the general integrity of brain structures will cause some degree of executive impairment, with degree of impairment scaling with severity of injury and;
(2) Earlier injuries are associated with both worse outcomes and longer-lasting executive deficits, while acknowledging that there are certain critical periods of cortical development that potentially represent times of even greater vulnerability within an already vulnerable group.

Upon reading these two points, one might ask: Why are children at such a risk for developing deficits in executive functioning after TBI? The answer lies in the physical proportions of children and the physical properties of their developing brains. Compared to adults, children have disproportionately large and heavy heads while simultaneously having relatively underdeveloped neck muscles. This combination leads to children experiencing a greater magnitude of overall head movement (e.g., greater whiplash effects) when struck by a forceful impact, which elevates their risk for not only suffering a brain injury but a more serious one. Furthermore, children have thinner skulls and in the case of infants, cranial bones that have yet to fuse together. This leads to an added risk of fractures and increased force applied directly to the brain; and by extension, the potential for more serious damage to brain tissue. Compounding these risks is the pediatric brain itself, which is more likely to experience axonal tearing due to blood vessel elasticity. These risk factors culminate in a brain that is more likely to sustain whole brain injury as opposed to more focal injuries (Case, 2008). As discussed earlier, whole-brain involvement is necessary for executive functions and more complex injuries at developmentally critical periods will have proportionally greater impact on future functioning. Infants, in particular, fit this description and though these physical attributes become less obvious or pronounced as children age, they still remain relevant risk factors.

5.3.3 Severity of Injury and Executive Functioning

Due to the significant damage sustained in severe pediatric TBI, virtually every executive function is impacted. The following domains discussed in this section are among the most commonly affected areas of executive functioning in severe pediatric TBI and to a lesser degree, in moderate and mild TBI.

Attentional processes are one of the more sensitive areas to be impacted by severe pediatric TBI (Babikian & Asarnow, 2009; Gil, 2003; Li & Liu, 2013). Given the relatively early maturation of basic attentional control, age of injury, and follow-up becomes particularly relevant as studies with younger samples may not necessarily show differences between pediatric TBI and control groups that are in the early stages of development on both neuropsychological tasks (e.g., NEPSY Auditory Attention) and rating scales like the BRIEF (Crowe, Catroppa, Babl, & Anderson, 2013; Tonks, Williams, Yates, & Slate, 2011), whereas studies with older samples may demonstrate deficits in the domain due to slowed development of attentional processes (Tonks et al., 2011). In terms of more complex attention, it appears that tasks that measure divided attention (e.g., sustained attention in the Dual Task (Score DT) from the Test of Everyday Attention for Children—TEA-Ch) are more sensitive to TBI than more simple forms of attention (e.g., Sky Search from the TEA-Ch) with individuals impacted by severe TBI performing worse than non-TBI controls, even 5 years post-injury (Nadebaum, Anderson, & Catroppa, 2007). That being said, tasks of processing speed (e.g., Coding or Symbol Search) require some degree of focused attention and are sensitive to severe TBI (Nadebaum et al., 2007).

Pediatric patients who have experienced severe traumatic brain injuries have also been observed to develop secondary attention deficit hyperactivity disorder (ADHD). Children who suffer from any kind of TBI are three times more likely to be diagnosed with ADHD than uninjured peers (Schachar, Levin, Max, Purvis, & Chen, 2004), and it is expected that more severe injuries increase this likelihood. Despite many similarities with developmental ADHD in terms of behavioral presentation, a study comparing the neuropsychological performance of children who develop secondary ADHD due to TBI compared to those already with developmental ADHD and TBI-only controls, found significantly greater planning difficulties weaker working memory, and slow and imprecise divided attention for those in the secondary ADHD group (Ornstein et al., 2014).

Alongside issues of attentional control, difficulties with inhibition are commonly seen in pediatric TBI populations. Crowe et al. (2013), using the NEPSY Statue task, found that any degree of TBI led to significantly more difficulties with sustaining performance with a greater number of errors and lower total scores, even for mild pediatric TBI. In a 2-year prospective study of 65 children with severe TBI, using measures like the Stroop and the Statue task, inhibitory control deficits were observed at 2-years post-injury (Krasny-Pacini et al., 2017). Irrespective of age-at-injury Tavano et al. (2014) found that disinhibition was the main feature of TBI symptomatology when comparing children and adults who suffered from TBI.

Multiple reviews of the literature suggest that pediatric TBI, particularly severe TBI has an impact on working memory and on memory function as a whole (e.g., Ashton, 2010; Babikian & Asarnow, 2009; Gil, 2003; Levin & Hanten, 2005). Performance on measures such as the Children's Memory Scale—Attention and Concentration Index have shown observable deficits up to 2 years post-injury (Krasny-Pacini et al., 2017). Even after 10-years post-injury, deficits are observed in tasks like Digit Span, the Rey Auditory Verbal Learning Task, and Token Test for those impacted by severe pediatric TBI (Horneman & Emanuelson, 2009).

Planning and goal setting are higher-order processes that rely on less complex executive functions like attentional control, working memory, and inhibition. It should be no surprise then that given the impact of pediatric TBI on those foundational processes, that more complex executive functions would be affected as well. Perhaps reflecting the delayed onset of executive problems after TBI, Tonks et al. (2011) found that while children under the age of 10 did not show any deficits in Delis–Kaplan Executive Function System (DKEFS) Tower Test performance compared to controls, differences were found in children older than 10. In a sample of 36 adolescents and young adults who suffered mild-to-severe pediatric TBI nearly a decade prior, large effect sizes were observed for the DKEFS Sorting Task ($d = 0.82$), errors made on the DKEFS Tower Test ($d = 1.43$), and the Rey Complex Figure Task—Copy Condition ($d = 0.82$); in this study, those who suffered moderate-to-severe TBI performed worse than individuals who were diagnosed with mild TBI (Muscara, Catroppa, & Anderson, 2008).

One particularly interesting study used a virtual reality anticipation of consequences task in a sample of typically developing adolescents and adolescents that suffered from moderate-to-severe TBI. These researchers found that those with TBI were less likely to think about long-term consequences and more likely to consider only the immediate consequences of an action (Cook et al., 2013). Perhaps even more telling is a study by Wade et al. (2017) where 153 adolescents with moderate-to-severe TBI were assessed on their problem-solving abilities using the Social Problem-Solving Inventory (SPSI) and Dodge Social Information Processing Short Stories. Not only did this group of adolescents report lower levels of rational problem-solving, but they also reported lower levels of negative problem orientations, impulsivity, and avoidance compared to the mean of the normative sample of the SPSI, indicating a relative disengagement from any problem-solving activity. This self-reporting pattern suggests that those suffering from pediatric TBI may lack awareness or underestimate the challenges of problem-solving. Tangentially related to this point, while there is generally a lack of strong evidence suggesting an increase in aggression after TBI, it is suggested that observed increases in aggression may stem from deficits sustained in areas of social problem-solving (Li & Liu, 2013). Aggression may be also manifested as emotional dysregulation and defensiveness as in Sam's case.

One of the defining characteristics of the executive system is cognitive flexibility and it too is impacted by pediatric TBI. Muscara et al. (2008) observed large effect sizes for Trails B ($d = 1.55$), Colour-Word Interference—Time ($d = 0.85$) and Errors ($d = 0.98$), where those diagnosed with moderate-to-severe TBI performed more slowly and with more errors than those diagnosed with mild TBI. Krasny-Pacini et al. (2017) found that performance on tasks like the Wisconsin Card Sorting Task, Design Fluency, and the total number of trials completed in the Tower of London was most impaired at 3-months post-injury but showed rapid recovery by 12 months post-injury. In examinations of executive dysfunction and pediatric TBI at the behavioral level, the BRIEF has been used in much of the literature and has shown good sensitivity of executive deficits (Crowe et al., 2013; Karver et al., 2012; Krasny-Pacini et al., 2017; Mangeot, Armstrong, Colvin, Yates, & Taylor, 2002; Muscara et al., 2008; Nadebaum et al., 2007). However, the BRIEF is not the only measure that has been used to assess more ecologically valid executive deficits. Using an executive behavior screener derived from the Behavior Assessment System for Children (BASC-2) rating scales, Direnfeld (2017) found that adolescents with mild-to-severe TBI demonstrated greater difficulties in behavioral and emotional control than adolescents with neuropsychiatric or neurodevelopmental conditions.

5.3.4 Severe Versus Moderate Pediatric TBI

Often due to small sample size, much of the research tends to place both moderate and severe pediatric TBI in the same categories for analysis but in studies where this is not the case, differences are often observed. Those who have suffered a severe brain injury in childhood go on to have far more significant deficits and show slowed trajectories of recovery compared to moderate TBI (Babikian & Asarnow, 2009). As demonstrated in a study by Karver et al. (2012), children who suffered from severe TBI continue to exhibit higher levels of parent-reported internalizing and externalizing problems using the CBCL as well as increased executive deficit using the BRIEF two years post-injury, whereas children with moderate or complicated mild TBI were more similar to controls who suffered from orthopedic injuries. Gerrard-Morris et al. (2010) followed a group of 3–6-year-olds who had suffered mild-to-severe TBI or orthopedic injuries as a control, finding that, after 18 months post-injury, the children with severe TBI continued to exhibit greater deficits in cognitive ability on neuropsychological measures like the Stroop or Digit Span and developed (or recover) at a slower rate than the other groups during the study period. In a 4-year prospective study of 189 children suffering from orthopedic injuries or moderate-to-severe TBI, chronic adaptive functioning deficits were observed, with moderate TBI showing fewer deficits than severe injuries (Taylor, Yeates, Wade, Drotar, Stancin, & Minich, 2002). Similarly, a 5-year prospective study of 98 children diagnosed with moderate TBI, severe TBI, or orthopedic injuries not only showed that the degree of executive dysfunction, as rated with the BRIEF, was related to the degree of injury, but also showed pediatric TBI in general leads to a chronic pattern of executive deficits (Mangeot et al., 2002). After 10 years post-injury, compared to severe TBI, individuals who suffered moderate TBI showed less impairment in the domains of attention and working memory, verbal learning and memory, visual organization, and cognitive flexibility (Horneman & Emanuelson, 2009).

5.3.5 *Mild Pediatric TBI and Executive Functioning*

While there is some evidence for the long-term impact of complicated (i.e., more severe) mild TBI on divided attention (Papoutsis, Stargatt, & Catroppa, 2014), in stark contrast to severe or even moderate TBI, uncomplicated mild pediatric TBI is generally characterized by relatively minor executive functioning impairments and few (if any) observable long-term impacts (Babikian & Asarnow, 2009). Those who present with long-term difficulties form only a small subset of the injured population (McCrory et al., 2017; Zemek, Farion, Sampson, & McGahern, 2013). Predicting children who go on to develop lingering concussion symptomatology is difficult, and some measures designed for this purpose, while outperforming physician judgment alone, have modest predictive capacity and require further refinement (Zemek et al., 2016). In fact, external factors may be more relevant in this group in terms of post-TBI symptom presentation. For example, it has been observed that executive difficulties post-TBI only emerged in a sample of preschoolers who had insufficient sleep (Landry-Roy, Bernier, Gravel, & Beauchamp, 2018). Physical exercise has been shown to reduce the overall likelihood of developing post-TBI symptomatology (Chrismas & Rivera, 2016; Grool et al., 2016). As children who suffer from mild TBI tend to recover fully, lingering deficits are generally attributed to environmental or pre-injury factors like genetics, premorbid ability, or family characteristics (Babikian, McArthur, & Asarnow, 2013; Chapman & McKinnon, 2000; Durish et al., 2018; Sesma et al., 2008).

5.3.6 *Adolescence and mTBI*

After discussing the typical findings in pediatric TBI and executive functioning, there appears to be an age-group and injury group that exhibits an atypical trajectory of recovery; adolescents who suffer from mild TBI. Among researchers, there is a general consensus that the foundations for most executive systems are in place by the time a child reaches adolescence, theoretically making executive functioning more resistant to long-term damage; however, and as discussed earlier, our systematic review of meta-analyses examining the effects of mild traumatic brain injury on cognition, identified that adolescents are the most vulnerable to the negative cognitive effects of mild traumatic brain injury and suffered particularly when it comes to executive functioning (Karr et al., 2014b). While these negative effects are far less than what a child might experience in a severe or moderate traumatic brain injury, it does appear for mild TBI at least, and it is adolescents who may be more impacted relative to other pediatric age groups. One may be prompted to ask: What could be the reason for this?

From a developmental perspective, adolescence is a time of physical, social, and neurological change. One of these changes is the finding that cognitive capacities are increasing throughout childhood and into adolescence, and there is an increase in activation within subcortical systems during adolescence, which has implications for emotion processing and regulation (Galvan et al., 2006). It has been suggested that while adolescents have an executive capacity that is similar to adults, their performance is impacted in situations where emotionally salient content is present (Crone, 2009). In support of this developmental executive functioning perspective, Prencipe et al. (2011) found that while performance on executive functioning tasks improved as children age, improvements in less emotionally salient executive functioning tasks (e.g., Stroop task) occurred earlier and were more robust, whereas performance on more emotionally salient executive functioning tasks (e.g., Iowa Gambling Task) did not improve until mid-adolescence. Indeed, it is in areas of emotional or psychological distress where researchers tend to find the most evidence for the impacts of mild TBI in adolescence as opposed to standardized or computerized measures of cognitive functioning (Brooks et al., 2013). Mild TBI may impact an adolescent's ability to modulate their emotions and through this emotional dysregulation, executive function performance is reduced.

5.4 TBI in Adults and Executive Functioning

5.4.1 Occupational TBI Statistics and Trends

Occupational TBI, and particularly mTBI, is a burdening and costly issue for employees, employers, and compensation cooperatives. Reports for the province of British Columbia where we are located revealed that of the 4800 annual survivors of TBI, 3800 are estimated to be cases of mTBI (Martin, 2003). Cumulative evidence has demonstrated a group of variables that seem to serve as risk factors for experiencing an mTBI, and consequently, compensation claims, including, gender, age, and field of work. The concussion rates in female employees is about half of the prevalence rate for males, particularly for workers aged 15–24 years. However, the rate of employment of females between the ages of 25 and 64 years is not disparate from that of their counterpart males, demonstrating a higher risk for males to suffer a concussion in our province even when rate of employment by gender is taken into account. In terms of age, within the age range of 25–64, it appears that males aged between of 25–44 years are at a higher risk of occupational concussion. Similarly, a prospective cohort study on Ontarian workers being compensated for mTBI found that most mTBIs (i.e., 80%) involved workers between the ages of 20–49, with a majority of males (i.e., 68.3%) being affected (Kristman et al., 2010). Thus, these prevalence rates may be consistent at least across Canadian regions.

There are also known moderators of the capacity of the injured employee to return to work. For instance, there is a positive correlation between age and the amount of time spent on disability leave from work (Martin, 2003; Kristman et al., 2010). Also, individuals with mTBI holding professional or managerial positions return to work significantly faster than their counterparts in manual/labor occupations. These findings have been consistent across several studies conducted in other samples (e.g., Cancelliere et al., 2014). Despite the steadily increasing reports of mixed-mechanism mTBI (e.g., from falls, sports, motor vehicle accidents), work-related mTBI is prone to both under- and over-diagnosis, because injuries may go unreported, or symptoms unrelated to mTBI may be misattributed to the injury, especially in delayed recovery situations (Chang, Lonbard, & Greher, 2011), making it difficult to have a clear picture of the current statistics.

5.4.2 Occupational Versus Sports-Related MTBI in Adults

5.4.2.1 Differences in Cognitive Outcomes

The preponderance of research on mTBI has occurred within athletic settings (Comper, Hutchinson, Magrys, Mainwaring, & Richards, 2010; Dougan, Horswill, & Geffen, 2013), but a large amount of research has also explored non-sports-related mechanisms of head injury and its neurological and cognitive sequelae (Belanger et al., 2005). These injuries have been historically amalgamated into a non-athletic category, often referred to as mixed-mechanism mTBI, with injury etiologies ranging from falls to motor vehicle accidents. Previous research has documented key differences between sports-related and mixed-mechanism injuries, with many variables differentiating athletes from the general population, including fitness and incentives for quick recovery (i.e., return-to-play; Belanger & Vanderploeg, 2005). In turn, although past research has extrapolated from sports-related concussion research into other injury types (e.g., military concussion; Lew, Thomander, Chew, & Bleiberg, 2007), mixed-mechanism mTBI may present as a unique style injury, with unique sequelae compared to sports-related head injury (Karr et al., 2014b). As such, the cognitive effects of mixed-mechanism mTBI (i.e., range: 0.07–0.61) differ from that of sports-related concussion, as these injuries produce smaller acute effect sizes than sports-related head injuries across meta-analyses (Karr et al., 2014b), but persist for much longer following injury (Belanger et al., 2005). The minor head injuries experienced by workers may present unique cognitive outcomes, and further, some of these differences contribute to the discrepancy noted between workers and "general population."

Some of the differences in cognitive performance observed after sports-related concussions versus occupational and mixed-mechanism injuries are associated with executive functioning (Karr et al., 2014b). Cumulative evidence using randomized studies (avoiding self-selection effects) has demonstrated that physical exercise is beneficial to us (Hillman, Erickson, & Kramer, 2008), particularly, to our executive functioning (Chang Labban, Gapin, & Etnier, 2012; Tomporowski, Lambourne, & Okumura, 2011; Verburgh, Königs, Scherder, & Oosterlaan, 2013). There are at least three mechanisms through which physical exercise enhances executive functioning (Best, 2010): (1) the executive demands inherent to the type of goal-directed exercise, (2) the neurophysiological changes induced by exercise, including up-regulation of growth factors such as the insulin-like growth factor-1 (for neuronal growth and survival), and the brain-derived neurotrophic factor (activity-dependent modulator of exercise-induced plasticity), and (3) the greater cardiovascular capacity associated with physical fitness, which enhances the efficiency with which oxygen and nutrients are supplied to the brain. Further, variables moderating these effects include exercise intensity and duration (higher effects for higher intensity and longer duration), type of cognitive task (highest effects on higher-order tasks), and fitness level (higher effects observed for higher fitness level). Most research examining the effects of exercise on cognition focuses on interventions involving acute bouts of physical activity. These effects may be short-lived and not necessarily comparable to the effects of long-term physical activity (Padilla, Pérez, & Andrés, 2014). Thus, researchers have pushed for longitudinal evaluation of the effects of exercise on behavior, cognition, and executive neural systems (Voss, Nagamatsu, Liu-Ambrose, & Kramer, 2011). Positive effects of long-term physical exercise on executive attention (Pérez, Padilla, Parmentier, & Andrés, 2014) and inhibitory control (Padilla et al., 2014) have been demonstrated. Although research is still scarce, differences in executive structural and functional neural connectivity (Huang, Lu, Song, & Wang, 2015; Marks et al., 2007) between athletes and controls have been shown, with most research being conducted in young adult athletes.

5.4.2.2 Differences in Recovery Times

Sports-related concussions present a more rapid average recovery rate than mixed mechanism mTBI. Although athletes typically recover from sports-related concussion within seven days of injury (Belanger & Vanderploeg, 2005), the rate of recovery following mixed-mechanism mTBI appears far less clear. Notably, nearly all cognitive abilities present significant effect sizes following 90 days; however, compensation seeking moderates this phenomenon, with non-forensic participants presenting a more rapid recovery before 90 days (Belanger et al., 2005). Past researchers have posited the existence of a "miserable minority" (Ruff et al., 1994; Ruff, Camenzuli, & Mueller, 1996), a term used to describe a small portion of individuals with mTBI that do not reach full recovery by 90 days. Researchers have debated the existence of such persistent symptoms (Rohling et al., 2011), attributing their existence to, in part, feigned symptoms or limited effort on testing (Rohling, Larrabee, & Millis, 2012). Curiously, merely bringing mTBI to the attention of a head-injured individual actually worsens their neuropsychological performance, even outside of situations involving external incentives and/or low effort (Suhr & Gunstad, 2002, 2005). In turn, concussed individuals may experience expectancy effects and misattribute general fatigue to persistent post-concussive symptoms.

5.4.2.3 Differences in Effort (e.g., The "Sandbagging" Phenomenon)

Malingering following mTBI in litigation settings occurs at a roughly 40% base rate, indicating that nearly half of concussed individuals feign symptoms when involved in compensation-seeking claims (Mittenberg, Patton, Canyock, & Condit, 2002). In athletic settings, effort has inversely affected cognitive performance, where low effort at baseline testing will result in what appears to be a less severe deficit at post-concussion testing (Erdal, 2012). Termed "sandbagging", this technique allows players to quickly return to play following injury, as a coach or sports trainer may misinterpret the athlete as recovered. Contrarily, workers may have less tangible incentives to return to work, benefiting from extended time-off, increased rest, and continued pay. As such, they may present an opposite trend, with limited effort at post-injury testing.

One variable that may have an effect on the motivation of workers to return to work is the presence of posttraumatic Stress disorder (PTSD) symptoms. The context in which an occupational mTBI can occur (e.g., falling off a roof, being struck by an everyday tool) in association with the possibility of near-death experiences may increase the incidence of PTSD symptoms. Unfortunately, the rate at which mTBI and PTSD co-occur appears unclear to date, with estimates ranging from 5 to 39% (Carlson et al., 2011). Early research has identified that PTSD is associated with increased post-concussive symptom reporting following mTBI (Bryant & Harvey, 1999). However, the majority of research on mTBI and PTSD has occurred among active duty soldiers and veterans (e.g., Amick et al., 2013; Nelson et al., 2012; Verfaellie, Lafleche, Avron Spiro, & Bousquet, 2014), with no known studies evaluating posttraumatic psychiatric symptoms following workplace mTBI. A past systematic review evaluating the quality of past concussion research recommended that future researchers use a musculoskeletal or orthopedic injury group for comparison in order to control for the aspects of an injury event extraneous to neurological injury (Comper et al., 2010). These extraneous components of injury likely include the trauma surrounding the event and the sequential pain and hardship of recovering from an injury.

5.4.3 Military TBI and Executive Functioning

Since the United States Department of Defense began tracking the frequency of TBI among Service Members in 2000, 383,947 TBIs have been documented through the first quarter of 2018 (U.S. Department of Defense, 2019). The majority of such injuries are mild (82.3%), with far fewer falling within the moderate (9.7%) to severe (1.1%) range. An entire system of care has been developed within the US Veterans Health Administration (VHA) to address polytrauma, which is inclusive of assessment, treatment, and rehabilitation for mTBI and co-occurring mental health needs (Belanger, Uomoto, & Vanderploeg, 2009). TBI has become a significant area of health care cost within the US VHA. In 2009, veterans with TBI diagnosis had four times the healthcare costs than veterans without TBI, and those veterans with the highest costs had comorbid TBI, PTSD, and pain (Taylor et al., 2012). In 2012, veterans with comorbid TBI and PTSD incurred greater healthcare costs than Veterans with PTSD or TBI alone (Kehle-Forbes, Campbell, Taylor, Scholten, & Sayer, 2017). Specific to mild injury, veterans diagnosed with mTBI in 2010 had two to three times higher VHA healthcare costs than veterans who screened negative for TBI over a 3-year period, with the most service utilization concentrated in mental health (Taylor et al., 2017b).

Because most military TBIs are mild in severity, the majority of TBI research on veterans has focused exclusively on mTBI. A growing emphasis has also focused on blast-related mTBI, which is a unique mechanism of injury among primarily military populations (Cernak & Noble-Haeusslein, 2010; Rosenfeld et al., 2013). Researchers have compared the cognitive sequelae of mTBI due to blast and blunt trauma, finding no empirical differences in outcome (Belanger et al., 2011; Lange et al., 2012; Luethcke, Bryan, Morrow, & Isler, 2011). Nonetheless, multiple studies have specifically examined blast-related mTBI among military samples (Amick et al., 2013; Kontos et al., 2013; Nelson et al., 2012, 2010; Peskind et al., 2011; Scheibel et al., 2012; Shandera-Ochsner et al., 2013; Vakhtin et al., 2013; Verfaellie et al., 2014). The cognitive effects of blast-related mTBI are, at most, subtle, with a recent meta-analysis finding evidence of very small group differences based on cross-sectional studies comparing veterans with and without a remote history of blast-related mTBI (Karr, Areshenkoff, Duggan, & Garcia-Barrera, 2014a). The overall effect size (plus highest density interval in parentheses) was $d = -0.12$ (−0.21, −0.04). Many specific cognitive domains were rarely measured and did not provide precise estimates of group differences. Executive function was more regularly evaluated and demonstrated an overall effect of $d = -0.16$ (−0.31, 0.00). When separated based on executive-related constructs (Karr et al., 2018; Miyake et al., 2000), the only negative effect of blast-related mTBI was observed for set shifting: $d = -0.33$ (−0.55, −0.05).

Despite the subtle effects of blast-related mTBI on cognitive functioning, the majority of veterans screening positive for TBI report moderate to very severe cognitive complaints, including forgetfulness (83%), poor concentration (76%), slowed thinking, difficulty, organizing, and difficulty finishing things (64%), and difficulty making decisions (55%); and interestingly, these cognitive complaints are common among veterans without TBI as well, but occur at lower frequencies: forgetfulness (68%), poor concentration (62%), slowed thinking, difficulty, organizing, and difficulty finishing things (50%), and difficulty making decisions (43%) (Scholten, Sayer, Vanderploeg, Bidelspach, & Cifu, 2012). A recent study examined subjective change in executive function among veterans with a remote history of mTBI, retrospectively rated on the Frontal Systems Behavior Scale (FrSBe) (Karr, Rau, Shofer, Hendrickson, Peskind, & Pagulayan, 2019). Veterans reported significant increases in executive dysfunction post-mTBI. Only 11% of the sample reported clinically significant executive dysfunction prior to their mTBI, whereas 82% reported clinically significant executive dysfunction following their mTBI. Pre-injury characteristics (e.g., age, premorbid intelligence), injury-related characteristics (e.g., number of blast exposures), sleep quality, and neuropsychological test performances failed to predict subjective change on the FrSBe, and PTSD emerged as the sole independently significant predictor of subjective decline in executive function post mTBI. Another study on Active Duty Service Members found minimal correspondence between post-mTBI FrSBe and objective cognitive performances, but found significant correspondence between post-mTBI FrSBe ratings and depression symptoms (Schiehser et al., 2011). Perceived executive dysfunction following mTBI may be closely related to mental health symptomatology as opposed to objective impairment on executive function tests.

The psychiatric complexity of TBI among veterans makes the injury unique in comparison to other populations that experience PTSD at a lower prevalence. Among veterans of operations Enduring Freedom and Iraqi Freedom, PTSD prevalence has been estimated at 23% (Fulton et al., 2015). It is the most common co-occurring psychiatric disorder among Iraq and Afghanistan Veterans with TBI: 73% of Veterans with TBI had PTSD, 45% had depression, and 22% had anxiety (Taylor et al., 2012). Considering the high comorbidity of TBI and PTSD among veterans, and the high healthcare costs associated with these co-occurring conditions, the effects of mTBI cannot be fully appreciated without closely considering the effects of PTSD as well. When comparing meta-analytic effects of remote blast-related mTBI and PTSD, the significantly greater impact of PTSD on executive function becomes evident. A large-scale meta-analysis on the cognitive effects of PTSD found medium effect sizes for executive functions ($d = -0.45$) and attention/working memory ($d = -0.50$). These effect sizes of current PTSD diagnosis, albeit medium in magnitude, dwarf those effects associated with cross-sectional studies on remote blast-related mTBI (Karr et al., 2014a). Although these conclusions demonstrate a greater impact of PTSD on executive function than mTBI, they do not necessarily indicate that mTBI has no meaningful impact on cognitive functioning or neurological structure.

Traumatic axonal injury is a common neurological injury linked to mTBI (Hurley, McGowan, Arfanakis, & Taber, 2014), and multiple past studies have examined changes in brain white matter associated with a history of blast-related mTBI (Bazarian et al., 2013; Jorge et al., 2012; MacDonald et al., 2013, 2011; Matthews, Spadoni, Lohr, Strigo, & Simmons, 2012; Matthews et al., 2011; Petrie et al., 2013; Sponheim et al., 2011). Some of these past studies have shown evidence for concentrated anterior damage that may be associated with executive function deficits (Jorge et al., 2012; Sorg et al., 2014; Sponheim et al., 2011; Yeh et al., 2013). Despite evidence for potential cognitive and neurological changes associated with blast-related mTBI, the act of disentangling the effects of mTBI and PTSD has been an area of ongoing scientific investigation (Rosenfeld et al., 2013). Researchers have even proposed that mTBI and PTSD possibly involve similar underlying mechanisms, or independent pathophysiological mechanisms that result in a shared symptomatology (Hendrickson, Schindler, & Pagulayan, 2018). Cognitive concerns, often related to both mTBI and PTSD, are common among veterans, and regardless of etiology, evidence-based interventions that reduce such concerns have the capacity to improve quality of life among returning service members. Cognitive rehabilitation interventions have been developed to address such concerns in veterans with mTBI (Storzbach et al.,

2017), and other trauma-focused interventions have shown generalized benefits on post-concussion symptoms and cognitive concerns (Wolf et al., 2018). Future interventions that aim to address both PTSD and cognitive functioning may be attractive to veterans seeking to address both mental and cognitive health problems.

5.4.4 Executive Dysfunction After Adult TBI

Among the models that are used to discuss executive functioning (see Chap. 1 for a review), Stuss's approach to the conceptual fractionation of executive components has resonated in the clinical settings, particularly useful in examining the aftermath of TBI affecting the frontal and prefrontal areas. Stuss and his colleagues proposed a conceptualization of executive function that includes an aspect of unity, represented by attention, the cognitive foundation of all other processes, and an aspect of diversity, corresponding to three processes: (1) **energization**, associated with bilateral superior medial regions, is the process of initiation and sustaining behavioral responses, particularly in the absence of external triggers or motivators; (2) **task setting**, associated with left lateral frontal areas, particularly involving ventrolateral regions, is the ability to set a stimulus-response, starting from an a priori association and progressing to a trial and error-based learned association; and (3) **monitoring**, associated with right lateral prefrontal areas, is the process of inspecting the task performance over time, making adjustments to behavior as needed (Stuss & Alexander, 2007). They applied this approach in a review of the literature and concluded that while there is no undifferentiated, unifying, dysexecutive syndrome, lesions to specific regions of the frontal lobes produce specific dysexecutive problems. For instance, damage to bilateral (but mostly right) superior medial frontal areas (and their connection to anterior cingulate cortex and supplementary motor areas), appears to be associated with deficient energization (e.g., apathy, unmotivation, problems with initiation, concentration and task maintenance, verbal fluency, impaired interference control in the Stroop test). Damage to left lateral frontal areas, particularly ventral components, was associated with impaired task setting (e.g., problems with task analysis, setting task criterion toward producing correct responses, set lost in the Wisconsin Card Sorting Test, false-positive responses in memory tests—i.e., identifying non-listed words as correct, false alarms in go/no-go tasks—i.e., incorrect responses to the no-go stimulus, and inability to use verbal task instructions to guide behavior). Further, damage to the right lateral frontal regions was associated with impaired monitoring (e.g., problems with modulation of expectancy and time estimation in reaction time tasks, monitoring of temporal information in self-timed conditions, poor error checking and monitoring performance overtime, double recalls in memory tasks—i.e., recalling the same word twice; Stuss & Alexander, 2007).

Cumulative research has consistently demonstrated the vulnerability of executive functioning to TBI, regardless of the level of severity (Lezak et al., 2012; Roebuck-Spencer & Sherer, 2008), but certainly with large variability on presentation. On mTBI, common executive-related difficulties reported include attentional deficits and difficulty in speed of processing, associated with the diffuse axonal damage commonly observed after mTBI (Krpan, Levine, Stuss, & Dawson, 2007). Our meta-analysis identified that executive functions are the most susceptible to the impacts of multiple mTBIs (Karr et al., 2014b), but there is consensus in that the great majority of cases recover function within 90 days after injury, with neuropsychological testing findings being unable to detect impairments past three months in most cases (Dikmen, Machamer, & Temkin, 2001; Lange, Iverson & Franzen, 2009; Schretlen & Shapiro, 2003). These findings do not vary as a function of positive neuroimaging findings. In the absence of a global reduction in functioning, patients with complicated mTBI show a greater proportion of low scores than the uncomplicated mTBI during the acute phase of recovery (first two months), and these small differences are no longer significant after 3 months (Lange et al., 2009). This report is consistent with Sam's presentation.

A few patients may present with long-term difficulties and persistent post-concussion symptoms, particularly in relation to emotional dysregulation (e.g., anxiety, depression symptoms). There is ongoing examination trying to clarify the nature of this vulnerability to persistence of symptom reporting. A prospective biopsychological study by Wäljas et al. (2015) demonstrated that persistence of symptom presentation was not associated with level of severity of injury (e.g., complicated mTBI) but rather, with a prior history of mental health problems. A longitudinal study by Maruta et al. (2016) examined a group of patients at three months and then at 5 years post-injury and identified that the original mTBI retained associations with lower performance at a statistically significant level, even when variance associated with demographic variables (e.g., gender, race) and the development of depression and PTSD symptoms post-injury was accounted for in the model.

Almost every aspect of executive functioning has been reported as vulnerable to impairment after moderate and severe TBI. Deficits on planning, cognitive flexibility, working memory, attention, processing of information, poor judgment and impaired decision making, reduced capacity for self-evaluation and task monitoring, lack of initiation and motivation issues (e.g., apathy), impaired self-regulation and aggressive behavior, emotional and affect dysregulation, are on the top of the lists (Krpan et al., 2007; Langlois et al., 2006; Lezak et al., 2012; Maas et al., 2008; Roebuck-Spencer & Sherer, 2008; Stuss & Alexander, 2007). Executive dysfunctions are quite impairing and are critical in determining patients' ability to return to independent living and their jobs (Roebuck-Spencer & Sherer, 2008). They are difficult to treat, particularly as one of the key difficulties observed after moderate and severe TBI is impaired self-awareness (Prigatano, 2009). Self-awareness is associated not only with the drive to participate in rehabilitation, but also with empathy and insight (Lezak et al., 2012). As such, it is of great relevance in any intervention aiming to rehabilitate executive functions after TBI. The following section discusses rehabilitation approaches that have been deemed effective in gaining self-awareness and facilitating recovery of function post-injury.

5.5 Rehabilitation of Executive Dysfunctions After TBI

Despite the potential multitude of impairments associated with executive functioning following TBI, there are interventions that have shown to be effective for restitution of function. While Miyake and colleagues' (2000) approach offers a well-supported framework for studying executive functions, we will use Stuss' (2011) clinical–neuroanatomical–evolutionary model to lay out the different areas of executive dysfunction following insult to frontal regions in the brain that are commonly observed following TBI. Specifically, we will cover deficits relating to energization, executive cognitive functions, behavioral self-regulation, and metacognitive processes (Stuss, 2011). To address these areas, we will limit our discussion to interventions aimed at regaining self-awareness and remediating attention, problem-solving, and metacognition. Of note, the material in this section will be brief, highlighting only a few of the most used, supported, and promising treatments for executive-related dysfunctions.

5.5.1 Awareness Deficits and Associated Intervention Strategies

Self-awareness is characterized by an individual's ability to recognize cognitive, behavioral and emotional difficulties that may have occurred following brain injury (Crosson et al., 1989). It is common for there to be deficits in self-awareness following TBI, occurring 45–97% of the time (Sherer et al., 1998), and such impairment can be problematic in several ways. Unawareness of one's deficits negatively impacts the course of neurorehabilitation (e.g., of executive functioning), through its impairment of volition (Lezak et al., 2012), often reducing the effectiveness of treatment through noncompliance. It can be either neurogenic (i.e., anosognosia) or psychological (i.e., defensive denial), or some combination of both, with no existing gold standard assessments to discriminate between the two (Prigatano, 2005). Self-awareness can fluctuate throughout the course of rehabilitation, even moment to moment, and should therefore be frequently assessed in order to determine appropriate treatment.

Although empirically supported interventions for self-awareness deficits are lacking (Cicerone et al., 2005), we will briefly discuss two of the most commonly applied approaches. Giacino and Cicerone (1998) proposed a variety of interventions for different types of unawareness. For unawareness that is due to a specific cognitive deficit, intervention should target such deficit. In cases of amnesia, for instance, this could entail incorporating reminders about one's impairment. For dense unawareness due to organic brain dysfunction (i.e., anosognosia), treatment could entail structuring the environment to minimize the deficit, or training in task-specific routines (e.g., using procedural memory) without reliance on appreciation of deficits. Lastly, Giacino and Cicerone (1998) recommend that to treat unawareness from psychological (defensive) denial, a combination of supportive psychotherapy and other techniques like motivational interviewing could be effective; here, discrepancies between perceived abilities and actual performance should be gently highlighted.

Crosson and colleagues (1989) proposed a tripartite, hierarchical model of awareness, its deficits, and related recommended interventions (see Table 5.1). For impairment in *intellectual* awareness, which is the knowledge that one has a particular deficit, they recommend providing psychoeducation through review of materials such as medical charts, neuroimaging, and brain injury fact sheets. To treat deficits in *emergent* awareness, which is the more complex ability to recognize a problem as

Table 5.1 Awareness types (according to Crosson et al., 1989), cognitive domains influencing EF, and corresponding intervention strategies

Type of awareness	Impairment	Intervention
Intellectual—acknowledging that one has a particular deficit	Patient has not been told, or cannot remember, understand, or conceptualize that they have a particular deficit	Provide psychoeducation through review of neuroimaging, medical chart notes, brain injury fact sheets, etc
Emergent—recognizing a problem (due to their deficit) as it occurs	Patient understands they have a deficit, but is not aware of the problem "in the moment"	Experiential; error prediction and monitoring
Anticipatory—knowing where/when a problem is likely to occur, and planning to minimize its occurrence	Patient cannot make accommodations or compensations for a problem due to lack of skill-knowledge in implementing an appropriate plan	Train task-specific routines through procedural learning or metacognitive strategies (focus of traditional EF rehabilitation interventions)
Cognitive domain influencing executive functioning	**Impairment**	**Intervention**
Attention	Patient has difficulty concentrating on a task, often getting sidetracked	*Mindfulness training (MT)*: self-directed attention regulation through focused attention and open monitoring
Metacognition	Patient has difficulty carrying out a task, making several mistakes	*Self-instructional training (SIT)*: verbalization of thought process during task *Metacognitive skills training (MST):* explicit reflection of performance during task, and generation of solutions to encountered obstacles
Problem-solving	Patient has difficulty carrying out a task, making several mistakes	*Goal management training (GMT)*: formulation of steps to reach a goal, followed by frequent monitoring of action-goal congruency

it occurs, error prediction and monitoring may be beneficial. In addition, the experiential techniques may simply be effective, such as the experience of undergoing neuropsychological testing. Lastly, the most complex type of awareness that Crosson and colleagues (1989) propose is *anticipatory* awareness, which is undergoing planning to minimize the occurrence of deficits. Impairment in this area might benefit from training of task-specific routines through procedural learning or metacognitive strategies.

5.5.2 Attention Training

As with awareness, attention heavily influences higher-level executive functioning, thus making it an important area for rehabilitation following TBI. A recently developed intervention for attention that has shown promise is mindfulness training (MT). Self-directed attention regulation, specifically, is a major component of MT. MT typically begins with sessions involving focused attention, where an individual attempt to direct their attention toward a specific object. Often times, focused attention might be directed toward an individual's body (e.g., their lower abdomen), while they attempt to tune out external distractors. Following focused attention, individuals may practice open monitoring, in which they allow themselves to be aware of all experiences, external or internal, responding to sensations and thoughts with an open, receptive and non-judgmental attitude (Fox et al., 2014). MT allows for ecologically relevant practice and has several aims, including improvement of self-monitoring and attention.

The efficacy of mindfulness practices has recently been supported in the literature. A meta-analysis by Sedlmeier and colleagues (2012) found mindfulness meditation to be generally associated with medium effect sizes on attention. Further, mindfulness training has shown promise for individuals who have experienced a brain injury. In a pilot study conducted by Azulay and colleagues (2013), 22 patients who experienced a mild TBI underwent a 10-week program of mindfulness-based stress reduction (MBSR), a type of mindfulness practice involving body scans (i.e., somatically focused mindfulness practice), sitting and walking meditation, and yoga (Azulay, Smart, Mott, & Cicerone, 2013). Results demonstrated significant improvement in measures of attention, including sustained attention and attentional control.

5.5.3 Metacognitive Strategy Training

While behaviorally training patients to perform specific tasks involving executive functions (e.g., planning, sequencing, and organization) can be effective, metacognitive strategy training can have a more overarching and generalizable impact by improving executive functions themselves. Metacognition likely represents the most highly developed of the executive functions. Often defined as "thinking about thinking," metacognition relates to an individual's ability to self-monitor and evaluate, have appreciation of their abilities and limitations, and be able to flexibly implement strategies and supports when they are operating within an area of relative weakness. As such, interventions in the area of metacognition typically involve training in self-monitoring and self-regulation. Compared to behavioral training aimed at executing specific tasks, metacognitive strategy training requires a greater degree of awareness on the part of the individual.

A commonly used, and empirically supported, technique for metacognitive training is self-instructional training (SIT). Initially developed by Donald Meichenbaum for use with children, (e.g., Meichenbaum & Goodman, 1971), SIT involves explicitly verbalizing the problem-solving process as a means to make one's "thinking about thinking" more overt. This would include verbalizing what one is doing, how one is moving through the various steps, guiding oneself when the task at hand becomes difficult, and reinforcing oneself for task completion. Studies examining SIT have found it to be a particularly effective treatment following acquired brain injury (like in TBI), involving executive deficits, finding significant decreases in task-related errors and task-irrelevant behaviors (Cicerone & Giacino, 1992; Cicerone & Wood, 1987). However, Dawson and colleagues (2009) found that SIT might be better suited for specific tasks, as this approach did not appear to be effective for participants in their study who had more complex task goals.

In terms of other metacognitive interventions, a study was conducted by Ownsworth and colleagues (2010) to examine the impact of metacognitive skills training (MST) in error self-regulation following TBI (Ownsworth, Quinn, Fleming, Kendall, & Shum, 2010). Here, MST involved explicit reflection on prior performance of making a meal, errors made, and how those errors might be averted in the future. Individuals were also encouraged to generate their own solutions to problems rather than relying on therapist input. Results showed that individuals who underwent MST showed a significant reduction in the frequency of both errors made and checks (i.e., asking for therapist advice), and a significant increase in self-corrections from baseline (Ownsworth et al., 2010).

5.5.4 Problem-Solving Training

As per our opening case, Sam was recommended a problem-solving approach to her rehabilitation of the lingering executive impairments observed during the neuropsychological assessment. Problem-solving rehabilitation incorporates aspects of both attention and metacognitive training. Several interventions have been developed to train individuals with TBI-related executive dysfunctions in structured, systematic approaches to problem-solving. However, we will focus on the most well-known, and hitherto most empirically supported, treatment: goal management training (GMT; Levine et al., 2000, 2011; Novakovic-Agopian et al., 2010). This intervention was theoretically derived based on Duncan's (1986) theory of goal neglect (i.e., failure to maintain action in service of goals) following frontal brain injury. GMT is a five-stage process that involves (1) directing attention toward a goal, (2) selection of a particular goal, (3) parsing that goal into steps or sub-goals, (4) learning the necessary steps, and (5) during the implementation of these steps, continually monitoring to ensure that the outcome of action matches the desired goal. In this last step, patients are trained to stop their action, focus (i.e., return from mind-wandering), and check that their action is goal-relevant (often referred to as "updating their mental blackboard"). To assist with the focusing aspect, patients practice mindfulness aimed at improving their attention. These stages are repeated in an iterative fashion wherever there is a mismatch between the current action and the goal to be accomplished (Levine et al., 2000).

Like metacognitive strategy training, GMT provides the patient with generalizable skills that can be applied to any novel problem-solving situation, greatly increasing the likelihood of transfer of training to different contexts. Aside from helping with problem-solving, GMT can be useful in developing anticipatory awareness, where individuals recognize that they have a problem-solving deficit and work proactively to implement plans to approach that problem if and when it arises. However, like metacognitive strategy training, GMT and other problem-solving approaches are limited in that they require an awareness of deficits, at least at the intellectual level, in order for the strategies to be effective, as well as motivation to implement behavioral changes.

GMT has received empirical support for its effectiveness. A recent meta-analysis by Stamenova and Levine (2018) examined the effectiveness of GMT in various clinical samples, including TBI. Specifically, they looked at how well GMT treated cognition in a multitude of domains, including executive functioning, speed of processing, long-term memory, subjective ratings, and functional tasks like instrumental activities of daily living. They found that GMT produced small to medium effect sizes for all cognitive domains except for processing speed and that these effects were maintained at follow-up, except for subjective ratings. Medium effects were seen specifically for executive functioning tasks (Stamenova & Levine, 2018). Further support for GMT has come from a systematic review by Krasny-Pacini and colleagues (2014), who examined the problem-solving treatment in patients recovering from brain injury (Krasny-Pacini, Chevignard, & Evans, 2014). They found that comprehensive treatment plans including GMT, while integrating other approaches, are effective in executive function rehabilitation. However, they determined that there is not sufficient evidence yet to support GMT as an effective stand-alone treatment (Krasny-Pacini et al., 2014).

In summary, cognitive rehabilitation interventions can treat a variety of executive-related dysfunctions in people who have experienced a TBI. This chapter section discussed a handful of techniques targeting impairments in awareness, attention, metacognition, and problem-solving (summarized in Table 5.1). For deficits in awareness, various techniques can be employed depending on the type of awareness affected; these can range from reminder and psychoeducation about one's deficits to task-specific training and use of metacognitive strategies. Mindfulness training has shown some promise in treating attention, specifically sustained attention, attentional control and self-monitoring. Two types of interventions that have been supported for treating metacognition are self-instructional training (SIT) and metacognitive skills training (MST), both of which have helped improved task performance. Similar to metacognitive training, goal management training (GMT) has been effective in improving problem-solving skills, emphasizing a stepwise approach for selecting and attending to goals.

References

Amick, M. M., Clark, A., Fortier, C. B., Esterman, M., Rasmusson, A. M., Kenna, A., ... McGlinchey, R. (2013). PTSD modifies performance on a task of affective executive control among deployed OEF/OIF veterans with mild traumatic brain injury. *Journal of the International Neuropsychological Society, 19*(7), 792–801. https://doi.org/10.1017/S1355617713000544.

Angus Reid Institute. (2015, December 16). *Opinion poll on sports concussion in Canada.* Retrieved from http://angusreid.org/concussion-in-sport/.

Ashton, R. (2010). Practitioner review: Beyond shaken baby syndrome: What influences the outcomes for infants following traumatic brain injury? *Journal of Child Psychology and Psychiatry, 51*(9), 967–980.

Azulay, J., Smart, C. M., Mott, T., & Cicerone, K. D. (2013). A pilot study examining the effect of mindfulness-based stress reduction on symptoms of chronic mild traumatic brain injury/postconcussive syndrome. *The Journal of Head Trauma Rehabilitation, 28*(4), 323–331.

Babikian, T., & Asarnow, R. (2009). Neurocognitive outcomes and recovery after pediatric TBI: Meta-analytic review of the literature. *Neuropsychology, 23*(3), 283.

Babikian, T., McArthur, D., & Asarnow, R. F. (2013). Predictors of 1-month and 1-year neurocognitive functioning from the UCLA longitudinal mild, uncomplicated, pediatric traumatic brain injury study. *Journal of the International Neuropsychological Society, 19*(2), 145–154.

Bazarian, J. J., Donnelly, K., Peterson, D. R., Warner, G. C., Zhu, T., & Zhong, J. (2013). The relation between posttraumatic stress disorder and mild traumatic brain injury acquired during operations enduring freedom and Iraqi freedom. *Journal of Head Trauma Rehabilitation, 28*(1), 1–12. https://doi.org/10.1097/HTR.0b013e318256d3d3.

Belanger, H. G., Curtiss, G., Demery, J. A., Lebowitz, B. K., & Vanderploeg, R. D. (2005). Factors moderating neuropsychological outcomes following mild traumatic brain injury: A meta-analysis. *Journal of the International Neuropsychological Society, 11*(3), 215–227.

Belanger, H. G., Proctor-Weber, Z., Kretzmer, T., Kim, M., French, L. M., & Vanderploeg, R. D. (2011). Symptom complaints following reports of blast versus non-blast mild TBI: Does mechanism of injury matter? *The Clinical Neuropsychologist, 25*(5), 702–715. https://doi.org/10.1080/13854046.2011.566892.

Belanger, H. G., Spiegel, E., & Vanderploeg, R. (2010). Neuropsychological performance following a history of multiple self-reported concussions: A meta-analysis. *Journal of the International Neuropsychological Society, 16*(2), 262–267.

Belanger, H. G., Uomoto, J. M., & Vanderploeg, R. D. (2009). The veterans health administration system of care for mild traumatic brain injury: Costs, benefits, and controversies. *Journal of Head Trauma Rehabilitation, 24*(1), 4–13.

Belanger, H. G., & Vanderploeg, R. D. (2005). The neuropsychological impact of sports-related concussion: A meta-analysis. *Journal of the International Neuropsychological Society, 11*(4), 345–357.

Best, J. R. (2010). Effects of physical activity on children's executive function: Contributions of experimental research on aerobic exercise. *Developmental Review, 30*(4), 331–351.

Binder, L. M., Rohling, M. L., & Larrabee, G. J. (1997). A review of mild head trauma: I. Meta-analytic review of neuropsychological studies. *Journal of Clinical and Experimental Neuropsychology, 19*(3), 421–431. https://doi.org/10.1080/01688639708403870.

Brooks, B. L., McKay, C. D., Mrazik, M., Barlow, K. M., Meeuwisse, W. H., & Emery, C. A. (2013). Subjective, but not objective, lingering effects of multiple past concussions in adolescents. *Journal of Neurotrauma, 30*(17), 1469–1475.
Bruns, J., & Hauser, W. A. (2003). The epidemiology of traumatic brain injury: A review. *Epilepsia, 44*(s10), 2–10.
Bryant, R. A., & Harvey, A. G. (1999). Postconcussive symptoms and posttraumatic stress disorder after mild traumatic brain injury. *The Journal of Nervous and Mental Disease, 187*(5), 302–305.
Bullmore, E., & Sporns, O. (2009). Complex brain networks: graph theoretical analysis of structural and functional systems. *Nature Review Neurosciences, 10*(3), 186–198.
Caeyenberghs, K., Leemans, A., Leunissen, I., Gooijers, J., Michiels, K., Sunaert, S., et al. (2014). Altered structural networks and executive deficits in traumatic brain injury patients. *Brain Structure and Function, 219,* 193–209.
Canadian Institute for Health Information. (2016). *National ambulatory care reporting system.* Retrieved from https://www.cihi.ca/en/how-many-er-visits-forsport-related-brain-injuries-receive-a-concussion-diagnosis.
Cancelliere, D. C., Kristman, V. L., Cassidy, J., Hincapie, C. A., Cote, P., Boyle, E., … Borg, J. (2014). Systematic review of return to work after mild traumatic brain injury: Results of the international collaboration of mild traumatic brain injury prognosis. *Archives of Physical Medicine and Rehabilitation, 95*(3 Supplement 2), S201–S209.
Carlson, K. F., Kehle, S. M., Meis, L. A., Greer, N., MacDonald, R., Rutks, I., … Wilt, T. J. (2011). Prevalence, assessment, and treatment of mild traumatic brain injury and posttraumatic stress disorder: A systematic review of the evidence. *The Journal of Head Trauma Rehabilitation, 26*(2), 103–115.
Case, M. E. (2008). Accidental traumatic head injury in infants and young children. *Brain Pathology, 18*(4), 583–589.
Cernak, I., & Noble-Haeusslein, L. J. (2010). Traumatic brain injury: An overview of pathobiology with emphasis on military populations. *Journal of Cerebral Blood Flow and Metabolism, 30*(2), 255–266. https://doi.org/10.1038/jcbfm.2009.203.
Chang, Y. K., Labban, J. D., Gapin, J. I., & Etnier, J. L. (2012). The effects of acute exercise on cognitive performance: A meta-analysis. *Brain Research, 1453,* 87–101.
Chang, V. H., Lonbard, L. A., & Greher, M. R. (2011). Mild traumatic brain injury in the occupational setting. *Physical Medicine and Rehabilitation, 3*(10 Supplement 2), S387–S395.
Chapman, S. B., & McKinnon, L. (2000). Discussion of developmental plasticity: Factors affecting cognitive outcome after pediatric traumatic brain injury. *Journal of Communication Disorders, 33*(4), 333–344.
Chrisman, S. P., & Rivara, F. P. (2016). Physical activity or rest after concussion in youth: questions about timing and potential benefit. *JAMA, 316*(23), 2491–2492.
Cicerone, K. D., Dahlberg, C., Malec, J. F., Langenbahn, D. M., Felicetti, T., Kneipp, S., … Catanese, J. (2005). Evidence-based cognitive rehabilitation: Updated review of the literature from 1998 through 2002. *Archives of Physical Medicine and Rehabilitation, 86*, 1681–1692.
Cicerone, K. D., & Giacino, J. T. (1992). Remediation of executive function deficits after traumatic brain injury. *Neuropsychological Rehabilitation, 2,* 12–22.
Cicerone, K. D., & Wood, J. C. (1987). Planning disorder after closed head injury: A case study. *Archives of Physical Medicine and Rehabilitation, 68,* 111–115.
Cole, M. W., Pathak, S., & Schneider, W. (2010). Identifying the brain's most globally connected regions. *NeuroImage, 49,* 3132–3148.
Collie, A., McCrory, P., & Makdissi, M. (2006). Does history of concussion affect current cognitive status? *British Journal of Sports Medicine, 40*(6), 550–551. https://doi.org/10.1017/S1355617709991287.
Comper, P., Hutchison, M., Magrys, S., Mainwaring, L., & Richards, D. (2010). Evaluating the methodological quality of sports neuropsychology concussion research: A systematic review. *Brain Injury, 24*(11), 1257–1271. https://doi.org/10.3109/02699052.2010.506854.

Cook, L. G., Hanten, G., Orsten, K. D., Chapman, S. B., Li, X., Wilde, E. A., … Levin, H. S. (2013). Effects of moderate to severe traumatic brain injury on anticipating consequences of actions in adolescents: A preliminary study. *Journal of the International Neuropsychological Society, 19*(5), 508–517.

Coronado, V. G., Haileyesus, T., Cheng, T. A., Bell, J. M., Haarbauer-Krupa, J., Lionbarger, M. R., et al. (2015). Trends in sports- and recreation-related traumatic brain injuries treated in US emergency departments: The National Electronic Injury Surveillance System-All Injury Program (NEISS-AIP) 2001-2012. *Journal of Head Trauma Rehabilitation, 30*(3), 185–197.

Crone, E. A. (2009). Executive functions in adolescence: Inferences from brain and behavior. *Developmental Science, 12*(6), 825–830. https://doi.org/10.1111/j.1467-7687.2009.00918.x.

Crosson, B., Barco, P. P., Velozo, C. A., Bolesta, M. M., Cooper, P. V., Werts, D., et al. (1989). Awareness and compensation in post-acute head injury rehabilitation. *Journal of Head Trauma Rehabilitation, 4,* 46–54.

Crowe, L. M., Catroppa, C., Babl, F. E., & Anderson, V. (2013). Executive function outcomes of children with traumatic brain injury sustained before three years. *Child Neuropsychology, 19*(2), 113–126.

Cubon, V. A., Putukian, M., Boyer, C., & Dettwiler, A. (2011). A diffusion tensor imaging study on the white matter skeleton in individuals with sports-related concussion. *Journal of Neurotrauma, 28,* 189–201.

Cysique, L., Franklin, D., Abramson, I., Ellis, R., Letendre, S., Collier, A., … Heaton, R. K. (2011). Normative data and validation of a regression based summary score for assessing meaningful neuropsychological change. *Journal of Clinical and Experimental Neuropsychology, 33*(5), 505–522.

Dawson, D. R., Gaya, A., Hunt, A., Levine, B., Lemsky, C., & Polatajko, H. J. (2009). Using the cognitive orientation to occupational performance (CO-OP) with adults with executive dysfunction following traumatic brain injury. *Canadian Journal of Occupational Therapy, 76*(2), 115–127.

Devries, K. M., Mak, J. Y. T., García-Moreno, C., Petzold, M., Child, J. C., Falder, G., … Watts, C. H. (2013). The global prevalence of intimate partner violence against women. *Science, 340,* 1527–1528. https://doi.org/10.1126/science.1240937.

Diamond, A. (2013). Executive functions. *Annual Review of Psychology, 64,* 135–168. https://doi.org/10.1146/annurev-psych-113011-143750.

Dikmen, S., Machamer, J., & Temkin, N. (2001). Mild head injury: Facts and artifacts. *Journal of Clinical and Experimental Neuropsychology, 23*(6), 729–738.

Direnfeld, E. Y. (2017). *Validation of an executive function screener in a sample of adolescents with neurological disorders* (Doctoral dissertation). University of Victoria, Department of Psychology.

Dolan, R. J. (2008). Neuroimaging of cognition: Past, present, and future. *Neuron, 60,* 496–502.

Dougan, B. K., Horswill, M. S., & Geffen, G. M. (2013). Athletes' age, sex, and years of education moderate the acute neuropsychological impact of sports-related concussion: A meta-analysis. *Journal of the International Neuropsychological Society, 19,* 1–17.

Duncan, J. (1986). Disorganization of behavior after frontal lobe damage. *Cognitive Neuropsychology, 3,* 271–290.

Durish, C. L., Yeates, K. O., Stancin, T., Taylor, H. G., Walz, N. C., & Wade, S. L. (2018). Home environment as a predictor of long-term executive functioning following early childhood traumatic brain injury. *Journal of the International Neuropsychological Society, 24*(1), 11–21.

Eierud, C., Craddock, R. C., Fletcher, S., Aulakh, M., King-Casa, B., Kuehl, D., & LaConte, S. M. (2014). Neuroimaging after mild traumatic brain injury: Review and meta-analysis. *Neuroimage: Clinical, 4,* 283–295.

Erdal, K. (2012). Neuropsychological testing for sports-related concussion: How athletes can sandbag their baseline testing without detection. *Archives of Clinical Neuropsychology, 27*(5), 473–479.

Faul, M., Xu, L., Wald, M. M., Coronado, V. G. (2010). Traumatic brain injury in the United States: Emergency department visits, hospitalizations and deaths 2002–2006. Atlanta (GA): Centers for disease control and prevention, national center for injury prevention and control.

Fair, D. A., Dosenbach, N. U. F., Church, J. A., Cohen, A. L., & Brahmbhatt, S. (2007). Development of distinct control net- works through segregation and integration. *Proceedings of the National Academy of Sciences, USA, 104,* 13507–13512.

Fox, K. C., Nijeboer, S., Dixon, M. L., Floman, J. L., Ellamil, M., Rumak, S. P., … Christoff, K. (2014). Is meditation associated with altered brain structure? A systematic review and meta-analysis of morphometric neuroimaging in meditation practitioners. *Neuroscience & Biobehavioral Reviews, 43,* 48–73.

Frencham, K. A., Fox, A. M., & Maybery, M. (2005). Neuropsychological studies of mild traumatic brain injury: A meta-analytic review of research since 1995. *Journal of Clinical and Experimental Neuropsychology, 27*(3), 334–351.

Frost, R. B., Farrer, T. J., Primosch, M., & Hedges, D. W. (2013). Prevalence of traumatic brain injury in the general adult population: A meta-analysis. *Neuroepidemiology, 40*(3), 154–159.

Fulton, J. J., Calhoun, P. S., Wagner, H. R., Schry, A. R., Hair, L. P., Feeling, N., … Beckham, J. C. (2015). The prevalence of posttraumatic stress disorder in Operation Enduring Freedom/Operation Iraqi Freedom (OEF/OIF) Veterans: A meta-analysis. *Journal of Anxiety Disorders, 31,* 98–107. https://doi.org/10.1016/j.janxdis.2015.02.003.

Galvan, A., Hare, T. A., Parra, C. E., Penn, J., Voss, H., Glover, G., et al. (2006). Earlier development of the accumbens relative to orbitofrontal cortex might underlie risk-taking behavior in adolescents. *Journal of Neuroscience, 26*(25), 6885–6892.

Gerrard-Morris, A., Taylor, H. G., Yeates, K. O., Walz, N. C., Stancin, T., Minich, N., et al. (2010). Cognitive development after traumatic brain injury in young children. *Journal of the International Neuropsychological Society, 16*(1), 157–168.

Giacino, J. T., & Cicerone, K. D. (1998). Varieties of deficit unawareness after brain injury. *Journal of Head Trauma Rehabilitation, 13,* 1–15.

Gil, A. M. (2003). Neurocognitive outcomes following pediatric brain injury: A developmental approach. *Journal of School Psychology, 41*(5), 337–353.

Government of Canada. (2018, October 11). Sports and recreation related concussions and other traumatic brain injuries among Canada's children and youth. Retrieved March 10, 2019 from https://infobase.phac-aspc.gc.ca/datalab/head-injury-interactive-en.html.

Grool, A. M., Aglipay, M., Momoli, F., Meehan, W. P., Freedman, S. B., Yeates, K. O., … Barrowman, N. (2016). Association between early participation in physical activity following acute concussion and persistent postconcussive symptoms in children and adolescents. *JAMA, 316*(23), 2504–2514.

Haller, S., & Bartsch, A. J. (2009). Pitfalls in fMRI. *European Radiology, 19,* 2689–2706.

Heaton, R. K., Akshoomoff, N., Tulsky, D., Mungas, D., Weintraub, S., Dikmen, S., … Gershon, R. (2014). Reliability and validity of composite scores from the NIH toolbox cognition battery in adults. *Journal of the International Neuropsychological Society, 20,* 588–598.

Hendrickson, R. C., Schindler, A. G., & Pagulayan, K. F. (2018). Untangling PTSD and TBI: Challenges and strategies in clinical care and research. *Current Neurology and Neuroscience Reports, 18*(12). https://doi.org/10.1007/s11910-018-0908-5.

Hillman, C. H., Erickson, K. I., & Kramer, A. F. (2008). Be smart, exercise your heart: Exercise effects on brain and cognition. *Nature Reviews Neuroscience, 9*(1), 58–65.

Horneman, G., & Emanuelson, I. (2009). Cognitive outcome in children and young adults who sustained severe and moderate traumatic brain injury 10 years earlier. *Brain Injury, 23*(11), 907–914.

Huang, R., Lu, M., Song, Z., & Wang, J. (2015). Long-term intensive training induced brain structural changes in world class gymnasts. *Brain Structure and Function, 220*(2), 625–644.

Hurley, R. A., McGowan, J. C., Arfanakis, K., & Taber, K. H. (2014). Traumatic axonal injury: Novel insights into evolution and identification. *The Journal of Neuropsychiatry and Clinical Neurosciences, 16*(1), 1–7. https://doi.org/10.1176/jnp.16.1.1.

Inglese, M., Makani, S., Johnson, G., Cohen, B. A., Silver, J. A., Gonen, O., et al. (2005). Diffuse axonal injury in mild traumatic brain injury: A diffusion tensor imaging study. *Journal of Neurosurgery, 103*(2), 298–303.

Iverson, G. L., Brooks, B. L., Lovell, M. R., & Collins, M. W. (2006). No cumulative effects for one or two previous concussions. *British Journal of Sports Medicine, 40*(1), 72–75. https://doi.org/10.1136/bjsm.2005.020651.

Jennett, B., & Bond, M. (1975). Assessment of outcome after severe brain damage: A practical scale. *The Lancet, 305*(7905), 480–484.

Jorge, R. E., Acion, L., White, T., Tordesillas-Gutierrez, D., Pierson, R., Crespo-Facorro, B., et al. (2012). White matter abnormalities in veterans with mild traumatic brain injury. *American Journal of Psychiatry, 169*(12), 1284–1291. https://doi.org/10.1176/appi.ajp.2012.12050600.

Jurado, M. B., & Rosselli, M. (2007). The elusive nature of executive functions: A review of our current understanding. *Neuropsychology Review, 17*(3), 213–233. https://doi.org/10.1007/s11065-007-9040-z.

Karr, J. E., Areshenkoff, C. N., Duggan, E. C., & Garcia-Barrera, M. A. (2014a). Blast-related mild traumatic brain injury: A Bayesian random-effects meta-analysis on the cognitive outcomes of concussion among military personnel. *Neuropsychology Review, 24*(4), 428–444. https://doi.org/10.1007/s11065-014-9271-8.

Karr, J. E., Areshenkoff, C. N., & Garcia-Barrera, M. A. (2014b). The neuropsychological outcomes of concussion: A systematic review of meta-analyses on the cognitive sequelae of mild traumatic brain injury. *Neuropsychology, 28*(3), 321–336.

Karr, J. E., Areshenkoff, C. N., Rast, P., Hofer, S. M., Iverson, G. L., & Garcia-Barrera, M. A. (2018). The unity and diversity of executive functions: A systematic review and re-analysis of latent variable studies. *Psychological Bulletin, 144*(11), 1147–1185.

Karr, J. E., Rau, H. K., Shofer, J. B., Hendrickson, R. C., Peskind, E. R., & Pagulayan, K. F. (2019). Variables associated with subjective cognitive change among Iraq and Afghanistan war veterans with blast-related mild traumatic brain injury. *Journal of Clinical and Experimental Neuropsychology, 41*(7), 680–693. http://dx.doi.org/10.1080/13803395.2019.1611740.

Karver, C. L., Wade, S. L., Cassedy, A., Taylor, H. G., Stancin, T., Yeates, K. O., et al. (2012). Age at injury and long-term behavior problems after traumatic brain injury in young children. *Rehabilitation Psychology, 57*(3), 256.

Kehle-Forbes, S. M., Campbell, E. H., Taylor, B. C., Scholten, J., & Sayer, N. (2017). Does co-occurring traumatic brain injury affect VHA outpatient health service utilization and associated costs among veterans with posttraumatic stress disorder? An examination based on VHA administrative data. *Journal of Head Trauma Rehabilitation, 32*(1), E16–E23. https://doi.org/10.1097/HTR.0000000000000227.

Kinnunen, K. M., Greenwood, R., Powell, J. H., Leech, R., Hawkins, P. C., Bonnelle, V., … Sharp, D. J. (2010). White matter damage and cognitive impairment after traumatic brain injury. *Brain, 134*, 449–463.

Kontos, A. P., Kotwal, R. S., Elbin, R. J., Lutz, R. H., Forsten, R. D., Benson, P. J., et al. (2013). Residual effects of combat-related mild traumatic brain injury. *Journal of Neurotrauma, 30*(8), 680–686. https://doi.org/10.1089/neu.2012.2506.

Krasny-Pacini, A., Chevignard, M., & Evans, J. (2014). Goal management training for rehabilitation of executive functions: A systematic review of effectiveness in patients with acquired brain injury. *Disability and Rehabilitation, 36*(2), 105–116.

Krasny-Pacini, A., Chevignard, M., Lancien, S., Escolano, S., Laurent-Vannier, A., De Agostini, M., et al. (2017). Executive function after severe childhood traumatic brain injury–Age-at-injury vulnerability periods: The TGE prospective longitudinal study. *Annals of Physical and Rehabilitation Medicine, 60*(2), 74–82.

Kristman, V. L., Borg, J., Godbolt, A. K., Salmi, L. R., Cancelliere, C., Carroll, L. J., … Cassidy, J. D. (2014). Methodological issues and research recommendations for prognosis after mild traumatic brain injury: Results from the international collaboration on mild traumatic brain injury prognosis. *Archives of Physical Medicine and Rehabilitation, 95*(3 Supplement 2), S265–S277.

Kristman, V. L., Côté, P., Hogg-Johnson, S., Cassidy, J. D., Eerd, D. V., Vidmar, M., … Wennberg, R. A. (2010). The burden of work disability associated with mild traumatic brain injury in Ontario compensated workers: A prospective cohort study. *The Open Occupational Health & Safety Journal, 2*(1), 1–8.

Krpan, K. M., Levine, B., Stuss, D. T., & Dawson, D. R. (2007). Executive function and coping at one-year post traumatic brain injury. *Journal of Clinical and Experimental Neuropsychology, 29*(1), 36–46.

Landry-Roy, C., Bernier, A., Gravel, J., & Beauchamp, M. H. (2018). Executive functions and their relation to sleep following mild traumatic brain injury in preschoolers. *Journal of the International Neuropsychological Society, 24*(8), 769–780.

Lange, R. T., Iverson, G. L., & Franzen, M. D. (2009). Neuropsychological functioning following complicated vs. uncomplicated mild traumatic brain injury. *Brain Injury, 23*(2), 83–91.

Lange, R. T., Pancholi, S., Brickell, T. A., Sakura, S., Bhagwat, A., Merritt, V., & French, L. M. (2012). Neuropsychological outcome from blast versus non-blast: Mild traumatic brain injury in U.S. military service members. *Journal of the International Neuropsychological Society, 18*(3), 595–605. https://doi.org/10.1017/S1355617712000239.

Langlois, J. A., Rutland-Brown, W., & Wald, M. M. (2006). The epidemiology and impact of traumatic brain injury: A brief overview. *The Journal of Head Trauma Rehabilitation, 21*(5), 375–378.

Levin, H. S., & Hanten, G. (2005). Executive functions after traumatic brain injury in children. *Pediatric Neurology, 33*(2), 79–93.

Levine, B., Robertson, I. H., Clare, L., Carter, G., Hong, J., Wilson, B. A., et al. (2000). Rehabilitation of executive function: An experimental-clinical validation of goal management training. *Journal of the International Neuropsychological Society, 6,* 299–312.

Levine, B., Schweizer, T. A., O'Connor, C., Turner, G., Gillingham, S., Stuss, D. T., … Robertson, I. H. (2011). Rehabilitation of executive functioning in patients with frontal lobe brain damage with goal management training. *Frontiers in Human Neuroscience, 5.* https://doi.org/10.3389/fnhum.2011.00009.

Lew, H., Thomander, D., Chew, K., & Bleiberg, J. (2007). Review of sports-related concussion: Potential for application in military settings. *Journal of Rehabilitation Research and Development, 44*(7), 963–973. https://doi.org/10.1682/JRRD.2006.12.0169.

Lezak, M. D., Howieson, D. B., Loring, D. W., & Fischer, J. S. (2004). *Neuropsychological assessment* (4th ed.). USA: Oxford University Press.

Lezak, M. D., Howieson, D. B., Bigler, E. D., & Tranel, D. (2012). *Neuropsychological assessment* (5th ed.). USA: Oxford University Press.

Li, L., & Liu, J. (2013). The effect of pediatric traumatic brain injury on behavioral outcomes: A systematic review. *Developmental Medicine and Child Neurology, 55*(1), 37–45.

Lipton, M., Gulko, E., Zimmerman, M., Friedman, B., Kim, M., Gellella, E., … Branch, C. (2009). Diffusion-tensor imaging implicates prefrontal axonal injury in executive function impairment following very mild traumatic brain injury. *Radiology, 252*(3), 816–824. https://doi.org/10.1148/radiol.2523081584.

Luethcke, C. A., Bryan, C. J., Morrow, C. E., & Isler, W. C. (2011). Comparison of concussive symptoms, cognitive performance, and psychological symptoms between acute blast-versus nonblast-induced mild traumatic brain injury. *Journal of the International Neuropsychological Society, 17*(1), 36–45. https://doi.org/10.1017/S1355617710001207.

Lumba-Brown, A., Yeates, K. O., Sarmiento, K., Breiding, M. J., Haegerich, T. M., Gioia, G. A., … Joseph, M. (2018). Centers for disease control and prevention guideline on the diagnosis and management of mild traumatic brain injury among children. *JAMA Pediatrics, 172*(11), e182853–e182853.

Maas, A. I., Stocchetti, N., & Bullock, R. (2008). Moderate and severe traumatic brain injury in adults. *The Lancet Neurology, 7*(8), 728–741.

MacDonald, C. L., Johnson, A., Cooper, D., Malone, T., Sorrell, J., Shimony, J., … Brody, D. L. (2013). Cerebellar white matter abnormalities following primary blast injury in US military personnel. *PLoS ONE, 8*(2). https://doi.org/10.1371/journal.pone.0055823.

MacDonald, C. L., Johnson, A. M., Cooper, D., Nelson, E. C., Werner, N. J., Shimony, J. S., … Brody, D. L. (2011). Detection of blast-related traumatic brain injury in U.S. military personnel. *New England Journal of Medicine, 364*(22), 2091–2100. https://doi.org/10.1056/NEJMoa1008069.

Mangeot, S., Armstrong, K., Colvin, A. N., Yeates, K. O., & Taylor, H. G. (2002). Long-term executive function deficits in children with traumatic brain injuries: Assessment using the Behavior Rating Inventory of Executive Function (BRIEF). *Child Neuropsychology, 8*(4), 271–284.

Mannix, R., O'Brien, M. J., & Meehan, W. P., III. (2013). The epidemiology of outpatient visits for minor head injury: 2005 to 2009. *Neurosurgery, 73*(1), 129–134.

Marks, B. L., Madden, D. J., Bucur, B., Provenzale, J. M., White, L. E., Cabeza, R., et al. (2007). Role of aerobic fitness and aging on cerebral white matter integrity. *Annals of the New York Academy of Sciences, 1097*(1), 171–174.

Martin, C.W., & WCB Evidence Based Practice Group. (2003). Mild traumatic brain injury: Review of the literature and a look at the WCB of BC data. Retrieved from the WorkSafeBC website: http://www.worksafebc.com/health_care_providers/Assets/PDF/MTBI.pdf.

Maruta, J., Spielman, L. A., Yarusi, B. B., Wang, Y., Silver, J. M., & Ghajar, J. (2016). Chronic post-concussion neurocognitive deficits. II. Relationship with persistent symptoms. *Frontiers in human neuroscience, 10*(45), 1–10. https://doi.org/10.3389/fnhum.2016.00045.

Matthews, S. C., Spadoni, A. D., Lohr, J. B., Strigo, I. A., & Simmons, A. N. (2012). Diffusion tensor imaging evidence of white matter disruption associated with loss versus alteration of consciousness in warfighters exposed to combat in operations enduring and Iraqi freedom. *Psychiatry Research—Neuroimaging, 204*(2–3), 149–154. https://doi.org/10.1016/j.pscychresns.2012.04.018.

Matthews, S. C., Strigo, I. A., Simmons, A. N., O'Connell, R. M., Reinhardt, L. E., & Moseley, S. A. (2011). A multimodal imaging study in U.S. veterans of operations Iraqi and enduring freedom with and without major depression after blast-related concussion. *NeuroImage, 54*(Suppl. 1), S69–S75. https://doi.org/10.1016/j.neuroimage.2010.04.269.

Mayer, A. R., Mannell, M. V., Ling, J., Gsparovic, C., & Yeo, R. A. (2011). Functional connectivity in mild traumatic brain injury. *Human Brain Mapping, 32,* 1825–1835.

McCrea, M., Hammeke, T., Olsen, G., Leo, P., & Guskiewicz, K. (2004). Unreported concussion in high school football players. *Clinical Journal of Sport Medicine, 14*(1), 13–17. https://doi.org/10.1097/00042752-200401000-00003.

McCrory, P., Meeuwisse, W., Dvorak, J., Aubry, M., Bailes, J., Broglio, S., … Davis, G. A. (2017). Consensus statement on concussion in sport—the 5th international conference on concussion in sport held in Berlin, October 2016. *British Journal of Sports Medicine, 51*(11), 838–847.

McDonald, B. C., Saykin, A. J., & McAllister, T. W. (2012). Functional MRI of mild traumatic brain injury (mTBI): Progress and perspectives from the first decade of studies. *Brain Imaging and Behavior, 6,* 193–207.

Meichenbaum, D. H., & Goodman, J. (1971). Training impulsive children to talk to themselves: A means of developing self-control. *Journal of Abnormal Psychology, 77,* 115–126.

Menon, D. K., Schwab, K., Wright, D. W., & Maas, A. I. (2010). Position statement: definition of traumatic brain injury. *Archives of Physical Medicine and Rehabilitation, 91*(11), 1637–1640.

Messé, A., Caplain, S., Paradot, G., Garrigue, D., Mineo, J. F., Soto Ares, G., … Lehéricy, S. (2011). Diffusion tensor imaging and white matter lesions at the subacute stage in mild traumatic brain injury with persistent neurobehavioral impairment. *Human Brain Mapping, 32*(6), 999–1011.

Mittenberg, W., Patton, C., Canyock, E., & Condit, D. (2002). Base rates of malingering and symptom exaggeration. *Journal of Clinical and Experimental Neuropsychology, 24,* 1094–1102.

Miyake, A., Friedman, N. P., Emerson, M. J., Witzki, A. H., Howerter, A., & Wager, T. D. (2000). The unity and diversity of executive functions and their contributions to complex "frontal lobe" tasks: A latent variable analysis. *Cognitive Psychology, 41*(1), 49–100. https://doi.org/10.1006/cogp.1999.0734.

Moffitt, T. E., Arseneault, L., Belsky, D., Dickson, N., Hancox, R. J., Harrington, H., … Sears, M. R. (2011). A gradient of childhood self-control predicts health, wealth, and public safety. *Proceedings of the National Academy of Sciences, 108*(7), 2693–2698.

Mungas, D., Heaton, R., Tulsky, D., Zelazo, P. D., Slotkin, J., Blitz, D., … Gershon, R. (2014). Factor structure, convergent validity, and discriminant validity of the NIH Toolbox Cognitive Health Battery (NIHTB-CHB) in adults. *Journal of the International Neuropsychological Society, 20*, 579–587.

Murugavel, M., Cubon, V., Putukian, M., Echemendia, R., Cabrera, J., Osherson, D., & Dettwiler, A. (2014). A longitudinal diffusion tensor imaging study assessing white matter fiber tracts after sports related concussion. *Journal of Neurotrauma*. Advance Online Publication. https://doi.org/10.1089/neu.2014.3368.

Muscara, F., Catroppa, C., & Anderson, V. (2008). The impact of injury severity on executive function 7–10 years following pediatric traumatic brain injury. *Developmental Neuropsychology, 33*(5), 623–636.

Nadebaum, C., Anderson, V., & Catroppa, C. (2007). Executive function outcomes following traumatic brain injury in young children: A five year follow-up. *Developmental Neuropsychology, 32*(2), 703–728.

Nakamura, T., Hillary, F. G., & Biswal, B. B. (2009). Resting network plasticity following brain injury. *PLoS One, 4*.

Nelson, N. W., Hoelzle, J. B., Doane, B. M., McGuire, K. A., Ferrier-Auerbach, A. G., Charlesworth, M. J., … Sponheim, S. R. (2012). Neuropsychological outcomes of U.S. veterans with report of remote blast-related concussion and current psychopathology. *Journal of the International Neuropsychological Society, 18*(5), 845–855. https://doi.org/10.1017/S1355617712000616.

Nelson, N. W., Hoelzle, J. B., McGuire, K. A., Ferrier-Auerbach, A. G., Charlesworth, M. J., & Sponheim, S. R. (2010). Evaluation context impacts neuropsychological performance of OEF/OIF veterans with reported combat-related concussion. *Archives of Clinical Neuropsychology, 25*(8), 713–723. https://doi.org/10.1093/arclin/acq075.

Novakovic-Agopian, T., Chen, A. J.-W., Rome, S., Abrams, G., Castelli, H., Rossi, A., … D'Esposito, M. (2010). Rehabilitation of executive functioning with training in attention regulation applied to individually defined goals: A pilot study bridging theory, assessment and treatment. *Journal of Head Trauma Rehabilitation*. https://doi.org/10.1097/htr.0b013e3181f1ead2.

Ogawa, S., Tank, D. W., Menon, R., Ellermann, J. M., Kim, S. G., Merkle, H., et al. (1992). Intrinsic signal changes accompanying sensory stimulation: Functional brain mapping with magnetic resonance imaging. *Proceedings of the National Academy of Sciences USA, 89*, 5951–5955.

Ornstein, T. J., Sagar, S., Schachar, R. J., Ewing-Cobbs, L., Chapman, S. B., Dennis, M., … Max, J. E. (2014). Neuropsychological performance of youth with secondary attention-deficit/hyperactivity disorder 6-and 12-months after traumatic brain injury. *Journal of the International Neuropsychological Society, 20*(10), 971–981.

Ownsworth, T., Quinn, H., Fleming, J., Kendall, M., & Shum, D. (2010). Error self-regulation following traumatic brain injury: A single case study evaluation of metacognitive skills training and behavioral practice interventions. *Neuropsychological Rehabilitation, 20*, 59–80.

Padilla, C., Pérez, L., & Andrés, P. (2014). Chronic exercise keeps working memory and inhibitory capacities fit. *Frontiers in behavioral neuroscience, 8*(49), 1–10. https://doi.org/10.3389/fnbeh.2014.00049.

Papoutsis, J., Stargatt, R., & Catroppa, C. (2014). Long-term executive functioning outcomes for complicated and uncomplicated mild traumatic brain injury sustained in early childhood. *Developmental Neuropsychology, 39*(8), 638–645.

Pandit, A. S., Expert, P., Lambiotte, R., Bonnelle, V., Leech, R., Turkheimer, F. E., et al. (2013). Traumatic brain injury impairs small-world topology. *Neurology, 80*(20), 1826–1833.

Parachute, Canada. (2015). *The cost of injury in Canada*. Toronto, ON: Parachute.

Pérez, L., Padilla, C., Parmentier, F. B., & Andrés, P. (2014). The effects of chronic exercise on attentional networks. *PLoS ONE, 9*(7), 1–8.

Peskind, E. R., Petrie, E. C., Cross, D. J., Pagulayan, K., McCraw, K., Hoff, D., … Minoshima, S. (2011). Cerebrocerebellar hypometabolism associated with repetitive blast exposure mild traumatic brain injury in 12 Iraq war veterans with persistent post-concussive symptoms. *NeuroImage, 54*(Suppl. 1), S76–S82. https://doi.org/10.1016/j.neuroimage.2010.04.008.

Petrie, E. C., Cross, D. J., Yarnykh, V. L., Richards, T., Martin, N. M., Pagulayan, K., … Peskind, E. R. (2013). Neuroimaging, behavioral, and psychological sequelae of repetitive combined blast/impact mild traumatic brain injury in Iraq and Afghanistan war veterans. *Journal of Neurotrauma, 31*(5), 425–436. https://doi.org/10.1089/neu.2013.2952.

Prencipe, A., Kesek, A., Cohen, J., Lamm, C., Lewis, M. D., & Zelazo, P. D. (2011). Development of hot and cool executive function during the transition to adolescence. *Journal of Experimental Child Psychology, 108*(3), 621–637.

Prigatano, G. P. (2005). Disturbances of self-awareness and rehabilitation of patients with traumatic brain injury: A 20-year perspective. *Journal of Head Trauma Rehabilitation, 20,* 19–29.

Prigatano, G. P. (2009). Anosognosia: Clinical and ethical considerations. *Current Opinion in Neurology, 22*(6), 606 611.

Rao, D. P., McFaull, S., Thompson, W., & Jayaraman, G. C. (2018). Traumatic brain injury management in Canada: Changing patterns of care. *Health Promotion and Chronic Disease Prevention in Canada, 38*(3), 147–150. https://doi.org/10.24095/hpcdp.38.3.05.

Roebuck-Spencer, T., & Sherer, M. (2008). Moderate and severe traumatic brain injury. In J. E. Morgan & J. H. Ricker (Eds.), *Textbook of clinical neuropsychology* (pp. 411–429). New York: Taylor & Francis.

Rohling, M. L., Binder, L. M., Demakis, G. J., Larrabee, G. J., Ploetz, D. M., & Langhinrichsen-Rohling, J. (2011). A meta-analysis of neuropsychological outcome after mild traumatic brain injury: Re-analyses and reconsiderations of Binder et al. (1997), Frencham et al. (2005), and Pertab et al. (2009). *The Clinical Neuropsychologist, 25*(4), 608–623. https://doi.org/10.1080/13854046.2011.565076.

Rohling, M. L., Larrabee, G. J., & Millis, S. R. (2012). The "miserable minority" following mild traumatic brain injury: Who are they and do meta-analyses hide them? *The Clinical Neuropsychologist, 26*(2), 197–213. https://doi.org/10.1080/13854046.2011.647085.

Rosen, B. R., Buckner, R. L., & Dale, A. M. (1998). Event-related functional MRI: Past, present, and future. *Proceedings of the National Academy of Sciences, USA, 95,* 773–780.

Rosenfeld, J. V., McFarlane, A. C., Bragge, P., Armonda, R. A., Grimes, J. B., & Ling, G. S. (2013). Blast-related traumatic brain injury. *The Lancet Neurology, 12*(9), 882–893. https://doi.org/10.1016/S1474-4422(13)70161-3.

Ruff, R. M., Camenzuli, L., & Mueller, J. (1996). Miserable minority: Emotional risk factors that influence the outcome of a mild traumatic brain injury. *Brain Injury, 10,* 551–565.

Ruff, R. M., Crouch, J. A., Troster, A. I., Marshall, L. F., Buchsbaum, M. S., Lottenberg, S., et al. (1994). Selected cases of poor outcome following a minor brain trauma: Comparing neuropsychological and positron emission tomography assessment. *Brain Injury, 8,* 297–308.

Ruff, R. M., Iverson, G. L., Barth, J. T., Bush, S. S., Broshek, D. K., Policy, N. A. N., et al. (2009). Recommendations for diagnosing a mild traumatic brain injury: A national academy of neuropsychology education paper. *Archives of Clinical Neuropsychology, 24*(1), 3–10.

Schachar, R., Levin, H. S., Max, J. E., Purvis, K., & Chen, S. (2004). Attention deficit hyperactivity disorder symptoms and response inhibition after closed head injury in children: Do preinjury behavior and injury severity predict outcome? *Developmental Neuropsychology, 25*(1–2), 179–198.

Scheibel, R. S., Newsome, M. R., Troyanskaya, M., Lin, X., Steinberg, J. L., Radaideh, M., et al. (2012). Altered brain activation in military personnel with one or more traumatic brain injuries following blast. *Journal of the International Neuropsychological Society, 18*(1), 89–100. https://doi.org/10.1017/S1355617711001433.

Schiehser, D. M., Delis, D. C., Filoteo, J. V., Delano-Wood, L., Han, S. D., Jak, A. J., … Bondi, M. W. (2011). Are self-reported symptoms of executive dysfunction associated with objective executive function performance following mild to moderate traumatic brain injury? *Journal of Clinical and Experimental Neuropsychology, 33*(6), 704–714. https://doi.org/10.1080/13803395.2011.553587.

Scholten, J. D., Sayer, N. A., Vanderploeg, R. D., Bidelspach, D. E., & Cifu, D. X. (2012). Analysis of US veterans health administration comprehensive evaluations for traumatic brain injury in operation enduring freedom and operation Iraqi freedom veterans. *Brain Injury, 26*(10), 1177–1184. https://doi.org/10.3109/02699052.2012.661914.

Schretlen, D. J., & Shapiro, A. M. (2003). A quantitative review of the effects of traumatic brain injury on cognitive functioning. *International review of psychiatry, 15*(4), 341–349.

Sedlmeier, P., Eberth, J., Schwarz, M., Zimmermann, D., Haarig, F., Jaeger, S., et al. (2012). The psychological effects of meditation: A meta-analysis. *Psychological Bulletin, 138*(6), 1139–1171.

Sesma, H. W., Slomine, B. S., Ding, R., & McCarthy, M. L. (2008). Executive functioning in the first year after pediatric traumatic brain injury. *Pediatrics, 121*(6), e1686–e1695.

Shandera-Ochsner, A. L., Berry, D. T. R., Harp, J. P., Edmundson, M., Graue, L. O., Roach, A., et al. (2013). Neuropsychological effects of self-reported deployment-related mild TBI and current PTSD in OIF/OEF veterans. *Clinical Neuropsychologist, 27*(6), 881–907. https://doi.org/10.1080/13854046.2013.802017.

Sharp, D. J., & Ham, T. E. (2011). Investigating white matter injury after mild traumatic brain injury. *Current Opinion in Neurology, 24*(6), 558–563.

Shenton, M. E., Hamoda, H. M., Schneiderman, J. S., Bouix, S. S., Pasternak, O. O., Rathi, Y. Y., … Zafonte, R. R. (2012). A review of magnetic resonance imaging and diffusion tensor imaging findings in mild traumatic brain injury. *Brain Imaging and Behavior, 6*(2), 137–192. https://doi.org/10.1007/s11682-012-9156-5.

Sherer, M., Bergloff, P., Levin, E., High, W. M., Jr., Oden, K. E., & Nick, T. G. (1998). Impaired awareness and employment outcome after traumatic brain injury. *Journal of Head Trauma Rehabilitation, 13,* 52–61.

Sherer, M., Novack, T. A., Sander, A. M., Struchen, M. A., Alderson, A., & Thompson, R. N. (2002). Neuropsychological assessment and employment outcome after traumatic brain injury: A review. *The Clinical Neuropsychologist, 16*(2), 157–178.

Sorg, S. F., Delano-Wood, L., Luc, N., Schiehser, D. M., Hanson, K. L., Nation, D. A., … Bondi, M. W. (2014). White matter integrity in veterans with mild traumatic brain injury: Associations with executive function and loss of consciousness. *Journal of Head Trauma Rehabilitation, 29*(1), 21–32. https://doi.org/10.1097/HTR.0b013e31828a1aa4.

Sosnoff, J. J., Broglio, S. P., Hillman, C. H., & Ferrara, M. S. (2007). Concussion does not impact intraindividual response time variability. *Neuropsychology, 21*(6), 796–802. https://doi.org/10.1037/0894-4105.21.6.796.

Sponheim, S. R., McGuire, K. A., Kang, S. S., Davenport, N. D., Aviyente, S., Bernat, E. M., et al. (2011). Evidence of disrupted functional connectivity in the brain after combat-related blast injury. *NeuroImage, 54*(Suppl. 1), S21–S29. https://doi.org/10.1016/j.neuroimage.2010.09.007.

Stamenova, V., & Levine, B. (2018). Effectiveness of goal management training® in improving executive functions: A meta-analysis. *Neuropsychological Rehabilitation*, 1–31.

Storzbach, D., Twamley, E. W., Roost, M. S., Golshan, S., Williams, R. M., O Neil, M., … Huckans, M. (2017). Compensatory cognitive training for operation enduring freedom/operation Iraqi freedom/operation new dawn veterans with mild traumatic brain injury. *Journal of Head Trauma Rehabilitation, 32*(1), 16–24. https://doi.org/10.1097/HTR.0000000000000228.

Stuss, D. T. (2011). Functions of the frontal lobes: Relation to executive functions. *Journal of the International Neuropsychological Society, 17*(5), 759–765.

Stuss, D. T., & Alexander, M. P. (2007). Is there a dysexecutive syndrome? *Philosophical Transactions of the Royal Society B: Biological Sciences, 362*(1481), 901–915.

Suhr, J. A., & Gunstad, J. (2002). "Diagnosis threat": The effect of negative expectations on cognitive performance in head injury. *Journal of Clinical and Experimental Neuropsychology, 24,* 448–457.

Suhr, J. A., & Gunstad, J. (2005). Further exploration of the effect of "diagnosis threat" on cognitive performance in individuals with mild head injury. *Journal of the International Neuropsychological Society, 11,* 23–29.

Tavano, A., Galbiati, S., Recla, M., Bardoni, A., Dominici, C., Pastore, V., et al. (2014). Cognitive recovery after severe traumatic brain injury in children/adolescents and adults: Similar positive outcome but different underlying pathways? *Brain Injury, 28*(7), 900–905.

Taylor, H. G., Yeates, K. O., Wade, S. L., Drotar, D., Stancin, T., & Minich, N. (2002). A prospective study of short-and long-term outcomes after traumatic brain injury in children: behavior and achievement. *Neuropsychology, 16*(1), 15–27.

Taylor, C. A., Bell, J. M., Breiding, M. J., & Xu, L. (2017a). Traumatic brain injury–related emergency department visits, hospitalizations, and deaths—United States, 2007 and 2013. MMWR Surveillance Summary, 66(SS-9):1–16. http://dx.doi.org/10.15585/mmwr.ss6609a1.

Taylor, B. C., Hagel Campbell, E., Nugent, S., Bidelspach, D. E., Kehle-Forbes, S. M., Scholten, J., … Sayer, N. A. (2017b). Three year trends in veterans health administration utilization and costs after traumatic brain injury screening among veterans with mild traumatic brain injury. *Journal of Neurotrauma, 34*(17), 2567–2574. https://doi.org/10.1089/neu.2016.4910.

Taylor, B. C., Hagel, E. M., Carlson, K. F., Cifu, D. X., Cutting, A., Bidelspach, D. E., et al. (2012). Prevalence and costs of co-occurring traumatic brain injury with and without psychiatric disturbance and pain among Afghanistan and Iraq war veteran VA users. *Medical Care, 50*(4), 342–346. https://doi.org/10.1097/MLR.0b013e318245a558.

Teasdale, G., & Jennett, B. (1974). Assessment of coma and impaired consciousness: A practical scale. *The Lancet, 304*(7872), 81–84.

Tomporowski, P. D., Lambourne, K., & Okumura, M. S. (2011). Physical activity interventions and children's mental function: An introduction and overview. *Preventive Medicine, 52,* S3–S9.

Tonks, J., Huw Williams, W., Yates, P., & Slater, A. (2011). Cognitive correlates of psychosocial outcome following traumatic brain injury in early childhood: Comparisons between groups of children aged under and over 10 years of age. *Clinical Child Psychology and Psychiatry, 16*(2), 185–194.

U.S. Department of Defense. (2019). DoD TBI worldwide numbers for TBI. Retrieved from http://dvbic.dcoe.mil/dod-worldwide-numbers-tbi.

Vakhtin, A. A., Calhoun, V. D., Jung, R. E., Prestopnik, J. L., Taylor, P. A., & Ford, C. C. (2013). Changes in intrinsic functional brain networks following blast-induced mild traumatic brain injury. *Brain Injury, 27*(11), 1304–1310. https://doi.org/10.3109/02699052.2013.823561.

Valera, E. M., Campbell, J., Gill, J., & Iverson, K. M. (2019). Correlates of brain injuries in women subjected to intimate partner violence: Identifying the dangers and raising awareness. *Journal of Aggression, Maltreatment & Trauma.* Advance online publication. https://doi.org/10.1080/10926771.2019.1581864.

Verburgh, L., Königs, M., Scherder, E. J., & Oosterlaan, J. (2013). Physical exercise and executive functions in preadolescent children, adolescents and young adults: A meta-analysis. *British Journal of Sports Medicine*, 2012.

Verfaellie, M., Lafleche, G., Spiro, Avron, & Bousquet, K. (2014). Neuropsychological outcomes in OEF/OIF veterans with self-report of blast exposure: Associations with mental health, but not mTBI. *Neuropsychology, 28*(3), 337–346. https://doi.org/10.1037/neu0000027.

Virji-Babul, N., Hilderman, C., Makan, N., Liu, A., Smith-Forrester, J., Franks, C., & Wang, J. Z. (2014). Changes in functional brain networks following sports related concussion in adolescents. *Journal of Neurotrauma*. Advance online publication. https://doi.org/10.1089/neu.2014.3450.

Voss, M. W., Nagamatsu, L. S., Liu-Ambrose, T., & Kramer, A. F. (2011). Exercise, brain, and cognition across the life span. *Journal of Applied Physiology, 111*(5), 1505–1513.

Wade, S. L., Cassedy, A. E., Fulks, L. E., Taylor, H. G., Stancin, T., Kirkwood, M. W., … Kurowski, B. G. (2017). Problem-solving after traumatic brain injury in adolescence: Associations with functional outcomes. *Archives of Physical Medicine and Rehabilitation*, *98*(8), 1614–1621.

Wäljas, M., Iverson, G. L., Lange, R. T., Hakulinen, U., Dastidar, P., Huhtala, H., … Öhman, J. (2015). A prospective biopsychosocial study of the persistent post-concussion symptoms following mild traumatic brain injury. *Journal of Neurotrauma*, *32*(8), 534–547.

Watts, D. J., & Strogatz, S. H. (1998). Collective dynamics of "small-world" networks. *Nature, 393,* 440–442.

Weintraub, S., Dikmen, S. S., Heaton, R. K., Tulsky, D. S., Zelazo, P. D., Slotkin, J., … Gershon, R. (2014). The Cognition Battery of the NIH Toolbox for assessment of neurological and behavioral function: Validation in an adult sample. *Journal of the International Neuropsychological Society, 20*, 567–578.

Wolf, G. K., Mauntel, G. J., Kretzmer, T., Crawford, E., Thors, C., Strom, T. Q., et al. (2018). Comorbid posttraumatic stress disorder and traumatic brain injury: Generalization of prolonged-exposure PTSD treatment outcomes to postconcussive symptoms, cognition, and self-efficacy in veterans and active duty service members. *Journal of Head Trauma Rehabilitation, 33*(2), E53–E63. https://doi.org/10.1097/HTR.0000000000000344.

Yeh, P.-H., Wang, B., Oakes, T. R., French, L. M., Pan, H., Graner, J., … Riedy, G. (2013). Post-concussional disorder and PTSD symptoms of military-related traumatic brain injury associated with compromised neurocircuitry. *Human Brain Mapping, 35*(6), 2652–2673. https://doi.org/10.1002/hbm.22358.

Zakzanis, K. K., Leach, L., & Kaplan, E. (1999). Mild traumatic brain injury. *Neuropsychological differential diagnosis* (pp. 163–171). Lisse Netherlands: Swets & Zeitlinger Pub.

Zemek, R., Barrowman, N., Freedman, S. B., Gravel, J., Gagnon, I., McGahern, C., … Craig, W. (2016). Clinical risk score for persistent postconcussion symptoms among children with acute concussion in the ED. *JAMA, 315*(10), 1014–1025.

Zemek, R. L., Farion, K. J., Sampson, M., & McGahern, C. (2013). Prognosticators of persistent symptoms following pediatric concussion: A systematic review. *JAMA Pediatrics, 167*(3), 259–265.

Chapter 6
Executive Dysfunction Associated with Substance Abuse

Olga Inozemtseva and Edgar Mejía Núñez

6.1 Introduction

Substance abuse and substance dependence have been defined by several authors, and most of them highlight characteristics related to alterations in the motivational component and executive control of behavior. Thus, George and Koob (2010) define substance use disorder as chronic relapsing disorder characterized by increased motivation to seek drugs, compulsive drug intake, and loss of control over drug intake. Diagnostic and Statistical Manual of Mental Disorders ([DSM5], American Psychiatric Association [APA], 2013) points out that an essential feature of a substance use disorder is a cluster of cognitive, behavioral, and physiological symptoms indicating that the individual continues using the substance despite significant substance-related problems. The cluster of cognitive and behavioral alterations includes the important executive dysfunction that disturbs motivated, goal-directed behavior, inducing significant social, family, and labor problems in patients with substance use disorder. Relevant executive alterations in substance dependents have been reported in many studies; however, these dysfunctions have not been conceptualized as dysexecutive syndrome itself.

Godefroy et al. (2010) define dysexecutive syndrome as alterations in executive functions concerning both behavioral and cognitive domains or dissociated between these two domains. Therefore, the main objective of this chapter is to provide evidence about deficit in executive functions in persons with substance use disorder, which could be compatible with the concept of dysexecutive syndrome. Additionally,

O. Inozemtseva (✉)
Instituto de Neurociencias, CUCBA; Departamento de Estudios En Educación, CUCSH, Universidad de Guadalajara, Guadalajara, Mexico
e-mail: oinozem@yahoo.com

E. Mejía Núñez
Instituto de Neurociencias, Universidad de Guadalajara, Guadalajara, Mexico

A. Ardila et al. (eds.), *Dysexecutive Syndromes*,
https://doi.org/10.1007/978-3-030-25077-5_6

this chapter reviews theoretical, genetics, and neurophysiological basis of executive disorder associated with substance misuse.

6.2 Theoretical Approach to Executive Dysfunction in Addictive Behavior

The deficit in executive functioning, including the control of behavior, has been hypothesized as one of principal mechanisms involved in the acquisition phase, maintenance phase of addiction, relapses, as well as in the transition from substance use and abuse to dependence. There are several theoretical approaches that have been attempted to explain the role of executive functioning in addictive behavior.

According to Jentsch's and Taylor's (1999) model, the essential characteristic of addiction is the frontal cortical cognitive dysfunction, resulting in an inability to inhibit inappropriate unconditioned or conditioned responses, this characteristic is the result of chronic drug use. This model is based on the evidence that repetitive drug use increases incentive motivational qualities of drugs through their ability to augment mesolimbic dopamine (DA) release, particularly in the shell of nucleus accumbens. The second related phenomenon is the associative learning between drugs intake and external and internal cues and impulsivity, due to limbic amygdalar dysfunction, and impaired inhibitory control due to frontal cortical dysfunction. This dysfunction is associated with different cognitive impairments, including the inhibitory control and salience attribution to relevant stimuli such as drugs.

In a similar manner, Volkow, Fowler, and Wang (2003) proposed the model of addictive behavior based on the network of four circuits related to: (1) stimuli saliency or reward, located in the nucleus accumbens and in the ventral pallidum; (2) internal state or motivation/drive, located in the orbitrofrontal cortex; (3) memory and learning associations, located in the amygdala and the hippocampus; and (4) conflict resolution or control, located in the prefrontal cortex and in the anterior cingulate gyrus. All of these circuits receive innervations from DA neurons and are connected with one another through direct and indirect projections. The balanced functioning of the four circuits is responsible for the deployment of a motivated and goal-directed behavior. In addiction state, the reward value of drug increases (giving their repeated self-administration), the saliency value of non-drug rewards decreases, and the motivation and associative memory circuits overcome the prefrontal cortex control, favoring a positive feedback loop. Based on these elements, Volkow et al. conceptualized addiction as the impaired response inhibition and salience attribution syndrome (I-RISA), which involves a disruption of incentive salience attribution for non-drug and primary reinforces with a redirection of salience to drug rewards, linked to deficit in response inhibition (Goldstein & Volkow, 2002).

The mechanism of salience attribution redirection was analyzed by Robinson and Berridge (1993). The authors mention that the spectrum of the addictive behavior is guided by the neuroadaptations in the mesolimbic–cortical dopamine system elicited by repeated drug use. These changes are manifested both neurochemically and behaviorally leading to increase in a drug effect. Main characteristics of addiction, such as *craving* and *relapse*, are due directly to drug-induced changes in the system functioning. The hypersensitized neural system and his activation mediate a psychological function involved in the process of incentive motivation, called *attribution of incentive salience*, that makes stimuli and their representations (e.g. drug paraphernalia) highly salient, attractive, and "wanted." This phenomenon is achieved through associative learning between unconditioned stimuli (UCS) and conditioned stimuli (CS), increasing the incentive salience of drug-related stimuli that becomes able to control behavior. The UCS, like the drugs, produces pleasure directly (pleasure integrator), but produces incentive salience and elicits goal-directed behavior indirectly (incentive salience attributor). The activation of incentive salience attributor by UCS results in incentive salience being assigned to the perception of CS, what makes them attractive, 'wanted' and able to elicit approach. The sensitization of the neural substrate by drug taking leads to pathological "wanting" (*craving*) for associated stimuli (CS) with its excessive activation. *Craving* is manifested behaviorally as compulsive drug seeking and drug taking. Importantly, these neuroadaptations are long-lasting and, in some cases, maybe permanent.

Another theoretical model that is adjusted to explain addictive behavior is dual-process model of cognitive control. This model proposes the existence of two semi-independent systems: a fast associative "impulsive" system, which includes automatic appraisal of stimuli in terms of their emotional and motivational significance; and slow "reflective" system, which includes controlled processes related to conscious deliberations, emotion regulation, and expected outcomes (Braver, 2012). These two systems are related to different neural networks, the impulsive system includes structures such as striatum, periaqueductal gray, amygdale, and other brainstem nuclei. The reflective system includes structures like ventromedial prefrontal cortex, anterior cingulated, insular cortex, dorsolateral prefrontal cortex, and lateral orbitofrontal/inferior frontal gyrus (Bechara, 2005). The balance between both behavior regulation systems allows to display a socially appropriate behavior.

In the addictive state, due to brain changes as a result of the continued substance use, the impulsive system becomes sensitized to the drug and to cues that predict use. Now the drug-related cues automatically capture attention. As the addictive behavior develops, automatic-impulsive processing of drug-related stimuli increases in strength, and the modulation of the impulses becomes more difficult due to two points: stronger automatic approach tendencies to drug stimuli and weaker abilities to moderate or inhibit the actions. The long-term effects of drugs impair the ability to inhibit and regulate impulsive action tendencies, making addictive behavior more "stimulus driven," and more unconscious (Wiers & Stacy, 2006).

The aforementioned theoretical models indicate that executive control processes are fundamental for the successful inhibition of different manifestations of addictive behavior, such as the compulsive seek and use of drugs, preferences for immediate rewards, exacerbated attention to drug stimuli, redirection of salience attribution to drug-related stimuli. Failures in behavioral control also may be responsible for the transition from recreational to dependent drug use and relapse even after prolonged periods of abstinence. Thus, executive dysfunction in substance dependents is well recognized, even the impulse control impairment may predispose some individuals to impulsive use of an illicit drug or to the transition from recreational to dependent use (Garavan & Hester, 2007). In this regard, Garavan and Hester posed that it would be highly relevant to clarify the fact that cognitive abilities, particularly executive function, can predict the development of drug problems or can predict relapse.

6.3 Genetics Basis of Executive Disorder in Addictive Behavior

It was reported by several authors (c.f. Ersche, Turton, Pradhan, Bullmore, & Robbins, 2010; Ersche et al., 2012, 2013; Gorwood et al., 2012; Han et al., 2008) that addiction is a disorder based on genetic causes, therefore, it would be very important to establish the endophenotypes that involve genetic alterations related to drug dependence and dysexecutive characteristics. There are several studies which attempt to identify genetic bases of cognitive and behavior disorders in substance dependents. Ersche et al. (2010) applied the Barratt Impulsiveness Scale-11(BIS-11) to 29 cocaine or amphetamine dependents, 30 siblings of the dependent individuals with no personal history of substance dependence, and 30 healthy controls with no history of drug use. Trait-impulsivity was not only increased in the drug users but also in their siblings, indicating that it could be an endophenotype or vulnerability trait predisposing to development of stimulant dependence. It has been observed that BIS scores are associated with neurochemical structural variations in brain areas that are implicated in the pathophysiology of addiction-like reduced striatal dopamine receptor availability, reduced gray matter volume in the orbitofrontal cortex. Increased levels of trait-impulsivity in the siblings of drug users suggest that this mechanism may constitute a biological predisposition for drug dependence.

In later study, Ersche et al., (2012) assessed with executive function tasks (spatial working memory, mental planning and motor reactive inhibition) 50 stimulant-dependent individuals, 50 of their biological siblings without a history of drug dependence, and 50 unrelated healthy volunteers. Task performance differed significantly across the three groups. Drug-dependent individuals performed lower than healthy volunteers in all executive function tasks. Siblings were significantly lower than healthy volunteers and did not differ from drug-dependent individuals in motor reactive inhibition domain. In the task related to mental planning, the siblings performed as well as the control group and significantly better than the drug-dependent individuals. These results suggest cognitive deficits, predominantly in inhibitory control, identified in both drug-dependent individuals and their siblings represent a shared trait in family members that predates the exposure to stimulant drugs and may be a predisposing risk factor for the development of drug dependence. Impaired regulatory abilities in siblings without a history of chronic drug abuse might indicate a developmental dysfunction of prefrontal control as a vulnerability trait for substance abuse.

Also, there were attempts to relate the alterations in the genes, predominantly associated with dopaminergic neurotransmission system and certain behavioral or cognitive traits in the substance dependents. Han et al., (2008) identified that methamphetamine dependents were carriers of the DRD2-TaqI A1 allele, DRD2-TaqI A1 (A1A1 + A1A2) more frequently than the control group. In the methamphetamine-dependent group, those with DRD2-TaqI A1 showed higher total Addiction Severity Index (ASI) scores and Temperament and Character Inventory (TCI) scores compared with participants without it. There was a marginal trend of difference in perseverative errors of Wisconsin Card Sorting Test (WCST) between patients with and without DRD2-TaqI A1. The presence or absence of DRD2 TaqI A1 in healthy volunteers was not related to differences in the temperament pattern and the neurocognitive function.

In addition to the DRD2 gene, there are several other dopaminergic system genes involved in addictions, such as DRD1, DRD3, and DRD4. These genes are coding the dopamine receptors D1, D3, D4, respectively, and it has been seen that these genes are associated with different types of addiction (Gorwood et al., 2012). Thus, DRD1 and DRD3 genes have been linked with opiate and nicotine dependence (Duaux et al., 1998; Huang, et al., 2008a, 2008b; Levran et al., 2009; Vandenbergh et al., 2007); the DRD2 gen has been involved in alcohol, nicotine, opiate and stimulant dependence (Dick et al., 2007; Doehring et al., 2009; Han et al., 2008; Uhl, Drgon, Johnson, & Rose, 2009). The DRD4 participation has been demonstrated in nicotine, stimulant dependence and in risk for heroin dependence (Chen et al., 2011; Shao et al., 2006; Vandenbergh et al., 2007). The association of the DRD4 gene with ADHD is well documented. The history of ADHD in childhood, or its current presence is a risk factor for the acquisition of addictive behavior. Moreover, these genes involved in the dopamine pathway are associated with one or more addictions, and related to deficits in impulse control expressed by impulsivity, risk taking and stress reactivity (Gorwood et al., 2012).

These studies indicate that the heritability of addictive disorder is high, several specific sets of genes are involved in different types of addictive behavior, and it is viable to identify the endophenotypes between gene expression and behavior, cognitive impairments, particularly in executive functions. However, the researches in this area are not conclusive yet given to the heterogeneity of designs, methods, recruited samples, etc. It is very meaningful to continue this type of studies due to their contribution to the clinical field for the treatment and prevention of addictions.

6.4 Executive Functioning Deficit in Persons with Substance Use Disorder

Substance use disorder is characterized by an impairment of the Central Nervous System (CNS) and significant cognitive decrease, mainly in executive functions. Executive functions were defined as capabilities that enable a person to engage successfully in independent, purposive, self-directed, and self-sufficient behavior, to respond in adaptive manner to novel situations. They are the basis of many cognitive, emotional, social skills, and necessary for appropriate, socially responsible, and effectively self-sufficient adult conduct (Lezak, Howieson, Bigler, & Tranel, 2012). Verdejo-García, López-Torrecillas, Aguilar de Arcos, and Pérez-García (2005) reported that 44.7% of the participants with substance use disorder presented clinically significant moderate impairment in their executive functioning. These participants obtained t scores below normative value in two or more executive functioning measures. Alterations in executive functioning were presented independently of the type of substance consumed by patients. On a meta-analysis Spronk, van Wel, Ramaekers, and Verkes (2013) demonstrated that long-term cocaine use was associated with executive impairments, with strongest and most convincing evidence applies to such domains as sustained attention, response inhibition, and reward-based decision-making. Consistent deficits in attentional and impulse control, decision-making, inhibition, verbal working memory, and cognitive flexibility have also been shown in users of alcohol, opiates, methamphetamine or polyabusers (Baldacchino, Balfour, Passetti, Humphris, & Matthews, 2012; Crews & Boettiger, 2009; Dean, Groman, Morales, & London, 2013; Hagen et al., 2016). These contributions were evidenced by different, specific tasks for executive clinical assessment, which in general have low ecological validity. To complete the executive disorder profile of substance users, researchers usually apply instruments that provide the data on behavior in everyday life. These instruments are self-reports questionnaires with high ecological validity. Thus, Inozemtseva, Pérez-Solís, Matute, and Juárez (2016) reported a significative executive impairment in cocaine dependents in their everyday life recorded by The Behavior Rating Inventory of Executive Function, Adult Version (BRIEF-A). Twenty-six cocaine-only dependents had significantly more dysfunctional executive behaviors than the control group, both in the subscale of behavior regulation and in the subscale of metacognition. Similar results were reported in the Spanish sample assessed by The Dysexecutive Questionnaire (DEX-Sp). Substance-dependent participants scored higher than healthy controls in all comparisons (higher scores reflect worse result) (Pedrero-Pérez et al., 2009). One of the strongest critiques of questionnaires use is the subjectivity of participant's answers. For this reason, The Behavioral Assessment of the Dysexecutive Syndrome—BADS test was developed by Wilson, Alderman, Burgess, Ernslie, & Evans (1996). This instrument allows the registering of observable responses in situations approximated to the everyday life, and hence it was considered the test with high ecological validity. Verdejo-García and Pérez-García (2007) assessed with BADS 37 poly-substance users and 37 matched controls, the results showed a global effect of drug use on five of the six subtests of the BADS, substance users performed significantly poorer than controls. Additionally, Fernández-Serrano, Pérez-García, Perales and Verdejo-García (2010) reported that the best discriminating task between substance users and controls for planning was Zoo Map and for multi-tasking was Six Elements, both from BADS.

These results suggest that the executive dysfunction profile of persons with substance use disorder is represented by deficit in both on executive tasks performance and on dysexecutive behavior in everyday life, which is compatible with the definition of the dysexecutive syndrome proposed by Godefroy et al., (2010).

The executive function deficits in persons with substance use disorder are associated with several factors. One of them is the length of abstinence. Several brain plastic changes occur at cellular, structural, and functional levels throughout the abstinence that can determinate cognitive deficit manifestation.

Based on meta-analysis study, Potvin, Stavro, Rizkallah, & Pelletier (2014) showed three abstinence groups according to their duration: short- (positive for drugs urine screening), intermediate- ($\leq$12 weeks), and long-term ($\geq$20 weeks) abstinence on cocaine abusers. This grouping was done on the basis of effect size estimation in 11 cognitive and executive domains. The results revealed moderate impairment across 8 cognitive and executive domains during intermediate abstinence. The most impaired executive domains were impulse control, working memory, and processing speed. In the short abstinence, the domains of executive functions, impulse control, and working memory showed small to moderate deficits, and the domain of processing speed small deficit. The effect size was smaller in the short abstinence that in the intermediate on all executive domains. For long-term abstinence, small effect size estimates were found. This study evidenced a greater cognitive deficit in intermediate phase (abstinence $\leq$12 weeks) than in the short phase (positive for drugs urine screening) or in the long-term phase ($\geq$20 weeks).

On the other hand, several studies reported that substance users had significant alterations in executive functioning even in the short abstinence phase. Thus, Tomasi et al. (2007) assessed with n-back task 16 cocaine abusers divided in two subgroups (8 subjects with 1–3 days of abstinence (positive urine) and 8 with 4–30 days of abstinence (negative urine) and 16 healthy controls. Cocaine users showed lower accuracy and longer reaction time than the control group in all conditions, but positive urine group obtained lower accuracy on the 2-back task than the negative group. In a similar manner, recreational cocaine users with 72 h of abstinence scored lower than controls in digit span measure (Rahman & Clarke, 2005). The persons with alcohol use disorder with 5 days of abstinence showed deficiency in planning ability and working memory compared with healthy controls (Pandey et al. 2018).

In regard to long-term abstinence, there are discrepancies in the results obtained in few longitudinal studies conducted on this topic with patients who had more than 12 weeks of abstinence. Some suggest significant improvement in executive functions at 3 months after entering rehabilitation (Inozemtseva et al., 2016) as well as in behavioral characteristics at 6 months' post-treatment follow-up (Brown, Seraganian & Tremblay, 1993) and 3 months after entering rehabilitation (Inozemtseva et al., 2016). But others describe a persistent deficit or only slight improvement at 6 months of abstinence, after beginning a treatment program (Di Sclafani, Tolou-

Shams, Price & Fein, 2002). The discrepancies may be attributable to the degree of executive dysfunction in which patients who finish treatment and achieve to maintain abstinence for a long time begin their treatment. In the study of Inozemtseva et al., (2016), the patients who eventually completed treatment and improved executive functioning showed a greater capacity for self-analysis and reflection, higher self-awareness, and better executive functions at the beginning of treatment than those who did not. This is important because self-awareness level has been related to the motivation of patients to achieve rehabilitation (Malec & Moessner, 2000), which leads to better adherence to treatment and treatment outcomes. Similar results on the association between treatment dropout rates and cognitive functioning were reported by Aharonovich, et al. (2006), who found that dropouts showed more severe cognitive impairment—mainly in attention, memory, and the executive functions—than completers at the onset of abstinence. The authors propose that their results are related to successful treatment outcomes. These findings suggest that the apparent improvement in the executive functions of substance dependents over time is not due only to the effectiveness of treatment and the duration of abstinence, but also to intrinsic cognitive characteristics of patients, especially to executive functioning.

The degree of executive dysfunction also led to severity of dependence. Usually, the substance dependents that evidence more severe cognitive or executive dysfunction and less treatment adherence, consume more dose of substance (Bolla, Brown, Eldreth, Tate & Cadet, 2002; Inozemtseva et al., 2016). Verdejo-García et al. (2005) recoded the severity of drug use for cannabis, cocaine, heroin MDMA, and alcohol consumption in 38 polysubstance abusers by The Interview for Research on Addictive Behavior. The results showed that severity of MDMA use was the best predictor of performance on the tasks that composed the working memory index and similarities index. Severity of the use of cocaine was inversely related to performance on the Stroop task. Severity of cannabis alcohol, MDMA, and heroin use was the important predictor of performance on changes task that is related with cognitive flexibility. Both linear and nonlinear dose–response effects in marijuana users were registered (more joints per week was associated with greater neurocognitive deficit). The heavy users performed worse than the light users on 69% of the neurocognitive performance measurements. Significant group differences were also found between the light and middle users on four of the tests, and between the middle and heavy users on two of the tests (in favor of the group with the least severity of consumption) (Bolla, et al., 2002).

The previously mentioned evidence allows to posit that the degree of executive dysfunction is associated with severity of substance consumption and must be considered as an important characteristic of patients for prevention and rehabilitation actions.

6.5 Inhibitory Control Deficit and Impulsivity Traits in Persons with Substance Use Disorder

As mentioned previously, the inhibitory control is a cognitive process that is intimately involved in addictive behavior, in its phases of acquisition, maintenance, relapses, and transition from recreational drug use to dependency. Therefore, this cognitive process has been studied extensively in the area of addictions. Based on the definitions made by different authors, we can say that inhibitory control is one of the fundamental cognitive processes of executive control over behavior regulation. It acts by means of the voluntary suppression of an unwanted action, or suppression of an internal or external distractor (Bari & Robins, 2013; Barkley, 1997; Dempster & Corkill, 1999; Fridman & Miyake, 2004; Nigg, 2000). Nigg (2000) proposed several types of inhibitory control divided in three groups: executive inhibition of motor or cognitive response (interference control, cognitive inhibition, behavioral inhibition and oculomotor inhibition); motivational inhibition (response to punishment cues, response to novelty); automatic inhibition of attention. The behavioral inhibition involved the motor suppression of prepotent response (prepared or initiated). Go/No-Go and Stop Signal (SST) are tasks that frequently used to assess this inhibitory control. The meta-analysis study realized by Smith, Mattick, Jamadar & Iredale (2014) used fixed-effects models to integrate results from 97 studies that compared groups with heavy substance use or addiction-like behaviors with healthy control participants on Go/No-Go task, and the SST. The measures of interest were commission errors to NoGo stimuli, stop-signal reaction time (SSRT) in the SST, omission errors to Go stimuli, and reaction time in both tasks. The analysis of the results shows the increase of commission errors to NoGo stimuli in substance-abusing groups on the whole, that is indicative of a deficit in response inhibition. In general, the effect size was small-to-medium, and differs based on the type of drug abused. Thus, significant deficit in response inhibition (high number of commission errors) was registered in cocaine users, MDMA users, and tobacco smokers. These groups did not display significant differences in Go reaction time, suggesting that poorer inhibitory performance is not the result of a speed–accuracy trade-off. Alcohol-dependent groups also displayed significantly increased omission errors, suggesting that this group may have problems with inattention or stimulus discrimination. The lack of a difference in omission errors for tobacco smokers also suggests that poorer performance in these groups is specific to inhibitory processing.

In regards to SST, the drug-dependent groups show consistently longer SSRT than control groups. Longer duration of the SSRT indicates lower speed to inhibit an unwanted response setup, and consequently lower capacities to response inhibition. The authors report medium–large deficits in SSRT for methamphetamine users and gamblers, and small–medium effects for cocaine, alcohol dependence and heavy drinking. There were no significant effects for Go RT for most analyses. The authors of this study demonstrated the high prevalence of the deficit in behavior inhibition in different substance dependents. However, substantial heterogeneity between studies is apparent in terms of behavior inhibition deficit.

Oculomotor inhibition is considered as more sensitive to measure the inhibitory processes that other types of inhibitory control because an automatic response is inhibited and not learned, the participation of other cognitive processes is low, and the brain systems involved in oculomotor inhibitory control (visual and motor) have been well studied (Nigg, 2000; Roberts, Fillmore, & Milich, 2011). However, there are still few studies where oculomotor inhibitory control is analyzing in substance users. Rosse, McCarthy, Alim, & Deutsch (1994) observed a higher number of anti-saccadic errors (faults in the voluntary suppression of automatic eye movement) coupled with a greater number of compulsive behaviors in cocaine-dependent individuals. Dias, et al., (2015) reported similar results, persons with cocaine-dependent disorder made more errors overall during anti-saccade trials across all stimuli, indicating a deficit in oculomotor inhibitory control. Moreover, significant within-group differences led to stimuli type were registered on cocaine-dependent group, where this group made more errors on cocaine-related stimulus versus neutral- and shape gray-stimulus trials. There were no differences within the control group. Pro-saccade trials (directing the glance to the same direction of the stimuli) did not reveal any main effect of group. The authors related the high anti-saccade error rates in cocaine dependents to impairment of voluntary inhibition control generated by saccadic circuitry disruption due to cocaine long-time use.

Cannabis users show longer latencies than control group on both pro-saccadic and anti-saccadic tasks. Probably the slowness in the responses in cannabis users is due to the decrease in the overall response speed that is common in cannabis use (Huestegge, Radach, & Kunert, 2008).

In a similar manner, a higher number of anticipatory saccades in both pro-saccadic and anti-saccadic tasks in psychostimulant dependents was reported in contrast to healthy controls, suggesting difficulty in oculomotor inhibitory control (Núñez Mejía & Inozemtseva, 2017). Also, the same results (high number of anticipatory saccades) were observed in cannabis users with abstinence minimum of 12 h (Núñez Carranza & Inozemtseva, 2018).

Interference behavior control allows to suppress the preponderant response that significantly interferes with the execution of the task. The task commonly used to measure this type of inhibitory control is the Stroop color and word task, where the person has to say the color with which the word is written, inhibiting the meaning. Several studies have reported significantly lower performance in Stroop color and word task by substance dependents versus healthy controls. In general, the dependent participants show longer execution time and greater number of errors to inhibit interference (Bolla et al., 2002; Hekmat, Alam Mehrjerdi, Moradi, Ekhtiari & Bakhshi, 2011; Inozemtseva et al., 2016; Núñez Carranza & Inozemtseva, 2018).

Failures in inhibitory interference control are exacerbated when the stimulus are of high motivational salience, for example, words or images related to drugs. This type of task has been called as the Addiction Stroop test and has been considered as an instrument which measures inhibitory motivational control (Nigg, 2000). There are multiple studies where difficulties to inhibit the effect of drug stimuli interference were reported in substance dependents (Cox, Fadardi, & Pothos, 2006). One of these studies was conducted on alcohol dependents in abstinence. There was a significant main effect of word type, where the abstinent alcoholic group was slower to color name alcohol words than control words, but there were no significant differences between these words types in the control group. There was a significant interference effect of alcohol-related words in abstinent alcoholic group, and it was absent in the control group (Field, Mogg, Mann, Bennett, & Bradley, 2013).

Motivational inhibitory control refers to the ability to inhibit a response to a highly relevant stimulus or to delay the immediate reinforcer. The Kirby's Delay Discounting Test allows to estimate the capability to postpone the immediate reinforcer by calculating the coefficient k (greater k values indicate higher levels of impulsivity and lower capability to delay the reinforcer). Taylor et al., (2016) reported that polydrug participants had significantly higher discounting scores than controls. The similar data were reported on alcohol-dependents patients (Bjork, Hommer, Grant, & Danube, 2004).

Motivational inhibitory deficit also was reported by using The Iowa Gambling Test (IGT). Several studies report a consistently low performance in IGT by substance dependents compared with healthy controls. The low performance consists of a significantly high incidence of choice of the immediate reinforcer independent of the punishment that this choice entails (Barry & Petry, 2008; Fridberg et al., 2010; Gonzalez et al., 2012; Quednow et al., 2006Salgado et al., 2009). Similar results were obtained on alcohol dependents (Salgado et al., 2009), cannabis users (Gonzalez et al., 2012; Fridberg et al., 2010), MDMA users (Quednow et al., 2006). Furthermore, IGT performance can be considered as predictive factor for severity of addiction. Thus, poorer IGT performance was associated with more DSM-IV symptoms for cannabis dependence (Gonzalez et al., 2012). IGT scores correlated with years of MDMA use and impulsivity scores in MDMA users (Quednow, et al., 2006).

Previously, it was mentioned that impulsive personality traits invariably go along with substance use disorder. Moreover, impulsive traits can be a risk factor for addictive behavior acquisition, relapse, or transition from recreational consumption to dependence. MacKillop et al., (2016) proposed the hypothesis that the construct of impulsivity is not homogenous and tested this hypothesis in patients with a mild addictive disorder. The authors confirmed by factor analysis the existence of three types of impulsivity: impulsive choice (measured via behavioral choices on decision-making tasks), impulsive action (measured via motor responses on inhibitory control tasks), and impulsive personality traits (ascertained via self-report on the Behavior Impulsivity Scale—BIS-11 and the Urgency, Premeditation, Perseverance, Sensation Seeking, Positive Urgency, Impulsive Behavior Scale—UPPS-P. The Impulsive Personality Traits significantly related to the consumption of alcohol, tobacco, and drugs.

Many other studies demonstrated the presence of high levels of impulsivity traits in individuals with substance dependence. Dougherty et al., (2012) compared 45 marijuana-using adolescents to non-users. The users showed significantly greater impulsivity traits, measured by attention, motor, and non-planning subscales of BIS-11. Johns, Wang, Straub, and Moeller (2018) compared young cocaine dependents (20–49 years) with old cocaine dependents (50–60 years) on impulsivity scores recoded by Immediate Memory Task (IMT) and BIS-11. Older cocaine-dependent participants had higher state impulsivity as evident through significantly higher commission errors on the IMT. This may suggest that the older brain may be more sensitive to damage produced by cocaine use. Younger users scored higher than older cocaine-dependent participants on motor impulsivity subscale of BIS-11. There were no differences in non-planning impulsivity, attentional impulsivity, and total scores on the BIS-11. Taylor, et al. (2016) demonstrated that alcohol and polydrug users had significantly higher scores than controls on BIS-11 and UPPS-P instruments. Moreover, shorter length of abstinence was associated with higher scores on non-planning impulsivity subscale of BIS-11 and Negative Urgency and Premeditation subscales of UPPS-P. Ersche et al., (2010) also reported higher levels of impulsivity (measured by BIS-11) in drug users than in control, and in siblings of drug users.

It is evident that substance-dependent people have higher levels of impulsivity than healthy controls. However, more research is needed to understand when impulsive traits manifest as a consequence of substance use or as a personality trait that can predispose the person to substance use.

6.6 Neurobiological Network of Executive Dysfunction in Addictive Behavior

The executive functions are based on the operation of a wide network of well-identified brain circuits. There are many neuroimaging studies that describe the network, specific areas, and brain functioning implicated in executive functions. The evidence suggests that a common network supports cognitive control and underlie a range of distinct executive functions, including initiation, inhibition, working memory, flexibility, planning and vigilance. The increased activity in this common network when participants performed executive function tasks includes areas of the dorsolateral prefrontal cortex, frontopolar cortex, orbitofrontal cortex, anterior cingulate, and additional regions like the superior and inferior parietal, occipital (BA 19), temporal (BAs 13, 22, 37), as well subcortical areas including caudate, putamen, thalamus and cerebellum (Niendam et al., 2012).

In addiction disorders, the toxic effect of drugs can cause alterations in the CNS at structural and functional level, which can be long-lasting or even permanent. Imaging studies have also showed the neurochemical and functional changes in the brain areas implicated to executive function. These brain changes are mostly implicated on the brain dopamine system that is considered to be the neurotransmitter which most drugs of abuse exert their reinforcing effects. It is important to mention that acute and chronic drug consumption have different effects in dopamine synaptic transmission. Acute drug administration is related to increases of dopamine transmission whereas chronic drug administration is related to a decrease in dopamine activity after detoxification (Volkow et al., 2003). The theoretical model I-RISA, described before by Volkow et al., 2003 proposed the network of four circuits involved in drug abuse and addiction that received direct innervations from dopamine neurons which regulate motivation and reinforcing effects. They are also connected with one another through direct or indirect projections with glutamatergic regions. The four circuits are: (1) reward, located in the nucleus accumbens and ventral pallidum, (2) motivation/drive, located in the orbitofrontal cortex and the subcalosal cortex, (3) memory and learning, located in the amygdala and the hippocampus, and (4) control, located in the prefrontal cortex and the anterior cingulated gyrus. The authors mentioned that abnormalities in the prefrontal cortex and anterior cingulated cortex (control circuit) in drug-addicted subjects are involved in decision-making, inhibitory control, judgment, and cognitive control. Moreover, disruptions of the prefrontal cortex could lead to loss of self-directed/willed behavior in favor of automatic sensory-driven behavior. There are many imaging studies that provide evidence of disruptions on prefrontal cortex, anterior cingulated, and other areas that are linked to executive functions in users, dependents, and consumers of distinct drugs. Methamphetamine dependents showed a dysfunction in connectivity and less activation of dorsolateral prefrontal cortex, likewise they showed a stronger activation in the ventral striatum compared with healthy participants while performing of the Balloon Analogue Risk Task (BART)—task related with risk taking. The dorsolateral prefrontal cortex activation was related to selection of choices, leading to large rewards in the future, and small immediate losses, whereas ventral striatal activation was related to short-term rewards. As modulation of activation was stronger in the ventral striatum but weaker in the dorsolateral prefrontal cortex, decision-making in methamphetamine users may reflect the influence of immediate reward on behavior (Kohno, Morales, Ghreman, Hellemann, & London, 2014).

Likewise, methamphetamine users differed from healthy participants in the relationships between sustained attention task performance and regional cerebral glucose metabolism. Meth users showed a low regional cerebral glucose metabolism in the bilateral infragenual, perigenual, and midcingulate gyrus cortices, right insula, lateral orbitofrontal gyrus, and also a deficit in hippocampal structure (areas involved in the sustained attention task performance) associated with higher errors rates, compared with non-users. (London, et al., 2005).

As well, chronic cannabis users showed abnormal functional connectivity between striatum (basal ganglia) and anterior cingulated cortex compared with non-users when they evaluated the valence and arousal of affective images from International Affective Picture System. The lower arousal in response to affective pictures was significantly associated with attenuated connectivity of the striatum-anterior cingulated cortex circuit in cannabis users (Blanco-Hinojo et al., 2016).

Cocaine abusers have shown different activation profile during the performance of n-back working memory task. This profile was characterized by lower activation in regions of the mesencephalon, thalamus, left cerebellum, putamen, anterior cingulated, parahippocampal gyrus and amygdala as well a higher activation in prefrontal, and parietal cortices, and postcentral gyrus compared with healthy participants. The high activation of prefrontal cortex by dysfunctional mesocortical dopamine pathway was associated with impaired working memory. Hyperactivation of parietal areas represents a larger recruitment of attention network resources to compensate deficits in executive function (Tomasi et al., 2007).

In studies of inhibitory control, abstinent cocaine patients showed an increased activation of the right insula which predicts the successful responses on inhibitory control task (Go/No-Go). This increased activation acts as a compensatory inhibition mechanism (Bell, Foxe, Ross, & Garavan, 2014). Hester, Bell, Foxe, and Garavan (2013) found a greater tonic activity in bilateral middle frontal, and dorsal cortex, anterior cingulate, left putamen, and left inferior frontal gyrus when a group of cocaine dependents were performing the punishment conditions of Go/No-Go task compared with controls. Cocaine dependents showed significantly impaired inhibitory control and were less able to improve their performance in response to punishment coupled with a greater tonic phasic inhibition-related BOLD activity. Consistently, Leland, Arce, Miller, & Paulus (2008) found that methamphetamine dependents showed anterior cingulate cortex activation in responses to cues that predict the need to inhibit responses in Go/No-Go tasks. Methamphetamine dependents have inhibitory difficulties that were attenuated when they received in advance warning.

Similarly, Pandey et al. (2018) found smaller volumes in left pars orbitalis, right medial orbitofrontal, right caudal middle frontal cortical regions, and bilateral hippocampus, in individuals with alcohol use disorder compared with non-alcohol-use disorder participants. Likewise, they found a positive correlation between prefrontal cortical, left hippocampal volumes, and fractional anisotropy in working memory regions during visuospatial and working memory performance, and a negative correlation with lower problem-solving ability was found, suggesting the role of prefrontal focused circuitry in these cognitive functions.

Similar findings were revealed on problematic drinkers and alcohol dependents which showed increased dorsolateral prefrontal cortex activity during cognitive flexibility task (Self-Paced Switch Task). This higher prefrontal activation in cognitive demanding tasks in presence of neural damage reflects a compensatory mechanism in alcohol consumers (Jansen, et al., 2014).

6.7 Conclusions

The executive dysfunction is common in substance use disorder. Mainly, it is manifested on such domains as sustained attention, response inhibition, reward-based decision-making, impulse control, working memory, and cognitive flexibility, registered in laboratory conditions and in everyday life. The executive disorder in substance users has been related to disruption in the functioning of areas involved on dopaminergic system, including prefrontal cortex, anterior cingulate, basal ganglia, among others. Also, the increase in subcortical structures activation associated with hypoactivation of the prefrontal areas was reported. This fact is compatible with theoretical models of addictive behavior, which propose the hypersensitization of the motivational processes related to lack in the behavioral control. The deficit in behavior control has been suggested as one of the central components of addictive behavior in several theoretical models. Many studies reported alterations in behavioral inhibitory control, oculomotor, motivational, and interference control. In addition, dependents are characterized by a high incidence of impulsive personality traits that can be a predisposing or risk factor for the acquisition, maintenance, relapse and transition from recreational drug use to dependence. The impulsivity is seen as a predisposing factor for addictive behavior, and then it is possible to assume that it may have the genetic basis, expressed through endophenotypes and gene defect. The determination of endophenotypes for substance dependents is very important for prevention and rehabilitation of addictions, but its existence is not yet clear. In a similar manner, it is important to continue studies on cognitive components and particularly executive functions in addictions, given that the degree of executive dysfunction is an aspect related with severity of the disorder and the effectiveness for its rehabilitation.

References

Aharonovich, E., Hasin, D. S., Brooks, A. C., Liu, X., Bisaga, A., & Nunes, E. V. (2006). Cognitive deficits predict low treatment retention in cocaine dependent patients. *Drug and Alcohol Dependence, 81*(3), 313–322. https://doi.org/10.1016/j.drugalcdep.2005.08.003.

American Psychiatric Association. (2013). *Diagnostic and statistical manual of mental disorders* (5th ed.). Arlington, VA: American Psychiatric Publishing.

Baldacchino, A., Balfour, D. J. K., Passetti, F., Humphris, G., & Matthews, K. (2012). Neuropsychological consequences of chronic opioid use: A quantitative review and meta-analysis. *Neuroscience and Biobehavioral Reviews, 36*(9), 2056–2068. https://doi.org/10.1016/j.neubiorev.2012.06.006.

Bari, A., & Robbins, T. W. (2013). Inhibition and impulsivity: Behavioral and neural basis of response control. *Progress in Neurobiology, 108,* 44–79. https://doi.org/10.1016/j.pneurobio.2013.06.005.

Barry, D., & Petry, N. M. (2008). Predictors of decision-making on the Iowa Gambling Task: Independent effects of life time history of substance use disorders and performance on the Trail Making Test. *Brain and Cognition, 66*(3), 243–252. https://doi.org/10.1016/j.bandc.2007.09.001.

Barkley, R. A. (1997). Behavioral inhibition, sustained attention, and executive functions: Constructing a unifying theory of ADHD. *Psychological Bulletin, 121*(1), 65–94. https://doi.org/10.1037/0033-2909.121.1.65.

Bechara, A. (2005). Decision making, impulse control and loss of willpower to resist drugs: A neurocognitive perspective. *Nature Neuroscience, 8*(11), 1458–1463. https://doi.org/10.1038/nn1584.

Bell, R. P., Foxe, J. J., Ross, L. A., & Garavan, H. (2014). Intact inhibitory control processes in abstinent drug abusers (I): A functional neuroimaging study in former cocaine addicts. *Neuropharmacology, 82,* 143–150. https://doi.org/10.1016/j.neuropharm.2013.02.018.

Bjork, J. M., Hommer, D. W., Grant, S. J., & Danube, C. (2004). Impulsivity in abstinent alcohol-dependent patients: Relation to control subjects and type 1–/type 2–like traits. *Alcohol, 34*(2–3), 133–150. https://doi.org/10.1016/j.alcohol.2004.06.012.

Blanco-Hinojo, L., Pujol, J., Harrison, B. J., Macià, D., Batalla, A., Nogué, S., et al. (2016). Attenuated frontal and sensory inputs to the basal ganglia in cannabis users. *Addiction Biology, 22*(4), 1036–1047. https://doi.org/10.1111/adb.12370.

Bolla, K. I., Brown, K., Eldreth, D., Tate, K., & Cadet, J. L. (2002). Dose-related neurocognitive effects of marijuana use. *Neurology, 59*(9), 1337–1343. https://doi.org/10.1212/01.wnl.0000031422.66442.4.

Braver, T. S. (2012). The variable nature of cognitive control: A dual mechanisms framework. *Trends in Cognitive Sciences, 16*(2), 106–113. https://doi.org/10.1016/j.tics.2011.12.010.

Brown, T. G., Seraganian, P., & Tremblay, J. (1993). Alcohol and cocaine abusers 6 months after traditional treatment: Do they fare as well as problem drinkers? *Journal of Substance Abuse Treatment, 10,* 545–552. https://doi.org/10.1016/07405472(93)90058-a.

Chen, D., Liu, F., Shang, Q., Song, X., Miao, X., & Wang, Z. (2011). Association between polymorphisms of DRD2 and DRD4 and opioid dependence: Evidence from the current studies. *American Journal of Medical Genetics Part B: Neuropsychiatric Genetics, 156B*(6), 661–670. https://doi.org/10.1002/ajmg.b.31208.

Crews, F. T., & Boettiger, C. A. (2009). Impulsivity, frontal lobes and risk for addiction. *Pharmacology, Biochemistry and Behavior, 93*(3), 237–247. https://doi.org/10.1016/j.pbb.2009.04.018.

Cox, W. M., Fadardi, J. S., & Pothos, E. M. (2006). The addiction-Stroop test: Theoretical considerations and procedural recommendations. *Psychological Bulletin, 132*(3), 443–476. https://doi.org/10.1037/0033-2909.132.3.443.

Dean, A. C., Groman, S. M., Morales, A. M., & London, E. D. (2013). An evaluation of the evidence that methamphetamine abuse causes cognitive decline in humans. *Neuropsychopharmacology, 38*(2), 259–274. https://doi.org/10.1038/npp.2012.179.

Dempster, F. N., & Corkill, A. J. (1999). Interference and inhibition in cognition and behavior: Unifying themes for educational psychology. *Educational Psychology Review, 11*(1), 1–88. https://doi.org/10.1023/a:1021992632168.

Di Sclafani, V., Tolou-Shams, M., Price, L. J., & Fein, G. (2002). Neuropsychological performance of individuals dependent on crack-cocaine, or crack-cocaine and alcohol, at 6 weeks and 6 months of abstinence. *Drug and Alcohol Dependence, 66,* 161–171. https://doi.org/10.1016/s0376-8716(01)00197-1.

Dias, N. R., Schmitz, J. M., Rathnayaka, N., Red, S. D., Sereno, A. B., Moeller, F. G., et al. (2015). Anti-saccade error rates as a measure of attentional bias in cocaine dependent subjects. *Behavioural Brain Research, 292,* 493–499. https://doi.org/10.1016/j.bbr.2015.07.006.

Dick, D. M., Wang, J. C., Plunkett, J., Aliev, F., Hinrichs, A., Bertelsen, S., Budde, J.P., Goldstein, E.L., Kaplan, D., Edenberg, H.J., Nurnberger, J. Jr., Hesselbrock, V., Schuckit, M., Kuperman, S., Tischfield, J., Porjesz, B., Begleiter, H., Bierut, L.J., & Goate, A. (2007). Family-based association analyses of alcohol dependence phenotypes across DRD2 and neighboring gene ANKK1. *Alcoholism: Clinical and Experimental Research, 31*(10), 1645–1653. https://doi.org/10.1111/j.1530-0277.2007.00470.x.

Doehring, A., von Hentig, N., Graff, J., Salamat, S., Schmidt, M., Geisslinger, G., et al. (2009). Genetic variants altering dopamine D2 receptor expression or function modulate the risk of opiate addiction and the dosage requirements of methadone substitution. *Pharmacogenetics and Genomics, 19*(6), 407–414. https://doi.org/10.1097/fpc.0b013e328320a3fd.

Dougherty, D. M., Mathias, C. W., Dawes, M. A., Furr, R. M., Charles, N. E., Liguori, A., et al. (2012). Impulsivity, attention, memory, and decision-making among adolescent marijuana users. *Psychopharmacology (Berl), 226*(2), 307–319. https://doi.org/10.1007/s00213-012-2908-5.

Duaux, E., Gorwood, P., Griffon, N., Bourdel, M. C., Sautel, F., Sokoloff, V. P., et al. (1998). Homozygosity at the dopamine D3 receptor gene is associated with opiate dependence. *Molecular Psychiatry, 1*(4), 333–336.

Ersche, K. D., Jones, P. S., Williams, G. B., Smith, D. G., Bullmore, E. T., & Robbins, T. W. (2013). Distinctive personality traits and neural correlates associated with stimulant drug use versus familial risk of stimulant dependence. *Biological Psychiatry, 74*(2), 137–144.

Ersche, K. D., Turton, A. J., Chamberlain, S. R., Müller, U., Bullmore, E. T., & Robbins, T. W. (2012). Cognitive dysfunction and anxious-impulsive personality traits are endophenotypes for drug dependence. *American Journal of Psychiatry, 169*(9), 926–936.

Ersche, K. D., Turton, A. J., Pradhan, S., Bullmore, E. T., & Robbins, T. W. (2010). Drug addiction endophenotypes: Impulsive versus sensation-seeking personality traits. *Biological Psychiatry, 68*(8), 770–773. https://doi.org/10.1016/j.biopsych.2010.06.015.

Fernández-Serrano, M. J., Pérez-García, M., Perales, J. C., & Verdejo-García, A. (2010). Prevalence of executive dysfunction in cocaine, heroin and alcohol users enrolled in therapeutic communities. *European Journal of Pharmacology, 626*(1), 104–112. https://doi.org/10.1016/j.ejphar.2009.10.019.

Field, M., Mogg, K., Mann, B., Bennett, G. A., & Bradley, B. P. (2013). Attentional biases in abstinent alcoholics and their association with craving. *Psychology of Addictive Behaviors, 27*(1), 71–80. https://doi.org/10.1037/a0029626.

Fridberg, D. J., Queller, S., Ahn, W.-Y., Kim, W., Bishara, A. J., Busemeyer, J. R., et al. (2010). Cognitive mechanisms underlying risky decision-making in chronic cannabis users. *Journal of Mathematical Psychology, 54*(1), 28–38. https://doi.org/10.1016/j.jmp.2009.10.002.

Friedman, N. P., & Miyake, A. (2004). The relations among inhibition and interference control functions: A latent-variable analysis. *Journal of Experimental Psychology: General, 133*(1), 101–135. https://doi.org/10.1037/0096-3445.133.1.101.

Garavan, H., & Hester, R. (2007). The role of cognitive control in cocaine dependence. *Neuropsychology Review, 17*(3), 337–345. https://doi.org/10.1007/s11065-007-9034-x.

George, O., & Koob, G. F. (2010). Individual differences in prefrontal cortex function and the transition from drug use to drug dependence. *Neuroscience and Biobehavioral Reviews, 35*(2), 232–247. https://doi.org/10.1016/j.neubiorev.2010.05.002.

Godefroy, O., Azouvi, P., Robert, P., Roussel, M., LeGall, D., & Meulemans, T. (2010). Dysexecutive syndrome: Diagnostic criteria and validation study. *Annals of Neurology, 68*(6), 855–864. https://doi.org/10.1002/ana.22117.

Goldstein, R. Z., & Volkow, N. D. (2002). Drug addiction and its underlying neurobiological basis: Neuroimaging evidence for the involvement of the frontal cortex. *American Journal of Psychiatry, 159*(10), 1642–1652. https://doi.org/10.1176/appi.ajp.159.10.1642.

Gonzalez, R., Schuster, R. M., Mermelstein, R. J., Vassileva, J., Martin, E. M., & Diviak, K. R. (2012). Performance of young adult cannabis users on neurocognitive measures of impulsive behavior and their relationship to symptoms of cannabis use disorders. *Journal of Clinical and Experimental Neuropsychology, 34*(9), 962–976. https://doi.org/10.1080/13803395.2012.703642.

Gorwood, P., Le Strat, Y., Ramoz, N., Dubertret, C., Moalic, J.-M., & Simonneau, M. (2012). Genetics of dopamine receptors and drug addiction. *Human Genetics, 131*(6), 803–822. https://doi.org/10.1007/s00439-012-1145-7.

Hagen, E., Erga, A. H., Hagen, K. P., Nesvåg, S. M., McKay, J. R., Lundervold, A. J., et al. (2016). Assessment of executive function in patients with substance use disorder: A comparison of inventory- and performance-based assessment. *Journal of Substance Abuse Treatment, 66,* 1–8. https://doi.org/10.1016/j.jsat.2016.02.010.

Han, D. H., Yoon, S. J., Sung, Y. H., Lee, Y. S., Kee, B. S., Lyoo, I. K., et al. (2008). A preliminary study: Novelty seeking, frontal executive function, and dopamine receptor (D2) TaqI A gene polymorphism in patients with methamphetamine dependence. *Comprehensive Psychiatry, 49*(4), 387–392.

Hekmat, S., Alam Mehrjerdi, Z., Moradi, A., Ekhtiari, H., & Bakhshi, S. (2011). Cognitive flexibility, attention and speed of mental processing in opioid and methamphetamine addicts in comparison with non-addicts. *Basic and Clinical Neuroscience, 2*(2), 12–19.

Hester, R., Bell, R. P., Foxe, J. J., & Garavan, H. (2013). The influence of monetary punishment on cognitive control in abstinent cocaine-users. *Drug and Alcohol Dependence, 133*(1), 86–93. https://doi.org/10.1016/j.drugalcdep.2013.05.027.

Huang, W., Ma, J. Z., Payne, T. J., Beuten, J., Dupont, R. T., & Li, M. D. (2008a). Significant association of DRD1 with nicotine dependence. *Human Genetics, 123*(2), 133–140. https://doi.org/10.1007/s00439-007-0453-9.

Huang, W., Payne, T. J., Ma, J. Z., & Li, M. D. (2008b). A functional polymorphism, rs6280, in DRD3is significantly associated with nicotine dependence in European-American smokers. *American Journal of Medical Genetics Part B: Neuropsychiatric Genetics, 147B*(7), 1109–1115. https://doi.org/10.1002/ajmg.b.30731.

Huestegge, L., Radach, R., & Kunert, H. (2008). Long-term effects of cannabis on oculomotor function in humans. *Journal of Psychopharmacology, 23*(6), 714–722. https://doi.org/10.1177/0269881108091601.

Inozemtseva, O., Pérez-Solís, L., Matute, E., & Juárez, J. (2016). Differential improvement of executive functions during abstinence in cocaine-dependent patients: A longitudinal study. *Substance Use and Misuse, 51*(11), 1428–1440. https://doi.org/10.1080/10826084.2016.1178293.

Jansen, J. M., van Holst, R. J., van den Brink, W., Veltman, D. J., Caan, M. W. A., & Goudriaan, A. E. (2014). Brain function during cognitive flexibility and white matter integrity in alcohol-dependent patients, problematic drinkers and healthy controls. *Addiction Biology, 20*(5), 979–989. https://doi.org/10.1111/adb.12199.

Jentsch, J. D., & Taylor, J. R. (1999). Impulsivity resulting from frontostriatal dysfunction in drug abuse: Implications for the control of behavior by reward-related stimuli. *Psychopharmacology (Berl), 146*(4), 373–390. https://doi.org/10.1007/pl00005483.

Johns, S. E., Wang, Q., Straub, L. K., & Moeller, F. G. (2018). Impulsivity and decision making in older and younger cocaine-dependent participants: A preliminary study. *The American Journal on Addictions, 27*(7), 557–559. https://doi.org/10.1111/ajad.12806.

Kohno, M., Morales, A. M., Ghahremani, D. G., Hellemann, G., & London, E. D. (2014). Risky decision making, prefrontal cortex, and mesocorticolimbic functional connectivity in methamphetamine dependence. *JAMA Psychiatry, 71*(7), 812. https://doi.org/10.1001/jamapsychiatry.2014.399.

Leland, D. S., Arce, E., Miller, D. A., & Paulus, M. P. (2008). Anterior cingulate cortex and benefit of predictive cueing on response inhibition in stimulant dependent individuals. *Biological Psychiatry, 63*(2), 184–190. https://doi.org/10.1016/j.biopsych.2007.04.031.

Levran, O., Londono, D., O'Hara, K., Randesi, M., Rotrosen, J., Casadonte, P., et al. (2009). Heroin addiction in African Americans: A hypothesis-driven association study. *Genes, Brain and Behavior, 8*(5), 531–540. https://doi.org/10.1111/j.1601-183x.2009.00501.x.

Lezak, M. D., Howieson, D. B., Bigler, E. D., & Tranel, D. (2012). *Neuropsychological Assessment* (5th ed.). New York, NY, US: Oxford University Press.

London, E. D., Berman, S. M., Voytek, B., Simon, S. L., Mandelkern, M. A., Monterosso, J., et al. (2005). Cerebral metabolic dysfunction and impaired vigilance in recently abstinent methamphetamine abusers. *Biological Psychiatry, 58*(10), 770–778. https://doi.org/10.1016/j.biopsych.2005.04.039.

MacKillop, J., Weafer, J., Gray, J. C., Oshri, A., Palmer, A., & de Wit, H. (2016). The latent structure of impulsivity: Impulsive choice, impulsive action, and impulsive personality traits. *Psychopharmacology (Berl), 233*(18), 3361–3370. https://doi.org/10.1007/s00213-016-4372-0.

Malec, J. F., & Moessner, A. M. (2000). Self-awareness, distress and postacute rehabilitation outcome. *Rehabilitation Psychology, 45,* 227–241. https://doi.org/10.1037/0090-5550.45.3.227.

Niendam, T. A., Laird, A. R., Ray, K. L., Dean, Y. M., Glahn, D. C., & Carter, C. S. (2012). Meta-analytic evidence for a super ordinate cognitive control network subserving diverse executive functions. *Cognitive, Affective, & Behavioral Neuroscience, 12*(2), 241–268. https://doi.org/10.3758/s13415-011-0083-5.

Nigg, J. T. (2000). On inhibition/disinhibition in developmental psychopathology: Views from cognitive and personality psychology and a working inhibition taxonomy. *Psychological Bulletin, 126*(2), 220–246. https://doi.org/10.1037/0033-2909.126.2.220.

Núñez Carranza, A. E. & Inozemtseva, O. (2018). Control inhibitorio motor, oculomotor y de interferencia en consumidores crónicos de cannabis (Phd thesis, Instituto de Neurociencias de la Universidad de Guadalajara, Guadalajara, México). From https://www.riudg.udg.mx/handle/20.500.12104/9.

Núñez Mejía, E. J. & Inozemtseva, O. (2017). Control inhibitorio oculomotor en dependientes a psicoestimulantes y su relación con los síntomas conductuales del TDAH en la niñez (Master thesis, Instituto de Neurociencias de la Universidad de Guadalajara, Guadalajara, México). From https://www.riudg.udg.mx/handle/20.500.12104/9.

Pandey, A. K., Ardekani, B. A., Kamarajan, C., Zhang, J., Chorlian, D. B., Byrne, K. N., Pandey, G., Leigh-Meyers, J., Kinreich, S., & Porjesz, B. (2018). Lower prefrontal and hippocampal volume and diffusion tensor imaging differences reflect structural and functional abnormalities in abstinent individuals with alcohol use disorder. *Alcoholism: Clinical and Experimental Research, 42*(10), 1883–1896 https://doi.org/10.1111/acer.13854.

Pedrero-Pérez, E. J., Ruiz-Sánchez de León, J. M., Rojo-Mota, G., Llanero-Luque, M., Olivar-Arroyo, A., Bouso-Saiz, J. C., et al. (2009). Spanish version of the dysexecutive questionnaire (DEX-Sp): Psychometric properties in addicts and non-clinical sample. *Adicciones, 21*(2), 155–166.

Potvin, S., Stavro, K., Rizkallah, É., & Pelletier, J. (2014). Cocaine and cognition: A systematic quantitative review. *Journal of Addiction Medicine, 8*(5), 368–376. https://doi.org/10.1097/adm.0000000000000066.

Quednow, B. B., Kühn, K.-U., Hoppe, C., Westheide, J., Maier, W., Daum, I., & Wagner, M. (2006). Elevated impulsivity and impaired decision-making cognition in heavy users of MDMA ("Ecstasy"). *Psychopharmacology*, *189*(4), 517–530. https://doi.org/10.1007/s00213-005-0256-4.

Rahman, Q., & Clarke, C. D. (2005). Sex differences in neurocognitive functioning among abstinent recreational cocaine users. *Psychopharmacology (Berl), 181*(2), 374–380. https://doi.org/10.1007/s00213-005-2257-8.

Roberts, W., Fillmore, M. T., & Milich, R. (2011). Linking impulsivity and inhibitory control using manual and oculomotor response inhibition tasks. *Acta Psychologica, 138*(3), 419–428. https://doi.org/10.1016/j.actpsy.2011.09.002.

Robinson, T. & Berridge, K. C. (1993). The neural basis of drug craving: An incentive-sensitization theory of addiction. *Brain Research Reviews, 18*(3), 247–291. https://doi.org/10.1016/0165-0173(93)90013-p.

Rosse, R. B., McCarthy, M. F., Alim, T. N., & Deutsch, S. I. (1994). Saccadic distractibility in cocaine dependent patients: A preliminary laboratory exploration of the cocaine-OCD hypothesis. *Drug and Alcohol Dependence, 35*(1), 25–30. https://doi.org/10.1016/0376-8716(94)90106-6.

Salgado, J. V., Malloy-Diniz, L. F., Campos, V. R., Abrantes, S. S. C., Fuentes, D., Bechara, A., et al. (2009). Neuropsychological assessment of impulsive behavior in abstinent alcohol-dependent subjects. *Revista Brasileira de Psiquiatria, 31*(1), 4–9. https://doi.org/10.1590/s1516-44462009000100003.

Shao, C., Li, Y., Jiang, K., Zhang, D., Xu, Y., Lin, L., et al. (2006). Dopamine D4 receptor polymorphism modulates cue-elicited heroin craving in Chinese. *Psychopharmacology (Berl), 186*(2), 185–190. https://doi.org/10.1007/s00213-006-0375-6.

Smith, J. L., Mattick, R. P., Jamadar, S. D., & Iredale, J. M. (2014). Deficits in behavioral inhibition in substance abuse and addiction: A meta-analysis. *Drug and Alcohol Dependence, 145,* 1–33. https://doi.org/10.1016/j.drugalcdep.2014.08.009.

Spronk, D. B., van Wel, J. H. P., Ramaekers, J. G., & Verkes, R. J. (2013). Characterizing the cognitive effects of cocaine: A comprehensive review. *Neuroscience and Biobehavioral Reviews, 37*(8), 1838–1859. https://doi.org/10.1016/j.neubiorev.2013.07.003.

Taylor, E. M., Murphy, A., Boyapati, V., Ersche, K. D., Flechais, R., Kuchibatla, S., et al. (2016). Impulsivity in abstinent alcohol and polydrug dependence: A multidimensional approach. *Psychopharmacology (Berl), 233*(8), 1487–1499. https://doi.org/10.1007/s00213-016-4245-6.

Tomasi, D., Goldstein, R. Z., Telang, F., Maloney, T., Alia-Klein, N., Caparelli, E. C., & Volkow, N. D. (2007). Widespread disruption in brain activation patterns to a working memory task during cocaine abstinence. *Brain Research, 1171*, 83–92. https://doi.org/10.1016/j.brainres.2007.06.102.

Uhl, G. R., Drgon, T., Johnson, C., & Rose, J. E. (2009). Nicotine abstinence genotyping: Assessing the impact on smoking cessation clinical trials. *The Pharmacogenomics Journal, 9*(2), 111–115. https://doi.org/10.1038/tpj.2008.10.

Vandenbergh, D. J., O'Connor, R. J., Grant, M. D., Jefferson, A. L., Vogler, G. P., Strasser, A. A., et al. (2007). Dopamine receptor genes (DRD2, DRD3 and DRD4) and gene-gene interactions associated with smoking-related behaviors. *Addiction Biology, 12*(1), 106–116. https://doi.org/10.1111/j.1369-1600.2007.00054.x.

Verdejo-García, A. J., López-Torrecillas, F., de Arcos, F. A., & Pérez-García, M. (2005). Differential effects of MDMA, cocaine, and cannabis use severity on distinctive components of the executive functions in polysubstance users: A multiple regression analysis. *Addictive Behaviors, 30*(1), 89–101.

Verdejo-García, A., & Pérez-García, M. (2007). Ecological assessment of executive functions in substance dependent individuals. *Drug and Alcohol Dependence, 90*(1), 48–55. https://doi.org/10.1016/j.drugalcdep.2007.02.010.

Volkow, N. D., Fowler, J. S., & Wang, G. J. (2003). The addicted human brain: Insights from imaging studies. *Journal of Clinical Investigation, 111*(10), 1444–1451. https://doi.org/10.1172/jci18533.

Wiers, R. W., & Stacy, A. W. (2006). Implicit cognition and addiction. *Current Directions in Psychological Science, 15,* 6.

Wilson, B. A., Alderman, N., Burgess, P. W., Emslie, H., & Evans, J. J. (1996). *Behavioral Assessment of the Dysexecutive Syndrome. Bury St.* Edmunds, UK: Thames Valley Test Company.

Chapter 7
Executive Dysfunction in Subcortical Diseases

Alfredo Ardila

7.1 Introduction

Executive functions depend on an extensive brain circuit (Ardila, Bernal & Rosselli, 2017; Mazoyer et al., 2001; Niendam et al., 2012). It includes not only several cortical areas, such as the prefrontal cortex, the supplementary motor area, and the parietal lobe, but also some subcortical areas, including the basal ganglia and the thalamus. It is not surprising to find that subcortical pathologies can be associated with executive functions disturbances (Kramer, Reed, Mungas, Weiner & Chui, 2002).

Frontal-subcortical circuits form one of the principal organizational networks of the brain and are central to brain–behavior relationships (Mega & Cummings, 1994). The executive deficits, noted in subcortical disorders, may reflect a disturbance in the frontal–subcortical integrity. Diseases that are subcortical and affect executive functioning include Huntington disease, Parkinson disease, progressive supranuclear palsy, multiple sclerosis, HIV, subcortical ischemic vascular disease, and Wilson disease (Domínguez et al., 2017; Elias & Treland, 1994; Jahanshahi et al., 2002; Martínez-Horta et al., 2013). Patients with multiple systems atrophy and progressive supranuclear palsy also present significant deficits in executive function (Lawrence et al., 1996; Robbins et al., 1994)

In the chapter, the involvement of some subcortical areas, including the basal ganglia, the thalamus, and the white matter, in executive functions will be examined. It is emphasized that they contribute to a complex brain functional system supporting diverse executive functions.

A. Ardila (✉)
Sechenov University, Moscow, Russia
e-mail: ardilaalfredo@gmail.com

Albizu University, Miami, FL, USA

A. Ardila et al. (eds.), *Dysexecutive Syndromes*,
https://doi.org/10.1007/978-3-030-25077-5_7

7.2 Basal Ganglia

Alexander, DeLong and Strick (1986) proposed that a crucial organizing principle of the brain is the corticostriatal circuitry, intimately linking regions of the frontal cortex to striatal structures, via the thalamus and globus pallidus. This model suggests a functional, as well as anatomical, connectivity between the frontal cortex and the striatum. Divac, Rosvold and Schwarcbart (1967) showed that lesions to the caudate nucleus in animals resulted in deficits that resemble those following prefrontal ablation. Executive function deficits, therefore, appear to be a genuine concomitant of basal ganglia damage. This has led to the suggestion that executive functions depend on not only the brain cortex, but on the intact functioning of the corticostriatal circuitry as well. Functional neuroimaging studies have also shown the involvement of the basal ganglia and particularly the putamen in executive functions (Lewis, Dove, Robbins, Barker & Owen, 2004; Monchi, Petrides, Strafella, Worsley, & Doyon, 2006; Owen, 2004; Rogers, Andrews, Grasby, Brooks & Robbins, 2000; Sylvester et al., 2003).

In the two most typical basal ganglia diseases, namely, Parkinson disease and Huntington disease, disturbances in executive functions have been extensively documented since several decades ago (e.g., Lawrence et al., 1996; Owen et al., 1992; Robbins et al., 1994; Taylor, Saint-Cyr, & Lang, 1986).

7.2.1 Parkinson Disease

It has been suggested that the various cognitive symptoms found in Parkinson disease are secondary to executive dysfunction (Higginson et al 2003) and probably due to impairments in frontostriatal circuits (Zgaljardic, Borod, Foldi & Mattis, 2003; Dirnberger et al 2005). Using PET, it has been documented that Parkinson disease patients have reduced activation of the dorsolateral, frontal, mesial frontal, and striatal areas during cognitive tasks (Antonini et al 1995). Defects in two different tests of executive function (planning and spatial working memory) have been shown to be associated with abnormal function in the globus pallidus (Owen, 1997, 2004). Is has been argued that striatal dysfunction affects the expression of frontal lobe functions by disrupting transmission through frontostriatal circuitry. Rowe et al. (2002) found that "attention to action," where subjects had to focus on forthcoming motor responses, was associated with enhanced effective connectivity between prefrontal and premotor regions in normal subjects. This enhanced connectivity was not seen in patients with Parkinson disease, suggesting a context-specific functional disconnection within cortical networks. Noteworthy, executive functions impairment represents a reliable predictor of dementia in Parkinson disease (Levy et al., 2002).

Using a large sample of 115 consecutive patients with newly diagnosed Parkinson disease, it has been reported that relative to controls, Parkinson disease patients perform significantly worse on most cognitive measures (Muslimovic, Post, Speelman,

& Schmand, 2005). However, further analysis revealed that group differences in cognitive performance could mainly be explained by measures of immediate memory and executive function. In an extensive multicenter sample of 1346 patients with Parkinson disease directed to analyze the prevalence of mild cognitive impairment, it was found that a total of 25.8% of subjects were classified as having mild cognitive impairment. Memory impairment was most common (13.3%), followed by visuospatial (11.0%), and attention/executive ability impairment (10.1%) (Aarsland et al., 2010). Regarding cognitive profiles, 11.3% of the patients were classified as nonamnestic single-domain mild cognitive impairment, 8.9%, as amnestic single-domain, 4.8% as amnestic multiple-domain, and 1.3% as nonamnestic multiple-domain mild cognitive impairment. Mild cognitive impairment was associated with older age at assessment and at disease onset, male gender, depression, more severe motor symptoms, and advanced disease stage.

In a meta-analytic report of 18 studies of executive functions in Parkinson disease using five different executive function tests, it was found evidence for cognitive difficulties across all five tests. The findings support the view that executive functions impairments are evident in Parkinson disease (Kudlicka, Clare & Hindle, 2011). In an attempt to pinpoint the specific characteristics of executive function impairment in Parkinson disease patients without dementia, McKinlay, Grace, Dalrymple-Alford, and Roger (2010) selected 40 Parkinson disease without dementia and compared to healthy controls. They used measures of attention and speed of processing plus a comprehensive set of executive function tests including working memory, planning, and problem-solving. Patients with Parkinson showed deficits on measures of executive function, problem-solving, and visuospatial skills. However, they were unimpaired on measures of planning, attention, and memory/learning. In a similar vein, Weintraub et al. (2005) selected 46 Parkinson disease patients and administered three executive function tests: the Tower of London-Drexel, the Trail-Making Test, and the Stroop Color and Word Test. Factor analysis was used to probe for dimensions of executive control, and linear regression models were used to explore the association between the generated factors and other clinical features. Factor analysis revealed two executive factors: one related to planning and the other to inhibitory control. In linear regression models, poorer planning was associated with increasing severity of apathy, and diminished inhibitory control was associated with increasing severity of parkinsonism and lower educational level. It was concluded that planning deficits and diminished inhibitory control are two dimensions of executive impairment in Parkinson disease, the former associated with decreased motivation and the latter associated with motor slowing.

7.2.2 Huntington Disease

Long time ago, it is well known that patients with Huntington disease present significant cognitive impairments, including executive functions disturbances (Rosselli, Rosselli, Penagos, & Ardila, 1987). For instance, Lawrence et al. (1996) selected

18 patients with early Huntington disease and administered the Cambridge Neuropsychological Test Automated Battery. Tests of pattern and spatial recognition memory, spatial span, spatial working memory, spatial planning and visual discrimination learning/attentional set shifting were employed. Patients with early Huntington disease were found to have a wide range of cognitive impairments encompassing both visuospatial memory and executive functions. In contrast to patients with more advanced Huntington disease, early Huntington disease patients were not impaired at simple reversal learning, but were impaired at performing an extradimensional shift.

Similarly, Lange, Sahakian, Quinn, Marsden and Robbins (1995) observed that patients with Huntington disease are significantly worse on tests of pattern and spatial recognition, simultaneous matching to sample, visuospatial paired associates, and on three tests sensitive to frontal lobe dysfunction–namely the Tower of London, a spatial working memory test, and a test of visual discrimination learning and reversal paradigm. The authors argued that their results are consistent with the hypothesis that patients with Huntington disease exhibit deficits in tests sensitive to frontostriatal dysfunction and that this form of intellectual deterioration is qualitatively distinct from that seen in Alzheimer's disease. Executive dysfunction in Huntington disease, on the other hand, has been associated with striatal and insular atrophy (Peinemann et al., 2005).

In an extensive international study, it was attempted to determine the stage in the Huntington disease prodrome that can be significantly differentiated from normal controls in a reliable way (Stout et al., 2011). Seven hundred and thirty-eight patients and 168 normal control participants were included. Nineteen cognitive tasks were used to assess attention, working memory, psychomotor functions, episodic memory, language, recognition of facial emotion, sensory-perceptual functions, and executive functions. Compared with the controls, the asymptomatic group showed significantly poorer performance on nearly all of the cognitive tests. The authors concluded that neurocognitive tests are robust clinical indicators of the disease process prior to reaching criteria for the motor diagnosis of Huntington disease.

In general, it is considered that tasks measuring mainly attention and executive functions adequately assess the progression of Huntington disease (Lemiere et al. 2004; Montoya et al., 2006). Nonetheless, semantic memory and delayed recall memory are relatively unaffected at early stages of the disease (Ho et al., 2003).

7.3 Thalamus

The thalamus is connected with the prefrontal cortex, and it is not surprising to find executive functions disturbances in cases of thalamic pathology. The mediodorsal thalamic nucleus represents an association hub mediating interconnections with several cortical areas but mainly the prefrontal cortex. Executive dysfunction has also been reported in case of anterior thalamic ischemia (Linek et al., 2005). There is also evidence that the thalamus participates in an executive functions brain system

(Alexander, DeLong, & Strick, 1986; Ardila et al., 2017). For instance, Van der Werf et al. (2003) found evidence of deficits of memory, executive functioning, and attention following infarction in the thalamus. Lesions including the medial dorsal nucleus, midline nuclei and/or intralaminar nuclei were accompanied by executive dysfunctioning. Radanovic, Azambuja, Mansur, Porto, and Scaff (2003) studied six patients with thalamic vascular lesions to characterize their communicative abilities as well as the interface between language alterations and other cognitive abilities such as attention, memory, and frontal executive. Results showed these patients present impairments in several cognitive domains, especially attention and executive functions.

To describe the pathways emerging from or projecting to the mediodorsal nucleus of the thalamus Jakab et al. (2012) collected diffusion tensor MR imaging data of 156 subjects. The Wechsler Abbreviated Scale of Intelligence and measures of Delis–Kaplan Executive Function System (D-KEFS) test was individually administered. Inter-subject variability in terms of connectivity-based cluster sizes was found and the relative sizes of the lateral mediodorsal area significantly correlated with the individuals' performance in the D-KEFS Sorting test.

Using deep brain stimulation, it has also been demonstrated the involvement of the thalamus in executive functions. Twelve patients having undergone anterior thalamic nuclei deep brain stimulation for intractable epilepsy participated in the study. Patients performed a computer-based executive reaction time test–that is, a go/no-go visual discrimination task with threat-related emotional distractors and rule switching, while the deep brain stimulation was switched ON and OFF every few minutes. The anterior thalamic nuclei deep stimulation increased the amount of commission errors. Furthermore, anterior thalamic nuclei deep brain stimulation slowed reaction time (Hartikainen et al., 2014).

In summary, thalamic damage can be associated with executive functions disturbances. Furthermore, the thalamus has been proposed to participate in the so-called executive functions brain system (Ardila et al., 2017). This is understandable considering the connections between the thalamus and the prefrontal cortex.

7.4 Other Subcortical Diseases

Executive dysfunction has been documented in a diversity of conditions, including subcortical vascular disease (Mok et al., 2004), and white matter disease (Arnett et al., 1997).

7.4.1 Subcortical Vascular Disease

Subcortical ischemic vascular disease can be associated with cognitive disturbances, eventually resulting in a subcortical vascular dementia (Tomimoto, 2011). Cognitive disturbances in these patients include overt executive functioning abnormalities. It has been suggested that difficulties with mental set, cognitive control, and mental manipulation of information, negatively impact the performance in diverse executive functioning tests (Lamar, Price, Giovannetti, Swenson & Libon, 2010).

Tullberg et al. (2004) selected 78 individuals with subcortical ischemic vascular disease and Alzheimer disease patients to analyze the effect of white matter lesions in different brain regions on regional cortical glucose metabolism, regional cortical atrophy, and cognitive function in a sample with a broad range of cerebrovascular disease and cognitive function. The authors used a method to define volumes of interest from high-resolution three-dimensional T1-weighted MR images. Volumetric measures of MRI segmented white matter signal hyperintensities (WMH) in five different brain regions, which ultimately were related to regional PET glucose metabolism (rCMRglc) in cerebral cortex, MRI measures of regional cortical atrophy, and neuropsychological assessment of executive and memory function. They found that WMH was significantly higher in the prefrontal region compared to the other brain regions. In all subjects, higher frontal and parietal WMH were associated with reduced frontal rCMRglc. These associations were stronger and more widely distributed in non-demented subjects where reduced frontal rCMRglc was correlated with WMH for all regions measured. In contrast, there was no relationship between WMH in any brain region and rCMRglc in either parietal or occipitotemporal regions. WMHs in all brain regions were associated with low executive scores in non-demented subjects. The authors concluded that the frontal lobes are most severely affected by subcortical ischemic vascular disease and that WMHs are more abundant in the frontal region. Regardless of where in the brain these WMHs are located, they are associated with frontal hypometabolism and executive dysfunction.

Kramer et al (2002) used a cross-sectional comparison between older control subjects and non-demented patients with one or more subcortical lacunes. All participants were administered a neuropsychological test battery incorporating measures of executive functioning. No group differences were found on measures of recent verbal memory, language, or spatial ability. Normal controls performed better than patients with lacunes in visual memory. On the Stroop interference test, patients with lacunes performed as well as controls on the color naming condition but slower on the interference condition. Executive measures were correlated with extent of white matter signal hyperintensity but not the number of lacunes. The authors concluded that subcortical ischemic vascular disease is associated with subtle declines in executive functioning and visual memory, even in non-demented patients.

In conclusion, subcortical ischemic vascular disease can be associated with diverse cognitive impairments, potentially resulting in a subcortical vascular dementia. Among the cognitive disturbances observed in these patients, executive functions abnormalities represent a major component.

7.4.2 White Matter Disease

A diversity of studies has indicated that white matter pathology is associated with cognitive disturbances, particularly with memory and executive function defects. Executive function impairments observed in patients with multiple sclerosis—taking the typical condition involving the white matter—include not only attention control difficulties and decreased reasoning ability, but also planning ability impairments (Arnett et al., 1997), suggesting an extensive disturbance in diverse executive functions abilities. It has been observed that the most frequent cognitive symptoms in multiple sclerosis include deficits in complex attention, efficiency of information processing, executive functioning, processing speed, and long-term memory (Chiaravalloti & DeLuca, 2008).

Foong et al. (1997) investigated the deficits in executive function and the relationship to frontal lesion load as detected on MRI in 42 multiple sclerosis patients. A battery of neuropsychological test examining different executive skills was administered. Performance on these tests was impaired in the patient group when compared with a group of matched controls, but not all executive skills were affected to the same extent. Executive test scores significantly correlated with the severity of frontal lesion load. Koini et al. (2016) selected 26 patients with relapsing–remitting multiple sclerosis and 32 healthy control subjects; they underwent structural and functional MR imaging, during different tasks including a go/no-go task and a general neuropsychological assessment. Compared to control subjects, patients showed increased activation in a frontoparietal network, including both thalami, during the execution of the go/no-go task. Patients had decreased thalamic volume. Among tested variables, thalamic volume, together with thalamic activation, were the best predictors of executive functions.

Furthermore, it has been suggested that cognitive decline during normal aging can be explained as a disruption of cerebral white matter. Kennedy and Raz (2009) used diffusion tensor imaging to examine the associations between white matter integrity and performance on different cognitive tests in a sample of 52 healthy adults aged 19–81 years. The authors reported that age and regional white matter integrity differentially influenced cognitive performance. Age-related degradation in anterior brain areas was associated with lower processing speed and decreased working memory ability. By the same token, decline in posterior brain areas was associated with inhibition defects and switching difficulties. Age-related decrease in central white matter regions, on the other hand, was associated with lower performance in episodic memory tests. Gunning-Dixon et al. (2009) reviews the findings from several MRI techniques, including morphometric approaches, study of white matter hyperintensities, diffusion tensor imaging, and magnetization transfer imaging, that have been used to examine aging of the cerebral white matter. A general pattern of age-related preservation and decline was found indicating that the prefrontal white matter is most susceptible to the influence of age. Studies combining MRI with cognitive measures suggested that such age-related reductions in white matter integrity may result in a disconnection state that underlies some of the age-related performance decline in different cognitive domains. The authors proposed that white matter aging may be associated with decline in episodic memory, executive functions, and information processing speed.

In a quite extensive study, De Groot et al. (2000) examined the relationship between periventricular and subcortical white matter lesions and cognitive functioning in 1077 elderly subjects randomly sampled from the general population. Cognitive function was evaluated by using several neuropsychological tests from which the authors constructed compound scores for psychomotor speed, memory performance, and global cognitive function. When analyzed separately, both periventricular and subcortical lesions were related to all neuropsychological measures. Subjects with most severe periventricular subcortical lesions performed nearly below average on tasks involving psychomotor speed, and below average for global cognitive function. Tasks that involve speed of cognitive processes appear to be more affected by subcortical subcortical lesions than memory tasks.

Undoubtedly, white matter impairments are associated with executive functions disturbances. This association is evident not only in typical white matter diseases such as multiple sclerosis, but also during normal aging.

7.5 Conclusion

Subcortical pathologies can be associated with executive functions disturbances. Functional as well as anatomical connectivity between frontal cortex and striatum via the thalamus and the globus pallidus have been demonstrated. A myriad of studies have supported that executive functional disorders can be found in a diversity of pathological conditions, including Parkinson disease and Huntington disease, thalamic pathology, subcortical vascular disease, and white matter disease. The general conclusion is that clinical and experimental evidence demonstrates that subcortical structures participate in the executive functions brain system, and executive disorders are associated not only with cortical, but also with subcortical pathology.

References

Aarsland, D., Bronnick, K., Williams-Gray, C., Weintraub, D., Marder, K., Kulisevsky, J., et al. (2010). Mild cognitive impairment in Parkinson disease: A multicenter pooled analysis. *Neurology, 75*(12), 1062–1069.

Alexander, G. E., DeLong, M. R., & Strick, P. L. (1986). Parallel organization of functionally segregated circuits linking basal ganglia and cortex. *Annual Review of Neuroscience, 9,* 357–381.

Antonini, A., Vontobel, P., Psylla, M., Günther, I., Maguire, P. R., Missimer, J., et al. (1995). Complementary positron emission tomographic studies of the striatal dopaminergic system in Parkinson's disease. *Archives of Neurology, 52,* 1183–1190.

Arnett, P. A., Rao, S. M., Grafman, J., Bernardin, L., Luchetta, T., Binder, J. R., & Lobeck, L. (1997). Executive functions in multiple sclerosis: An analysis of temporal ordering, semantic encoding, and planning abilities. *Neuropsychology, 11*(4), 535–44.

Ardila, A., Bernal, B., & Rosselli, M. (2017). Executive functions brain system: An activation likelihood estimation meta-analytic study. *Archives of Clinical Neuropsychology, 33*(4), 379–405.

Chiaravalloti, N. D., & DeLuca, J. (2008). Cognitive impairment in multiple sclerosis. *Lancet Neurology, 7*(12), 1139–1151.

de Groot, J. C., de Leeuw, F. E., Oudkerk, M., van Gijn, J., Hofman, A., Jolles, J., et al. (2000). Cerebral white matter lesions and cognitive function: The Rotterdam Scan Study. *Annals of Neurology, 47*(2), 145–151.

Dirnberger, G., Frith, C. D., & Jahanshahi, M. (2005). Executive dysfunction in Parkinson's disease is associated with altered pallidalfrontal processing. *Neuroimage, 25,* 588–599.

Divac, I., Rosvold, H. E., & Schwarcbart, M. K. (1967). Behavioural effects of selective ablation of the caudate nucleus. *Journal of Comparative & Physiological Psychology, 63,* 184–190.

Domínguez, D. J. F., Poudel, G., Stout, J. C., Gray, M., Chua, P., Borowsky, B., et al. (2017). Longitudinal changes in the fronto-striatal network are associated with executive dysfunctio-nand behavioral dysregulation in Huntington's disease: 30 months IMAGE-HD data. *Cortex, 92,* 139–149.

Elias, J. W., & Treland, J. E. (1994). Executive function in Parkinson's disease and subcortical disorders. *Seminars in Clinical Neuropsychiatry, 4,* 34–40.

Foong, J., Rozewicz, L., Quaghebeur, G., Davie, C. A., Kartsounis, L. D., Thompson, A. J., et al. (1997). Executive function in multiple sclerosis. The role of frontal lobe pathology. *Brain, 120*(Pt 1), 15–26.

Gunning-Dixon, F. M., Brickman, A. M., Cheng, J. C., & Alexopoulos, G. S. (2009). Aging of cerebral white matter: a review of MRI findings. *International Journal of Geriatric Psychiatry: A Journal of the Psychiatry of Late Life and Allied Sciences, 24*(2), 109–117.

Hartikainen, K. M., Sun, L., Polvivaara, M., Brause, M., Lehtimäki, K., Haapasalo, J., et al. (2014). Immediate effects of deep brain stimulation of anterior thalamic nuclei on executive functions and emotion-attention interaction in humans. *Journal of Clinical and Experimental Neuropsychology, 36*(5), 540–550.

Higginson, C. I., King, D. S., Levine, D., Wheelock, V. L., Khamphay, N. O., & Sigvardt, K. A. (2003). The relationship between executive function and verbal memory in Parkinson's disease. *Brain and Cognition, 52*(3), 343–352.

Ho, A. K., Sahakian, B. J., Brown, R. G., Barker, R. A., Hodges, J. R., Ané, M. N., et al. (2003). Profile of cognitive progression in early Huntington's disease. *Neurology., 61*(12), 1702–1706.

Jahanshahi, M., Rowe, J., Saleem, T., Brown, R. G., Limousin-Dowsey, P., Rothwell, J. C., et al. (2002). Striatal contribution to cognition: Working memory and executive function in Parkinson's disease before and after unilateral posteroventral pallidotomy. *Journal of Cognitive Neurosciences, 14,* 298–310.

Jakab, A., Blanc, R., & Berényi, E. L. (2012). Mapping changes of in vivo connectivity patterns in the human mediodorsal thalamus: Correlations with higher cognitive and executive functions. *Brain Imaging & Behavior, 6*(3), 472–483.

Kennedy, K. M., & Raz, N. (2009). Aging white matter and cognition: Differential effects of regional variations in diffusion properties on memory, executive functions, and speed. *Neuropsychologia, 47*(3), 916–927.

Koini, M., Filippi, M., Rocca, M.A., Yousry, T., Ciccarelli, O., Tedeschi, G., Gallo, A., Ropele, S., Valsasina, P., Riccitelli, G., Damjanovic, D., Muhlert, N., Mancini, L., Fazekas, F., Enzinger, C & MAGNIMS fMRI Study Group. (2016). Correlates of executive functions in multiple sclerosis based on structural and functional mr imaging: Insights from a multicenter study. *Radiology, 280*(3), 869–879.

Kramer, J. H., Reed, B. R., Mungas, D., Weiner, M. W., & Chui, H. C. (2002). Executive dysfunction in subcortical ischaemic vascular disease. *Journal of Neurology, Neurosurgery and Psychiatry, 72*(2), 217–220.

Kudlicka, A., Clare, L., & Hindle, J. V. (2011). Executive functions in Parkinson's disease: Systematic review and meta-analysis. *Movements Disorders, 26*(13), 2305–2315.

Lamar, M., Price, C. C., Giovannetti, T., Swenson, R., & Libon, D. J. (2010). Subcortical ischaemic vascular disease. *Behavioral Neurology, 22*(1–2), 53–62.

Lange, K. W., Sahakian, B. J., Quinn, N. P., Marsden, C. D., & Robbins, T. W. (1995). Comparison of executive and visuospatial memory function in Huntington's disease and dementia of Alzheimer type matched for degree of dementia. *Journal of Neurology, Neurosurgery and Psychiatry, 58*(5), 598–606.

Lawrence, A. D., Sahakian, B. J., Hodges, J. R., Rosser, A. E., Lange, K. W., & Robbins, T. W. (1996). Executive and mnemonic functions in early Huntington's disease. *Brain, 119*(Pt 5), 1633–1645.

Lemiere, J., Decruyenaere, M., Evers-Kiebooms, G., Vandenbussche, E., & Dom, R. J. (2004). Cognitive changes in patients with Huntington's disease (HD) and asymptomatic carriers of the HD mutation—A longitudinal follow-up study. *Neurology, 251*(8), 935–942.

Levy, G., Jacobs, D. M., Tang, M. X., Côté, L. J., Louis, E. D., Alfaro, B., et al. (2002). Memory and executive function impairment predict dementia in Parkinson's disease. *Movement Disorders, 17*(6), 1221–1226.

Lewis, S. J., Dove, A., Robbins, T. W., Barker, R. A., & Owen, A. M. (2004). Striatal contributions to working memory: A functional magnetic resonance imaging study in humans. *European Journal of Neuroscience, 19,* 755–760.

Linek, V., Sonka, K., & Bauer, J. (2005). Dysexecutive syndrome following anterior thalamic ischemia in the dominant hemisphere. *Journal of Neurological Sciences, 229–30,* 117–120.

Martínez-Horta, S., Pagonabarraga, J., Fernández de Bobadilla, R., García-Sanchez, C., & Kulisevsky, J. (2013). Apathy in Parkinson's disease: More than just executive dysfunction. *Journal of the International Neuropsychological Society, 21,* 1–12.

Mazoyer, B., Zago, L., Mellet, E., Bricogne, S., Etard, O., Houdé, O., et al. (2001). Cortical networks for working memory and executive functions sustain the conscious resting state in man. *Brain Research Bulletin, 54*(3), 287–298.

McKinlay, A., Grace, R. C., Dalrymple-Alford, J. C., & Roger, D. (2010). Characteristics of executive function impairment in Parkinson's disease patients without dementia. *Journal of the International Neuropsychological Society, 16*(2), 268–277.

Mega, M. S., & Cummings, J. L. (1994). Frontal-subcortical circuits and neuropsychiatric disorders. *Journal of Neuropsychiaty and Clinical Neurosciences, 16,* 358–370.

Mok, V. C., Wong, A., Lam, W. W., Tang, W. K., Kwok, T., Hui, A. C., et al. (2004). Cognitive impairment and functional outcome after stroke associated with small vessel disease. *Journal of Neurology, Neurosurgery and Psychiatry, 75*(4), 560–566.

Monchi, O., Petrides, M., Strafella, A. P., Worsley, K. J., & Doyon, J. (2006). Functional role of the basal ganglia in the planning and execution of actions. *Annals of Neurology, 59,* 257–264.

Montoya, A., Price, B. H., Menear, M., & Lepage, M. (2006). Brain imaging and cognitive dysfunctions in Huntington's disease. *Journal of Psychiatry & Neurosciences, 31*(1), 21–29.

Muslimovic, D., Post, B., Speelman, J. D., & Schmand, B. (2005). Cognitive profile of patients with newly diagnosed Parkinson disease. *Neurology, 65*(8), 1239–1245.

Niendam, T. A., Laird, A. R., Ray, K. L., Dean, Y. M., Glahn, D. C., & Carter, C. S. (2012). Meta-analytic evidence fora superordinate cognitive control network subserving diverse executive functions. *Cognitive, Affective, & Behavioral Neuroscience, 12*(2), 241–268.

Owen, A. M. (1997). Cognitive planning in humans: Neuropsychological, neuroanatomical and neuropharmacological perspectives. *Progress in Neurobiology, 53,* 431–450.

Owen, A. M. (2004). Cognitive dysfunction in Parkinson's disease: The role of frontostriatal circuitry. *The Neuroscientist, 10,* 525–537.

Owen, A. M., James, M., Leigh, P. N., Summers, B. A., Marsden, C. D., Quinn, N. A., et al. (1992). Fronto-striatal cognitive deficits at different stages of Parkinson's disease. *Brain, 115,* 1727–1751.

Peinemann, A., Schuller, S., Pohl, C., Jahn, T., Weindl, A., & Kassubek, J. (2005). Executive dysfunction in early stages of Huntington's disease is associated with striatal and insular atrophy:

A neuropsychological and voxel-based morphometric study. *Journal of Neurological Sciences, 239*(1), 111–119.

Radanovic, M., Azambuja, M., Mansur, L. L., Porto, C. S., & Scaff, M. (2003). Thalamus and language: Interface with attention, memory and executive functions. *Arquivos de Neuropsiquiatria, 61,* 34–42.

Robbins, T. W., James, M., Owen, A. M., Lange, K. W., Lees, A. J., & Leigh, P. N. (1994). Cognitive deficits in progressive supranuclear palsy, Parkinson's disease, and multiple system atrophy in tests sensitive to frontal lobe dysfunction. *Journal of Neurology, Neurosurgery and Psychiatry, 57,* 79–88.

Rogers, R. D., Andrews, T. C., Grasby, P. M., Brooks, D. J., & Robbins, T. W. (2000). Contrasting cortical and subcortical activations produced by attentional-set shifting and reversal learning in humans. *Journal of Cognitive Neuroscience, 12,* 142–162.

Rosselli, D., Rosselli, M., Penagos, B., & Ardila, A. (1987). Huntington's disease in Colombia: A neuropsychological analysis. *International Journal of Neurosciences, 32*(3–4), 933–942.

Rowe, J., Stephan, K. E., Fristonm, K., Frackowiak, R., Lees, A., & Passingham, R. (2002). Attention to action in Parkinson's disease: Impaired effective connectivity among frontal cortical regions. *Brain, 125,* 276–289.

Stout, J. C., Paulsen, J. S., Queller, S., Solomon, A. C., Whitlock, K. B., Campbell, J. C., et al. (2011). Neurocognitive signs in prodromal Huntington disease. *Neuropsychology, 25*(1), 1–14.

Sylvester, C. Y. C., Wager, T. D., Lacey, S. C., Hernandez, L., Nichols, T. E., & Smith, E. E. (2003). Switching attention and resolving interference: FMRI measures of executive functions. *Neuropsychologia, 41,* 357–370.

Taylor, A. E., Saint-Cyr, J. A., & Lang, A. E. (1986). Frontal lobe dysfunction in Parkinson's disease. *Brain, 109,* 845–883.

Tomimoto, H. (2011). Subcortical vascular dementia. *Neuroscience Research, 71*(3), 193–199.

Tullberg, M., Fletcher, E., DeCarli, C., Mungas, D., Reed, B. R., Harvey, D. J., et al. (2004). White matter lesions impair frontal lobe function regardless of their location. *Neurology, 63*(2), 246–253.

Van der Werf, Y. D., Scheltens, P., Lindeboom, J., Witter, M. P., Uylings, H. B., & Jolles, J. (2003). Deficits of memory, executive functioning and attention following infarction in the thalamus; A study of 22 cases with localized lesions. *Neuropsychologia, 41*(10), 1330–1344.

Weintraub, D., Moberg, P. J., Culbertson, W. C., Duda, J. E., Katz, I. R., & Stern, M. B. (2005). Dimensions of executive function in Parkinson's disease. *Dementia and Geriatric Cognitive Disorders, 20*(2–3), 140–144.

Zgaljardic, D. J., Borod, J. C., Foldi, N. S., & Mattis, P. (2003). A review of the cognitive and behavioral sequelae of Parkinson's disease: Relationship to frontostriatal circuitry. *Cognitive and Behavioral Neurology, 16*(4), 193–210.

Chapter 8
Executive Dysfunction During Normal and Abnormal Aging

Mónica Rosselli and Valeria L. Torres

8.1 Introduction

The neuroscience literature has established that the cognitive processes mediated by the frontal lobes undergo progressive changes as we age (Rosselli & Jurado, 2013). The vulnerability of the frontal lobe to aging and the parallel decline of executive and metacognitive functions are the bases for the frontal lobe hypothesis of aging (West, 1996). This hypothesis proposes that the prefrontal cortex (PFC) begins deteriorating before other regions (Rodríguez-Aranda & Sundet, 2006). The cerebral volume of the PFC (specifically, the orbitofrontal cortex) suffers a greater reduction compared to limbic areas and other brain regions (Lindberg, 2012). Kennedy and Raz (2015) also reported these changes in the PFC, as well as in the cerebellum and neostriatum. Shrinkage of the PFC, as well as the entorhinal cortex, has been linked to declines in cognitive performance or reduced ability to benefit from repeated testing (for a review, see Raz & Daugherty, 2018). The effects of aging have been demonstrated with interruptions of frontal tracks that connect the frontal lobe with other cortical and subcortical structures, such as the cortico–cortico and cortico–subcortical tracks (Sullivan, Rohlfing, & Pfefferbaum, 2010), with larger age effects in association tracks connecting frontal and parietal multimodal cortices than in projection fibers (Salat, 2014). This pattern of aging effects is in accordance to the first-in-last-out hypothesis (Raz & Daugherty, 2018): regions of the brain that develop later are more vulnerable to age-associated degeneration than those that evidence early growth.

The frontal lobe hypothesis of aging has been complemented with results from functional neuroimaging studies, showing that compared to young adults, older adults have reduced activity in some brain regions but increased activity in others (Cabeza,

M. Rosselli (✉) · V. L. Torres
Department of Psychology, Florida Atlantic University, Davie, FL, USA
e-mail: mrossell@fau.edu

V. L. Torres
e-mail: vtorres2015@fau.edu

A. Ardila et al. (eds.), *Dysexecutive Syndromes*,
https://doi.org/10.1007/978-3-030-25077-5_8

McIntosh, Tulving, Nyberg, & Grady, 1997). The age-related increases and decreases in neural activity are noticeable within the PFC (Cabeza, 2002). When comparing older and younger adults, older adults show a more bilateral pattern of activation of the PFC during tasks of verbal recall, implying a decreased activation of the left PFC and increased activation of the right PFC. These findings support the notion that cognitive processing in the aging brain differs from that of younger brains (Cabeza & Dennis, 2013).

The frontal lobes are the bases for executive functions (EFs). Age-related anatomical and functional changes of the frontal lobe are accompanied by EF changes. EF is an umbrella term covering cognitive and behavioral processes mediated by the frontal lobes (Rodríguez-Aranda & Sundet, 2006). EFs are regarded as a construct that includes numerous abilities required for the initiation and organization of activities and functions that contribute to the executive process of reaching a goal; these capabilities support various phases of the executive process, with the assumption that systematic monitoring of each phase provides insight into the overall process (Hanna-Pladdy, 2007). Intentionality seems to be an important component of EFs (Lezak, Howieson, & Loring, 2004), suggesting that the cognitive and behavioral processes of EFs are reflected in actions.

EFs can be separated into two processes: one relating to affective operations and the other to cognitive operations. EFs that have an affective/emotional component are considered "hot," while those that are relatively abstract and non-affective while relating to cognition (e.g., working memory and multitasking) are known as "cool" or "cold" (these include self-management skills without the involvement of emotion, such as updating, inhibition, and set-shifting; Ho, Hsu, Lu, Gossop, & Chen, 2018). "Hot" EFs include affective decision-making for events with emotionally significant consequences (i.e., meaningful rewards and/or losses; Kerr & Zelazo, 2004). Ardila (2013) suggested that cool EFs constitute a metacognitive group of EFs abilities, whereas hot EFs comprise the emotional/motivational EFs. The latter EFs include abilities required to fulfill basic impulses following socially accepted strategies in which inhibitory control plays a major role.

Failure to respond in a particular way during neuropsychological tasks or to environmental circumstances may reflect a dysexecutive syndrome (DES), a group of problems in inhibitory control, poor cognitive flexibility, and the inability to follow a plan. In the cognitive DES, deficits are found in metacognitive abilities (cool EFs), whereas in the behavioral DES, deficits are mainly observed in the form of behavioral disinhibition, global hypoactivity with apathy, perseverative behavior, and impulse control disorders (Godefroy et al., 2018). During complex interactions, the individual who wants to reach a goal may need to generate a plan while monitoring internal and external information. This individual must simultaneously maintain some information online and suppress inappropriate behaviors, as well as avoid distractions by irrelevant stimuli while initiating appropriate responses to changing environmental stimuli (Jurado & Rosselli, 2007). Therefore, adapting to a complex and changing environment requires a diverse range of EFs including problem-solving, set-shifting, self-monitoring, initiation, inhibition, planning, and sequencing. EF deficits in normal aging may affect behavior as well as cognition. In elderly individuals, cognitive deficits in planning, decision-making, organization, and self-control are expected to negatively affect their daily lives (Amieva, Phillips, & Della Sala, 2003).

Age-related deficits in EF can be observed by using standardized neuropsychological tests presumed to assess frontal function or in experimental paradigms focused on various executive processes (Cabeza & Dennis, 2013). The most studied EF processes are inhibitory control, cognitive flexibility, and set-shifting, planning, and initiation or self-generation (Hanna-Pladdy, 2007; Jurado & Rosselli, 2007). Age-related changes in these processes vary among individuals; some present with changes in only one process while others are affected in several domains (Byczewska-Konieczny, 2019). The effect of age on EFs may be a continuum, with the most extreme being the DES. Although there is no consensus regarding the diagnostic criteria for this syndrome, it may include objective changes in several behavioral and cognitive EF domains with preserved non-EF skills (Godefroy et al., 2018).

Baddeley and Wilson (1988) coined the term DES as a functional characterization of patients with deficits in the central executive component of working memory. This syndrome was later characterized in reference to a patient who had amnesia with confabulation after bilateral traumatic frontal damage (Baddeley & Wilson, 1988). This patient's DES included the following: (1) reduced performance and numerous perseverations on a test of cognitive flexibility (e.g., Wisconsin Card Sorting Test [WCST; Heaton, Chelune, Talley, Kay, & Curtis, 1993]); (2) poor thinking as reflected on their performance on the Cognitive Estimation Test (Shallice & Evans, 1978), and in other reasoning tests; (3) the inability to generate words in letter and semantic fluency tests; and (4) a change in behavior (from apathetic to charming and amusing).

The initial description of the DES was associated with focal frontal lobe pathology, but more recently, the field has recognized that it may arise from other neurological disorders, which explains why the term evolved to executive disorders (Godefroy et al., 2018; Hanna-Pladdy, 2007). Godefroy et al. (2018) stressed that the term "dysexecutive disorder" should be used to refer to all disorders related to decreased control of EFs, independent of their neurological etiology. Subsequently, "cognitive dysexecutive disorders" refer to the impairment of control processes that are assessed by cognitive tests and "behavioral dysexecutive disorders" refer to behavioral changes that are assessed by the direct examination of the subject's behavior or the use of behavioral inventories (Karzmark, Llanes, Tan, Deutsch, & Zeifert, 2012).

This chapter aims to review the findings that relate age to EF declines and to present evidence of the DES in abnormal aging. Dysfunctions in EF in cases of Mild Cognitive Impairment, different types of dementia, and other diseases are described. We highlight the idea that alterations of EFs in abnormal aging involve a neurological condition, whereas EF changes in healthy adults result from the normal processes of aging.

8.2 Dysexecutive Syndrome in Normal Aging

Consistent with the frontal lobe hypothesis, cognitive deficits in healthy older adults are greater for tasks that are highly dependent on executive control processes. These include inhibiting irrelevant information, switching in response to environmental changes, implementing planning strategies to achieve a goal, and initiating an action or response (Rosselli & Jurado, 2013).

8.2.1 Attentional Control/Response Inhibition

Attentional control is defined as the selective and inhibitory component of attention (Anderson, 2002) allowing us to focus our cognitive resources on specific aspects of the environment. The simultaneous inhibition of irrelevant information is essential in situations with high attentional demands. This control will vary depending on the length of the sustained attention and the depth of engagement with the source of information (Tas, Luck, & Hollingworth, 2016). Attentional control plays an important role in accomplishing goals by directing resources to systems related to the relevant task while inhibiting orientation to the irrelevant one.

Deficits in this ability can be explained by the inhibitory deficit hypothesis (Hasher & Zacks, 1988) which suggests that dysfunctions in the inhibitory mechanisms of attention are responsible for age-related cognitive deficits. The lack of inhibitory control would reduce working memory capacity due to the intrusion of irrelevant information, which will limit the processing capacity of relevant information. Because of this deficit, elderly individuals may get distracted easily, generate task errors, and increase the response processing time.

The Stroop test (Stroop, 1935) is the most common paradigm used to measure response inhibition. The Stroop requires participants to read color words (i.e., blue, green, red) printed in conflicting colored ink, which requires the suppression of reading while having to provide the color of the ink (e.g., the word "blue" printed in red ink). Previous research showed that elderly participants present inhibitory difficulties, as measured by response time. Older individuals appear to require more time to inhibit the automatic tendency to read the word compared to younger ones, thereby showing a larger Stroop effect (Van der Elst, Van Boxtel, Van Breukelen, & Jolles, 2006). Interestingly, West and Baylis (1998) found that the age-related increases in the Stroop effect were observed only when the proportion of incongruent trials was high, requiring a high demand of inhibitory processes, suggesting that older adults have a limited amount of inhibitory resources.

Although these outcomes support the idea of age-related declines in inhibitory processes, other research has suggested that general slowing can also explain the increases in the Stroop effect (Fisk & Warr, 1996). West and Alain (2000) tested this idea using Event Related Potentials (ERPs) and hypothesized that differences in the amplitude of ERP modulations between younger and older adults would reflect inhibitory attentional processes. Results showed an age-related decline in inhibitory processing resulting in a reduction in the amplitude of modulations differentiating incongruent trials from neutral and congruent trials over the midline frontocentral region and left parietal and bilateral frontal regions. Although older adults had a higher response time, age-related declines in inhibitory control contributed to the increased Stroop effect observed in the older adults of this study. Analyses of the response latency data revealed an age-related increase in the magnitude of the Stroop effect in older adults. The effect of age on incongruent trials remained significant after controlling for age-related differences in response latency on neutral trials. The authors concluded that there is a unique effect of age, beyond that of general slowing, that contributes to the larger Stroop effect observed in older adults.

Besides inhibitory control, vigilance, a type of sustained attention required for monitoring rare but critical events (Thomson & Hasher, 2017) also shows age-related changes. The alternating programs and go-no go paradigms that measure response inhibition are also sensitive to aging impairments (Gaál & Czigler, 2015).

8.2.2 Planning

Planning is essential for reaching a goal and includes the organization of behaviors in subgoals (Luria, 1976). A decreased capacity to make plans is seen in elderly individuals as early as age 60 and can be observed with the tower tests. After this age, adults being making errors in the Tower of London (Zook, Welsh, & Ewing, 2006) or the Tower of Hanoi (Sorel & Pennequin, 2008). These tests include the following detailed rules that need to be followed to successfully complete the final configuration: (1) only one disk can be moved at a time, and therefore, participants cannot hold more than one disk at a time; (2) smaller disks must always be placed above larger disks; and (3) the final configuration should be achieved in the least number of moves possible. Elderly adults make more moves and have higher completion times than younger adults (Andrés & Van der Linden, 2000; Sorel & Pennequin, 2008). Also, more rule-breaking is seen in the elderly (Passingham, 1993).

The effects of aging on planning tasks could also be influenced by the characteristics of the task and the participant's non-verbal abilities. Brennan, Welsh, and Fisher (1997) used two levels of complexity on the Hanoi tower test to compare three age groups: the young group, with a mean age of 19, the young old group, with a mean age of 65, and an old group, with a mean age of 75. Results showed no group differences when the task only used two disks, however, the performance of the young group was significantly better compared to the other groups when the number of disks was increased to four. These results underlined the interaction of aging effects with task difficulty. Similarly, Zook et al. (2006) found that low scores on the Tower of London test in elders over the age of 60 correlated with their non verbal skills; these are abilities traditionally included in the fluid intelligence category, which is very sensitive to aging (Jurado & Rosselli, 2007). Rönnlund, Lövdén, and Nilsson (2001) observed that the negative effects of aging on the Tower of Hanoi test were evident after the age of 65 and correlated with a greater number of moves and increased completion time. The same group of authors (Rönnlund et al., 2007) reported limited planning problems on the Tower of Hanoi test between the ages of 30 and 60 but a significant increase in the number of errors and in slowing after age 65.

Similarly, Allain et al. (2005) found that elderly participants (mean age of 80) made a greater number of errors when compared to younger participants (mean age of 29) in planning a visit to the zoo. Using ecologically valid tasks may be more appropriate for older adults, but age differences are not consistently reported in these types of studies (Phillips, Kliegel, & Martin, 2006).

In conclusion, research seems to suggest that healthy older adults have planning impairments when compared to younger healthy participants, with deficits appearing to subside with the use of ecologically valid tasks. Some research suggests that planning difficulties in normal aging result from issues in predetermining a complex course of action aimed at achieving a goal, more so than in guiding the execution of a sequence (Rosselli & Jurado, 2013).

8.2.3 Cognitive Flexibility/Set Shifting

Cognitive flexibility refers to the capacity to change a behavior or a mindset as a consequence of behavioral feedback (Jurado & Rosselli, 2007). This flexibility of the human mind allows us to appropriately adjust our behavior in response to environmental contingencies (Hanna-Pladdy, 2007). The most common neuropsychological tests used to study cognitive flexibility are the WCST and the Trail-Making Test-B (TMT-B; Reitan & Wolfson, 1993), with the go-no go paradigm occasionally included in this category (Hanna-Pladdy, 2007). This paradigm, despite being commonly used to measure response inhibitory control, requires cognitive flexibility.

The WCST, originally developed by Grant and Berg (Berg, 1948; Grant & Berg, 1948), is used to measure the ability to think in an abstract manner. The WCST assesses the capability of changing cognitive sets under shifting task demands that are unknown to the participants by employing cards that change in color, form, or number. Participants have to correctly sort the cards according to these three dimensions/categories using feedback (right or wrong) provided by the examiner. Dimensions are changed by the examiner without notice and participants must determine the rules of the test, understand when the rules have arbitrarily changed, and adjust their behavior accordingly (Bryan & Luszcz, 2000). Axelrod and Henry (1992) found a significant reduction in the number of correct categories and in an increase in the number of errors and perseverative responses (the continued incorrect response to one category despite receiving feedback) after the age of 60. Additionally, Daigneault, Braun, and Whitaker (1992) reported an increase in perseverative errors and a decrease in correct WCST categories at an earlier age (between 50 and 59 years). Bryan and Luszcz (2000) found a significant negative association ($r = -0.56$) between age and the number of categories on the WCST in a group of 60 older (aged between 65 and 88 years) and 60 younger (aged between 17 and 48 years) participants.

Several theories have attempted to explain these age effects on the WCST. Ridderinkhof, Span, and Van der Molen (2002) suggested that elders have an impaired ability to develop hypotheses when rules change constantly. Offenbach (1974) proposed that age affects the ability to use feedback information and consequently, working memory is impaired in tasks such as the WCST. Finally, Salthouse (1996) concluded that the decline in cognitive flexibility results from the slowing of the speed of processing, which reduces the amount of information that can be activated simultaneously.

Another neuropsychological test used to measure cognitive flexibility is the TMT-B, a visuomotor test in which the score corresponds to the time it takes to draw lines between alternating numbers and letters in consecutive order (Reitan & Wolfson, 1993). To be successful in this visuomotor test, conceptual flexibility is needed to alternate between numbers and letters (Kortte, Horner, & Windham, 2002). Typically, elderly participants make a greater number of errors and have longer completion times compared to younger participants (Ashendorf et al., 2008).

The influence of age on tests of cognitive flexibility is not always reported. For example, Mejía, Pineda, Alvarez, and Ardila (1998) did not observe differences on the WCST between two age groups of individuals between the ages of 55 and 70 and between 71 and 85. Surprisingly, Haaland, Vranes, Goodwin, and Garry (1987) reported a decrease in the number of perseverative errors along with an increase in the number of categories obtained by the older groups compared to younger groups. This group of authors only reported deficits in cognitive flexibility after 80 years of age.

In summary, most research on cognitive flexibility shows that increasing age is related to a higher number of perseverative errors and longer completion times (Bryan & Luszcz, 2000). However, other research does not support these results. These differences may be partially attributed to the variability of sample sizes and varying educational levels of the participants (Jurado & Rosselli, 2007). In addition, it is important to note that the cognitive flexibility tests mentioned above also require attentional control and working memory, and may have a motor component (e.g., the TMT-B).

The differences in cognitive flexibility that distinguish young adults from older adults have been correlated with variations in the activation level of prefrontal regions (Laguë-Beauvais, Brunet, Gagnon, Lesage, & Bherer, 2013). In general, studies of executive control using functional Magnetic Resonance Imaging (fMRI) show that older adults have increased activation in frontal regions, and this increase is positively correlated with task performance, suggesting that it plays a role as a compensatory mechanism. Madden et al. (2010) found that the pattern of event-related activation for task switching is similar for young and older adults, but older adults activate multiple prefrontal regions during task performance, not limiting the activation to regions specific to task switching. fMRI studies have shown that task switching involves activation of the frontoparietal network, although the regional patterns vary in response to individual task demand (Slagter et al., 2006). Additionally, differences in the integrity of the functional connectivity of the frontal lobe with other cortical areas have been observed, particularly with the parietal lobe (Gold, Powell, Xuan, Jicha, & Smith, 2010). Finally, Madden et al. (2010) compared the functional connectivity of a group of senile participants and a group of younger adults and reported that the senile group had less functional connectivity with other brain regions in tasks of cognitive flexibility, particularly when cue processing was involved. In this study, cueing indicated that a categorization decision needed to be made in relation to a target. Performance on this type of task is typically slower and less accurate when the categorization of the current trial switches from the previous trial, relative to when it repeats.

8.2.4 Initiation and Self-generation

The productivity of an individual is determined in part by his/her own behavioral initiative. Reduced initiation or latency in responding can modify the response efficiency. Tests that require the timed generation of items (verbal with phonological or semantic fluency or nonverbal with design fluency) with specific task constraints have been used to estimate the generational capacity of an individual (Lezak et al., 2004). To be successful on these tests, participants need to implement a recall strategy (words or designs), followed by an additional strategy to keep responses within the mandated category with the corresponding inhibition of irrelevant words, while also monitoring recall to avoid repetitions. Also, these tasks require the flexibility to move within the subcategories to have a more efficient word recall. For example, within the animal category, there are subcategories of mammals, birds, reptiles, etc. (Rosselli, Tappen, Williams, Salvatierra, & Zoller, 2009).

Research on the effects of age on fluency tests has produced contradictory results. Some authors have concluded that there are no age effects, while others suggest that young adults outperform older adults (Jurado & Rosselli, 2007). Fisk and Sharp (2004) found no evidence to support the theory of a negative effect of age on word fluency, however, these effects were found during paradigms that required the simultaneous manipulation of information. Similarly, Rodríguez-Aranda and Sundet (2006) found age differences in different types of EF tests, except for verbal fluency. Some researchers suggest that verbal fluency remains unchanged by age because it depends on a source of verbal knowledge that remains intact over the years (Crawford, Bryan, Luszcz, Obonsawin, & Stewart, 2000). In fact, several authors have found that the level of vocabulary is not sensitive to the passage of time and changes are evident only in the eighth decade of life (Emery, 1985). Bryan, Luszcz, and Crawford (1997) evaluated older adults whose ages ranged from 72 to 95 and found small age-related declines on phonological fluency, demonstrating that this ability is somewhat preserved in old age.

On the other hand, Brickman et al. (2005) reported a linear decline in verbal fluency function as age progressed. These authors replicated previous findings that suggest that semantic fluency is impaired before phonological fluency. Likewise,

Bolla, Lindgren, Bonaccorsy, and Bleecker (1990) found a significant age effect on phonological and semantic fluency when studying a group of elderly people with a high level of education.

Two meta-analyses demonstrated a slow deterioration of phonological fluency functions after the age of 40, which became faster after 60 (Rodríguez-Aranda & Martinussen, 2006; Loonstra, Tarlow, & Sellers, 2001). A recent longitudinal study shows the deterioration of both semantic and phonological fluidity in 96 patients with normal aging and with an average age of 74 years. The decrease in semantic fluency (number of recalled animals and supermarket items) over time was significantly faster than the decrease in phonological fluency (words beginning with F, A, and S) (Clark et al., 2009). It is unclear why there are divergent results, but it is possible that these are related to different education levels (Rosselli & Jurado, 2013). The effect of education on verbal fluency tests has been clearly established (Ardila, Ostrosky-Solis, Rosselli, & Gómez, 2000; Rosselli et al., 2009); these levels must be strictly controlled along with other socioeconomic variables (Jurado & Rosselli, 2007).

The performance of young and old adults on tasks of verbal fluency correlates with the activation of the frontal (inferior and medial portion) and temporal lobes (superior and medial turns) of the left hemisphere (Baldo, Schwartz, Wilkins, & Dronkers, 2006). It has been observed, however, that in old age, activation of these areas is more extensive and is accompanied by additional activation of the right frontal lobe (Cabeza & Dennis, 2013). This supplementary activation has been positively correlated with performance on memory tasks (Cabeza, Anderson, Locantore, & McIntosh, 2002) but negatively correlated with performance on verbal fluency tasks (particularly, semantic verbal fluency; Meinzer et al., 2009). That is, greater bilateral activation was associated with superior performance on memory tests (Cabeza et al., 2002), but worse performance on verbal fluency. Meinzer et al. (2012) reported that in phonological fluency tasks, but not semantic fluency, young adults can, like older adults, present activation in the right frontal lobe, but this activation is limited to one frontal region, in contrast to the broad activation observed in older adults. Additionally, this study found that the presence of negative bilateral activation (areas that are active during rest and are inhibited during the task) of anterior and posterior areas of the midline and temporal and parietal regions (especially the frontal lobe and precuneus during semantic fluency) during fluency tasks differed between young and older adults. During phonological fluency tasks, a pattern of negative activation was observed, very similar to that found in semantic fluency tasks. Compared with the young adults, the brains of the older adult sample in Meinzer et al.'s (2012) study were characterized by a much lower negative activation.

Nonverbal equivalents of the verbal fluency tasks include design fluency tasks such as the 5-Point Test (Regard, Strauss, & Knapp, 1982). This task requires participants to generate as many designs as possible in three minutes using 5-dot matrices. Participants have to connect two or more dots within the time frame without repetitions. This test appears to place greater demands on executive control mechanisms than semantic fluency tests (Foldi, Helm-Estabrooks, Redfield, & Nickel, 2003). Research on the influence of age on design fluency is mixed; some studies found no influence of age (Daigneault et al., 1992) and others report detrimental age effects

(Mittenberg, Seidenberg, O'Leary, & DiGiulio, 1989). It is possible that this test is sensitive to age only when comparing extreme age groups (Bryan & Luszcz, 2000).

8.2.5 Behavioral/Emotional Dysexecutive Syndrome

Problems with response inhibition can be evident in a patient's failure to inhibit inappropriate verbal or behavioral responses, and ideally, the assessment should be done by observing behavior during a clinical examination and using family reports. Response inhibition often presents as behavioral impulsivity, which can affect a wide range of everyday behaviors with significant consequences on effective functioning in the real world (Hanna-Pladdy, 2007). Most of the studies on dysexecutive functions associated with aging have analyzed cognitive abilities, while the behavioral component of the syndrome has rarely been investigated. The nature of behavioral dysexecutive symptoms in aging has been explored using the Dysexecutive Questionnaire (DEX; Burgess, Alderman, Evans, Emslie, & Wilson, 1998). This 20-item questionnaire assesses EF problems in four areas: personality, motivation, behavioral, and cognitive. Amieva et al. (2003) conducted a pilot study using the DEX with 20 elderly Scottish participants and identified five factors that accounted for 75.6% of the variance of DEX scores. The factors were related to intentionality/initiative (factor 1), coping with interfering events (factor 2), euphoria, perseveration, and confabulation (factor 3), planning and thinking ahead (factor 4), and social regulation (factor 5). All factors except for factor 4 correlated with EF measures; the strongest and most significant correlation ($r = 0.574, p = 0.008$) was found between factor 5 (social regulation) and completion time on the Zazzo Cancelation task. Byczewska-Konieczny (2019) replicated Amieva et al.'s (2003) study by administering the DEX to a larger sample of elderly Polish participants ($N = 40$). Additionally, DEX scores were correlated with performance on three neuropsychological measures of EF (Zazzo Cancelation task, Simon Task, and OSPAN task). Items from the DEX loaded onto three factors (F1, ability to plan and monitor of one's behavior; F2, emotional regulation; and F3, ability to cope with interfering events) that accounted for 43.38% of the total variance. The author did not find significant associations between these behavioral factors and scores on cognitive EF tasks in the sample of normally aging individuals. These findings are in contradiction to those by Chan (2001), who found significant correlations between cognitive EF tests and five factors from the DEX (F1, inhibition; F2, goal-directed behavior; F3, knowing-doing dissociation; F4, "in resistance" of both thinking processes and behavior; and F5, social regulation) in a sample of younger healthy Chinese adults. These age-discrepant results question the validity of the DEX with older individuals, as results have been obtained in younger samples. The limited theoretical validity across age groups makes the characterization of DES difficult in older groups; therefore, future research is needed to determine the relationship between cognitive and behavioral aspects of dysexecutive symptoms among elderly people from a nonclinical perspective.

Finally, since studies testing the validity of the DEX use samples from different cultures (Scottish, Polish, and Chinese), the potential contribution of cultural and socioeconomic factors on the reported results seems relevant.

The areas of the brain involved in emotional processing overlap with those associated with EF declines in aging. Therefore, van Reekum et al. (2018) suggested that the capacity to adaptively respond to emotional information declines with age. Recent evidence using neuroimaging suggests that when older adults process emotional facial expressions, they engage different cortical networks compared to younger adults. These networks involve dorsal areas in the medial PFC (mPFC; e.g., Williams et al., 2006) or ventrolateral PFC (VLPFC) when processing complex negative images (Dolcos, Wang, & Mather, 2014). van Reekum et al. (2018) demonstrated less activation in the left ventrolateral PFC (VLPFC) and greater ventromedial PFC (VMPFC) activity with increasing age during negative-picture viewing, while age was not correlated with amygdala activation (a structure for the acquisition and expression of emotions). The authors suggested that aging impacts activity in PFC systems that compute negative affect without necessarily altering the emotional response. This suggests that there is a compensatory mechanism with advancing age, reflected in greater engagement of medial rather than lateral PFC areas during the processing of emotion-laden information, preserving emotional reactivity.

8.3 Dysexecutive Syndrome in Abnormal Aging

As stated above, DES may be identified when there is frontal lobe damage as a result of disease (associated with aging) or injury (Poletti, Cavallo, & Adenzato, 2017) and includes cognitive impairment (dysregulation of EF) as well as emotional and behavioral concerns (Godefroy et al., 2010). It is important to note, however, that there is currently little consensus regarding the diagnosis and definition of DES, and terms are often used interchangeably to describe EF impairment (e.g., frontal lobe disorders or dysexecutive disorders; Godefroy et al., 2018).

It is essential to determine whether there are behavioral issues in DES, and it is important to assess cognitive changes with neuropsychological tests and behavioral changes with behavioral scales and by observing the patient (Hanna-Pladdy, 2007).

Within the EF disorders, Godefroy et al. (2018) described that the most common behavioral impairment is global hypoactivity with apathy, in which there is reduced motivation and activity, as well as disinhibition. The most commonly observed cognitive impairments were related to difficulties in self-initiating action.

8.3.1 Mild Cognitive Impairment and Dementia

While executive dysfunction (ED) is often seen as a sign of several dementia subtypes, it has also been described in amnestic Mild Cognitive Impairment (aMCI;

Blanco Martín et al., 2016) in which cognitive deficits are not severe enough to constitute functional impairment (Petersen et al., 1999). aMCI is considered a prodromal stage of dementia and is associated with a greater likelihood of progressing to dementia (Petersen et al., 2001). Blanco Martín et al. (2016) evaluated cognitively normal and aMCI individuals with neuropsychological and clinical tests. Their results suggest that executive changes are present in aMCI and that among the three tests included measuring EF, semantic fluency (specifically animals) was associated with progression from aMCI to dementia. Similarly, Peter et al. (2016) found that patients with aMCI perform significantly worse and use fewer strategies during semantic and design fluency compared to healthy controls (HC). Both groups, however, benefited equally from repeated assessment, highlighting the groups' abilities to increase performance with practice (fluency tasks were administered three times within two days). In aMCI, performance during semantic fluency was significantly predicted by design fluency performance, while in HC, it was significantly predicted by naming performance. These findings suggest that in aMCI, participants use an executive strategy rather than a semantic strategy. In HC, the volume of the superior frontal gyrus (SFG) significantly predicted semantic and design fluency performance and strategy use during design fluency. In aMCI, the SFG and the inferior frontal gyrus (IFG) predicted performance during semantic and design fluency. The IFG significantly predicted strategy use during semantic fluency in both groups. The authors concluded that the reduced semantic fluency performance in aMCI seems to be primarily due to dysfunctional executive control mechanisms rather than impaired semantic knowledge.

Similarly, in cases of non-amnestic dysexecutive vascular MCI (VaMCI), a review by Sudo et al. (2012) described the disconnection of the fronto-parietal-subcortical network. Sachdev et al. (2009) evaluated post-stroke patients with vaMCI between the ages of 45 and 87 who did not have a dementia diagnosis or other neurological disorders before vascular incidents. The authors used a neuropsychological battery that tested a wide range of domains and concluded that in vaMCI patients, EFs, assessed with the Controlled Oral Word Association Test (Benton & Hamsher, 1976; Morris et al., 1989) and language (tested with the shortened Boston Naming Test; Mack, Freed, Williams, & Henderson, 1992) declined more than other domains over three years.

ED is common in Alzheimer's disease (AD), but the main impairment in this case relates to memory deficits resulting from damage to medial temporal lobes. However, Godefroy et al. (2018) reported that in AD, over 75% of individuals have the behavioral and/or cognitive DES, while around 90% have some type of initial EF disorder (Godefroy et al., 2016). These individuals have impairments in planning, inhibition, and flexibility, as well as global hypoactivity apathy (Godefroy, Barbay, Andriuta, Tir, & Roussel, 2017).

Within AD, there are rare cases in which there may be a "frontal variant" of the disease (fvAD). This variant is also known as the behavioral/dysexecutive variant of AD (Ossenkoppele et al., 2015) which primarily presents with cognitive impairments (working memory, cognitive flexibility, planning, and problem-solving) and little behavioral concerns. In these patients, the atrophy mainly compromises the medial temporal lobes instead of the frontal lobes, which are significantly damaged in the behavioral variant of frontotemporal dementia (bvFTD). The damage in the behavioral/dysexecutive AD is in line with what is traditionally found in classical AD. However, due to the clinical similarities between fvAD and bvFAD, the differential diagnosis is challenging (Wong et al., 2019).

bvFTD is accompanied by changes in social cognition and EF, however, this impairment (particularly in the early stages of the disease) may only be observed using ecologically valid EF tests that include real-life EF and complex decision-making tasks (Torralva, Roca, Gleichgerrcht, Bekinschtein, & Manes, 2009). Specifically, bvFTD patients show impairments in planning, flexibility, complex decision-making, and organization. Similarly, Gansler, Huey, Pan, Wasserman, and Grafman (2017) evaluated patients with bvFTD, primary progressive aphasia (PPA), and corticobasal syndrome (CBS). The authors found that bvFTD patients had lower scores on EF tasks and a greater degree of dysexecutive behavior (DB) compared to the other two groups. Importantly, these authors emphasized the importance of combining EF as well as DB measures to assist in the diagnosis of the three disorders.

8.3.2 Subcortical Disorders

ED is also present in individuals with Parkinson's disease (PD), in which the hallmark symptoms are motor disturbances. This ED is reflected by worsened performance in several aspects of EF (e.g., set shifting, inhibitory control, reasoning, planning, and problem solving) which impacts the patients' daily lives (Kamei et al., 2008). This dysfunction includes behavioral as well as cognitive disturbances, whose impact should be carefully assessed (Ceravolo, Pagni, Tognoni, & Bonuccelli, 2012; Gruszka, Hampshire, Barker, & Owen, 2017).

Moreover, DES has been described at the early stages of PD (Foltynie, Brayne, Robbins, & Barker, 2004) and could include deficits of working memory, planning, attentional control, and set-shifting performance. However, one of the most common deficits is set-shifting difficulties which are evident in cognitive and motor tasks. These deficits are associated with hypoactivation in the inferior frontal sulcus (IFS), the striatum, and the anterior cingulate gyrus (ACC) (Gruszka et al., 2017).

Within PD, researchers also examined the incidence of dementia and explored whether certain variables could predict cognitive decline (Williams-Gray, Foltynie, Brayne, Robbins, & Barker, 2007). Their results suggested that 10% of their patients progressed to dementia after 3.5 years, while two-thirds developed cognitive deficits in this period. They additionally described that this rate may be influenced by age, the motor phenotype, and deficits in semantic fluency and a pentagon-copying task, all of which increased the risk of progressing to dementia.

DES has also been examined in nondemented PD patients (Roussel et al., 2017). The authors reported that DES was present in 81% of PD patients, with either cognitive or behavioral impairments observed in most patients. Behaviorally, these patients often presented global hypoactivity, while cognitive impairments included deficits in inhibition and flexibility.

8.3.3 Vascular Disorders

Besides neurological diseases in aging, ED has been identified as a factor for the risk of stroke in cognitively unimpaired individuals (Oveisgharan & Hachinski, 2015). Additionally, following a stroke, individuals may develop DES (Godefroy et al., 2018). More specifically, strokes in the thalamus (i.e., ischemic thalamic stroke) have also been shown to impair EF (Liebermann, Ploner, Kraft, Kopp, & Ostendorf, 2013). The authors found that their subjects, who mostly presented with ventral thalamic lesions, performed worse on the WCST while performance on other tests of EF (e.g., semantic and phonological fluency and the Stroop test) was normal. This suggests that different EF abilities may rely on diverse thalamic regions.

DES has also been characterized in individuals with ischemic vascular disease (IVD), in which patients exhibit difficulties in engaging in a certain task, inhibiting irrelevant answers, and continuing adequate behavior for the task (Lamar, Price, Giovannetti, Swenson, & Libon, 2010). These impairments were attributed to damage of the basal ganglia and thalamus and their connections to the frontal lobe.

8.4 Conclusion

In general, there is evidence suggesting that age-related changes in the frontal lobe (in volume and in the degree of functional connectivity with other regions) are associated with EF declines. These can be observed in healthy and abnormal aging and may influence several EF domains. DES appears to be the most severe manifestation of these deficits and is present in neurological disorders. Normally aging individuals suffer from deficits in attentional control and inhibiting unwanted responses, with impairments leading to greater distractibility and slower processing time during neuropsychological testing. Other theories propose that adulthood is characterized by general slowing, which may result in these deficits, however, there appears to be a unique effect beyond slowing accounting for inhibitory difficulties. Older adults also exhibit issues with planning for future actions to achieve a goal, particularly after the age of 65, as well as impairments in cognitive flexibility, possibly due to the inability to update hypotheses with constant rule changing, or, like inhibition, general slowing. Impairments in initiating behaviors are also seen in healthy adults, traditionally observed with fluency tests. Neuroimaging findings suggest that older adults use a compensatory mechanism during these tasks, resulting in greater activation than in younger adults.

Behavioral DES, unlike cognitive DES, is better captured using questionnaires and behavioral observations, however, the validity of these measures has yet to be established for aging populations. In older adults, there are emotional processing changes, with activation of different brain areas compared to younger adults. Conflicting results across cognitive and behavioral domains in aging may be related to different levels of education in the groups or the variety of the EF paradigms used, which tend to heavily rely on several lower-level functions.

Besides normal aging, DES (cognitive and behavioral) is present in several neurological diseases that are prevalent in older adults. In aMCI and VaMCI, EF is impaired, and this is reflected by deficits in fluency tests, highlighting the sensitivity of these measures in the early stages of AD and vascular dementia. In AD and in rare cases of a frontal variant, ED is present as well, resulting in difficulties with planning, cognitive flexibility, and other domains. In bvFTD, ED is reflected by impairments in planning, flexibility, complex decision-making, and organization. Lastly, the executive dysfunctions in PD have been described in the early stages of the disease (in working memory, planning, shifting, and attentional control) and in demented and nondemented PD patients. It appears that DES is prevalent in this condition and is associated with hypoactivation of the ACC, IFS, and striatum (brain regions associated with learning). Finally, the presence of DES in post-stroke patients has been identified in individuals with thalamic damage, emphasizing this structure and its numerous frontal connections as an important neural underpinning of EFs.

Overall, ED is prevalent in healthy older adults as well as in those with a wide range of neurological diseases. Cognitive impairments appear to be more accurately characterized with the use of ecologically valid tasks, which present participants with novel requirements, while behavioral impairments may only be observed with interviews and observations.

References

Allain, P., Nicoleau, S., Pinon, K., Etcharry-Bouyx, F., Barré, J., Berrut, G., … & Le Gall, D. (2005). Executive functioning in normal aging: A study of action planning using the Zoo Map Test. *Brain and cognition*, *57*(1), 4–7.

Amieva, H., Phillips, L., & Della Sala, S. (2003). Behavioral dysexecutive symptoms in normal aging. *Brain and Cognition, 53*(2), 129–132.

Anderson, P. (2002). Assessment and development of executive function (EF) during childhood. *Child Neuropsychology: A Journal on Normal and Abnormal Development in Childhood and Adolescence, 8*(2), 71–82. https://doi.org/10.1076/chin.8.2.71.8724.

Andrés, P., & Van der Linden, M. (2000). Age-related differences in supervisory attentional system functions. *The Journals of Gerontology Series B: Psychological Sciences and Social Sciences, 55*(6), P373–P380.

Ardila, A. (2013). There are two different dysexecutive syndromes. *Journal of Neurological Disorders*, *1*(1), 1–4. https://doi.org/10.4172/2329-6895.1000114.

Ardila, A., Ostrosky-Solis, F., Rosselli, M., & Gómez, C. (2000). Age-related cognitive decline during normal aging: the complex effect of education. *Archives of Clinical Neuropsychology: The Official Journal of the National Academy of Neuropsychologists, 15*(6), 495–513.

Ardila, A., & Rosselli, M. (in press). *Neuropsicologia clinica*. Mexico D.F.: Manual Moderno.

Ashendorf, L., Jefferson, A. L., O'Connor, M. K., Chaisson, C., Green, R. C., & Stern, R. A. (2008). Trail making test errors in normal aging, mild cognitive impairment, and dementia. *Archives of*

Clinical Neuropsychology: The Official Journal of the National Academy of Neuropsychologists, 23(2), 129–137. https://doi.org/10.1016/j.acn.2007.11.005.

Axelrod, B. N., & Henry, R. R. (1992). Age-related performance on the Wisconsin Card sorting, similarities, and controlled oral word association tests. *Clinical Neuropsychologist, 6*(1), 16–26. https://doi.org/10.1080/13854049208404113.

Baddeley, A., & Wilson, B. (1988). Frontal amnesia and the dysexecutive syndrome. *Brain and Cognition, 7*(2), 212–230.

Baldo, J. V., Schwartz, S., Wilkins, D., & Dronkers, N. F. (2006). Role of frontal versus temporal cortex in verbal fluency as revealed by voxel-based lesion symptom mapping. *Journal of the International Neuropsychological Society: JINS, 12*(6), 896–900. https://doi.org/10.1017/S1355617706061078.

Benton, A. L., & Hamsher, K. (1976). *Multilingual aphasia examination aphasia examination*. Iowa City, IA: University of Iowa.

Berg, E. A. (1948). A simple objective technique for measuring flexibility in thinking. *The Journal of General Psychology, 39*(1), 15–22.

Blanco Martín, E., Ugarriza Serrano, I., Elcoroaristizabal Martín, X., Galdos Alcelay, L., Molano Salazar, A., Bereincua Gandarias, R., et al. (2016). Dysexecutive syndrome in amnesic mild cognitive impairment: a multicenter study. *BMC Neurology, 16*(1), 88. https://doi.org/10.1186/s12883-016-0607-2.

Bolla, K. I., Lindgren, K. N., Bonaccorsy, C., & Bleecker, M. L. (1990). Predictors of verbal fluency (FAS) in the healthy elderly. *Journal of Clinical Psychology, 46*(5), 623–628.

Brennan, M., Welsh, M., & Fisher, C. (1997). Aging and executive function skills: An examination of a community-dwelling older adult population. *Perceptual and Motor Skills, 84,* 1187–1197.

Brickman, A. M., Paul, R. H., Cohen, R. A., Williams, L. M., MacGregor, K. L., Jefferson, A. L., … Gordon, E. (2005). Category and letter verbal fluency across the adult lifespan: relationship to EEG theta power. *Archives of Clinical Neuropsychology: The Official Journal of the National Academy of Neuropsychologists, 20*(5), 561–573. doi.org/https://doi.org/10.1016/j.acn.2004.12.006.

Bryan, J., & Luszcz, M. A. (2000). Measurement of executive function: Considerations for detecting adult age differences. *Journal of Clinical and Experimental Neuropsychology, 22*(1), 40–55.

Bryan, J., Luszcz, M. A., & Crawford, J. R. (1997). Verbal knowledge and speed of information processing as mediators of age differences in verbal fluency performance among older adults. *Psychology and Aging, 12*(3), 473–478.

Burgess, P. W., Alderman, N., Evans, J., Emslie, H., & Wilson, B. A. (1998). The ecological validity of tests of executive function. *Journal of the International Neuropsychological Society, 4*(6), 547–558.

Byczewska-Konieczny, K. (2019). Relation between cognitive and behavioral aspects of dysexecutive functioning in normal aging. *Applied Neuropsychology: Adult*, 1–11. https://doi.org/10.1080/23279095.2018.1550409.

Cabeza, R. (2002). Hemispheric asymmetry reduction in older adults: The HAROLD model. *Psychology of Aging, 17*(1), 85–100.

Cabeza, R., Anderson, N. D., Locantore, J. K., & McIntosh, A. R. (2002). Aging gracefully: Compensatory brain activity in high-performing older adults. *Neuroimage, 17*(3), 1394–1402.

Cabeza, R., & Dennis, N. A. (2013). In D. T. Stuss, R. T. Knight (Eds.), *Frontal lobes and aging: Deterioration and compensation in principles of frontal lobe function* (2nd ed.).

Cabeza, R., McIntosh, A. R., Tulving, E., Nyberg, L., & Grady, C. L. (1997). Age-related differences in effective neural connectivity during encoding and recall. *NeuroReport, 8,* 3479–3483.

Ceravolo, R., Pagni, C., Tognoni, G., & Bonuccelli, U. (2012). The epidemiology and clinical manifestations of dysexecutive syndrome in Parkinson's disease. *Frontiers in Neurology*, *3*. https://doi.org/10.3389/fneur.2012.00159.

Chan, R. C. (2001). Dysexecutive symptoms among a non-clinical sample: A study with the use of the Dysexecutive Questionnaire. *British Journal of Psychology, 92*(3), 551–565.

Clark, L. J., Gatz, M., Zheng, L., Chen, Y. L., McCleary, C., & Mack, W. J. (2009). Longitudinal verbal fluency in normal aging, preclinical, and prevalent Alzheimer's disease. *American Journal of Alzheimer's Disease & Other Dementias®, 24*(6), 461–468.

Crawford, J. R., Bryan, J., Luszcz, M. A., Obonsawin, M. C., & Stewart, L. (2000). The executive decline hypothesis of cognitive aging: Do executive deficits qualify as differential deficits and do they mediate age-related memory decline? *Aging, Neuropsychology, and Cognition, 7*(1), 9–31.

Daigneault, S., Braun, C. M., & Whitaker, H. A. (1992). Early effects of normal aging on perseverative and non-perseverative prefrontal measures. *Developmental Neuropsychology, 8*(1), 99–114.

Dolcos, F., Wang, L., & Mather, M. (2014). Current research and emerging directions in emotion-cognition interactions. *Frontiers in Integrative Neuroscience*, 8. https://doi.org/10.3389/fnint.2014.00083.

Emery, O. B. (1985). Language and aging. *Experimental Aging Research, 11*(1), 3–60.

Fisk, J. E., & Sharp, C. A. (2004). Age-related impairment in executive functioning: Updating, inhibition, shifting, and access. *Journal of Clinical and Experimental Neuropsychology, 26*(7), 874–890.

Fisk, J. E., & Warr, P. (1996). Age and working memory: The role of perceptual speed, the central executive, and the phonological loop. *Psychology and Aging, 11*(2), 316–323.

Foldi, N. S., Helm-Estabrooks, N., Redfield, J., & Nickel, D. G. (2003). Perseveration in normal aging: A comparison of perseveration rates on design fluency and verbal generative tasks. *Aging, Neuropsychology, and Cognition, 10*(4), 268–280. https://doi.org/10.1076/anec.10.4.268.28970.

Foltynie, T., Brayne, C. E. G., Robbins, T. W., & Barker, R. A. (2004). The cognitive ability of an incident cohort of Parkinson's patients in the UK. The CamPaIGN study. *Brain: A Journal of Neurology, 127*(Pt 3), 550–560. https://doi.org/10.1093/brain/awh067.

Gaál, Z. A., & Czigler, I. (2015). Age-related processing strategies and go–nogo effects in task-switching: an ERP study. *Frontiers in Human Neuroscience, 9*. https://doi.org/10.3389/fnhum.2015.00177.

Gansler, D. A., Huey, E. D., Pan, J. J., Wasserman, E., & Grafman, J. H. (2017). Assessing the dysexecutive syndrome in dementia. *Journal of Neurology, Neurosurgery and Psychiatry, 88*(3), 254–261. https://doi.org/10.1136/jnnp-2016-313576.

Godefroy, O., Azouvi, P., Robert, P., Roussel, M., LeGall, D., Meulemans, T., & Groupe de Réflexion sur l'Evaluation des Fonctions Exécutives Study Group. (2010). Dysexecutive syndrome: diagnostic criteria and validation study. *Annals of Neurology, 68*(6), 855–864. https://doi.org/10.1002/ana.22117.

Godefroy, O., Bakchine, S., Verny, M., Delabrousse-Mayoux, J.-P., Roussel, M., Pere, J.-J., & REFLEX study group (2016). Characteristics of Alzheimer's disease patients with severe executive disorders. *Journal of Alzheimer's Disease: JAD, 51*(3), 815–825. https://doi.org/10.3233/jad-150971.

Godefroy, O., Barbay, M., Andriuta, D., Tir, M., & Roussel, M. (2017). Global hypoactivity and apathy. In A. Verdelho & M. Gonçalves-Pereira (Eds.), *Neuropsychiatric symptoms of cognitive impairment and dementia* (pp. 71–91). Cham: Springer International Publishing. https://doi.org/10.1007/978-3-319-39138-0_5.

Godefroy, O., Martinaud, O., Narme, P., Joseph, P.-A., Mosca, C., Lhommée, E., … Roussel, M. (2018). Dysexecutive disorders and their diagnosis: A position paper. *Cortex, 109*, 322–335. https://doi.org/10.1016/j.cortex.2018.09.026.

Gold, B. T., Powell, D. K., Xuan, L., Jicha, G. A., & Smith, C. D. (2010). Age-related slowing of task switching is associated with decreased integrity of frontoparietal white matter. *Neurobiology of Aging, 31*(3), 512. https://doi.org/10.1016/j.neurobiolaging.2008.04.005.

Grant, D. A., & Berg, E. (1948). A behavioral analysis of degree of reinforcement and ease of shifting to new responses in a Weigl-type card-sorting problem. *Journal of Experimental Psychology, 38*(4), 404.

Gruszka, A., Hampshire, A., Barker, R. A., & Owen, A. M. (2017). Normal aging and Parkinson's disease are associated with the functional decline of distinct frontal-striatal circuits. *Cortex; a*

Journal Devoted to the Study of the Nervous System and Behavior, 93, 178–192. https://doi.org/10.1016/j.cortex.2017.05.020.
Haaland, K. Y., Vranes, L. F., Goodwin, J. S., & Garry, P. J. (1987). Wisconsin card sort test performance in a healthy elderly population. *Journal of Gerontology, 42*(3), 345–346.
Hanna-Pladdy, B. (2007). Dysexecutive syndromes in neurologic disease. *Journal of Neurologic Physical Therapy: JNPT, 31*(3), 119–127. https://doi.org/10.1097/NPT.0b013e31814a63c2.
Hasher, L., & Zacks, R. T. (1988). Working memory, comprehension, and aging: A review and a new view. In *Psychology of learning and motivation* (Vol. 22, pp. 193–225). Academic Press.
Heaton, R. K., Chelune, G. J., Talley, J. L., Kay, G. G., & Curtiss, G. (1993). *Wisconsin card sorting test manual: Revised and expanded.* Odessa, FL: Psychological Assessment Resources.
Ho, M. C., Hsu, Y. C., Lu, M. L., Gossop, M., & Chen, V. C. H. (2018). 'Cool' and 'Hot' executive functions in suicide attempters with major depressive disorder. *Journal of Affective Disorders, 235,* 332–340.
Jurado, M. B., & Rosselli, M. (2007). The elusive nature of executive functions: A review of our current understanding. *Neuropsychology Review, 17,* 213–233.
Kamei, S., Hara, M., Serizawa, K., Murakami, M., Mizutani, T., Ishiburo, M., … Hirayanagi, K. (2008). Executive dysfunction using behavioral assessment of the dysexecutive syndrome in Parkinson's disease. *Movement Disorders: Official Journal of the Movement Disorder Society, 23*(4), 566–573. https://doi.org/10.1002/mds.21890.
Karzmark, P., Llanes, S., Tan, S., Deutsch, G., & Zeifert, P. (2012). Comparison of the frontal systems behavior scale and neuropsychological tests of executive functioning in predicting instrumental activities of daily living. *Applied Neuropsychology: Adult, 19*(2), 81–85.
Kennedy, K. M., & Raz, N. (2015). Normal aging of the brain. *Brain mapping: An encyclopedic reference, 3,* 603–617.
Kerr, A., & Zelazo, P. D. (2004). Development of "hot" executive function: The children's gambling task. *Brain and Cognition, 55*(1), 148–157. https://doi.org/10.1016/S0278-2626(03)00275-6.
Kortte, K. B., Horner, M. D., & Windham, W. K. (2002). The trail making test, part B: cognitive flexibility or ability to maintain set? *Applied Neuropsychology, 9*(2), 106–109.
Laguë-Beauvais, M., Brunet, J., Gagnon, L., Lesage, F., & Bherer, L. (2013). A fNIRS investigation of switching and inhibition during the modified Stroop task in younger and older adults. *NeuroImage, 64,* 485–495. https://doi.org/10.1016/j.neuroimage.2012.09.042.
Lamar, M., Price, C. C., Giovannetti, T., Swenson, R., & Libon, D. J. (2010). The dysexecutive syndrome associated with ischaemic vascular disease and related subcortical neuropathology: A Boston process approach. *Behavioural Neurology, 22*(1–2), 53–62. https://doi.org/10.3233/BEN-2009-0237.
Lezak, M., Howieson, D. B., & Loring, D. W. (2004). *Executive functions and motor performance. Neuropsychological assessment* (pp. 611–646). Oxford: Oxford University Press.
Liebermann, D., Ploner, C. J., Kraft, A., Kopp, U. A., & Ostendorf, F. (2013). A dysexecutive syndrome of the medial thalamus. *Cortex; a Journal Devoted to the Study of the Nervous System and Behavior, 49*(1), 40–49. https://doi.org/10.1016/j.cortex.2011.11.005.
Lindberg, O. (2012). *The aging frontal lobe in health and disease: A structural magnetic resonance imaging study.* Inst för neurobiologi, vårdvetenskap och samhälle/Dept of Neurobiology, Care Sciences and Society.
Loonstra, A. S., Tarlow, A. R., & Sellers, A. H. (2001). COWAT metanorms across age, education, and gender. *Applied Neuropsychology, 8*(3), 161–166. https://doi.org/10.1207/S15324826AN0803_5.
Luria, A. R. (1976). *The working brain: An introduction to neuropsychology.* USA: Basic Books.
Mack, W. J., Freed, D. M., Williams, B. W., & Henderson, V. W. (1992). Boston naming test: Shortened versions for use in Alzheimer's disease. *Journal of Gerontology, 47*(3), P154–P158.
Madden, D. J., Costello, M. C., Dennis, N. A., Davis, S. W., Shepler, A. M., Spaniol, J., … & Cabeza, R. (2010). Adult age differences in functional connectivity during executive control. *Neuroimage, 52*(2), 643–657.

Meinzer, M., Flaisch, T., Wilser, L., Eulitz, C., Rockstroh, B., Conway, T., … & Crosson, B. (2009). Neural signatures of semantic and phonemic fluency in young and old adults. *Journal of Cognitive Neuroscience, 21*(10), 2007–2018.
Meinzer, M., Seeds, L., Flaisch, T., Harnish, S., Cohen, M. L., McGregor, K., … & Crosson, B. (2012). Impact of changed positive and negative task-related brain activity on word-retrieval in aging. *Neurobiology of Aging, 33*(4), 656–669.
Mejía, S., Pineda, D., Alvarez, L. M., & Ardila, A. (1998). Individual differences in memory Anid executive function abilities during normal aging. *International Journal ofNeuroscience, 95*(3–4), 271–284.
Mittenberg, W., Seidenberg, M., O'Leary, D. S., & DiGiulio, D. V. (1989). Changes in cerebral functioning associated with normal aging. *Journal of Clinical and Experimental Neuropsychology, 11,* 918–932.
Morris, J. C., Heyman, A., Mohs, R. C., Hughes, J. P., van Belle, G., Fillenbaum, G., … Clark, C. (1989). The consortium to establish a registry for Alzheimer's disease (CERAD). Part I. Clinical and neuropsychological assessment of Alzheimer's disease. *Neurology, 39*(9), 1159–1165. https://doi.org/10.1212/wnl.39.9.1159.
Offenbach, S. I. (1974). A developmental study of hypothesis testing and cue selection strategies. *Developmental Psychology, 10,* 484–490.
Ossenkoppele, R., Pijnenburg, Y. A. L., Perry, D. C., Cohn-Sheehy, B. I., Scheltens, N. M. E., Vogel, J. W., … Rabinovici, G. D. (2015). The behavioural/dysexecutive variant of Alzheimer's disease: clinical, neuroimaging and pathological features. *Brain: A Journal ofNeurology, 138*(Pt 9), 2732–2749. https://doi.org/10.1093/brain/awv191.
Oveisgharan, S., & Hachinski, V. (2015). Executive dysfunction is a strong stroke predictor. *Journal of the Neurological Sciences, 349*(1–2), 161–167. https://doi.org/10.1016/j.jns.2015.01.010.
Passingham, R. E. (1993). *Oxford psychology series, No. 21. The frontal lobes and voluntary action.* New York, NY, US: Oxford University Press.
Peter, J., Kaiser, J., Landerer, V., Köstering, L., Kaller, C. P., Heimbach, B., et al. (2016). Category and design fluency in mild cognitive impairment: Performance, strategy use, and neural correlates. *Neuropsychologia, 93,* 21–29.
Petersen, R. C., Doody, R., Kurz, A., Mohs, R. C., Morris, J. C., Rabins, P. V., et al. (2001). Current concepts in mild cognitive impairment. *Archives of Neurology, 58*(12), 1985–1992. https://doi.org/10.1001/archneur.58.12.1985.
Petersen, R. C., Smith, G. E., Waring, S. C., Ivnik, R. J., Tangalos, E. G., & Kokmen, E. (1999). Mild cognitive impairment: Clinical characterization and outcome. *Archives ofNeurology, 56*(3), 303–308.
Phillips, L. H., Kliegel, M., & Martin, M. (2006). Age and planning tasks: the influence of ecological validity. *International Journal of Aging and Human Development, 62*(2), 175–184. https://doi.org/10.2190/EM1W-HAYC-TMLM-WW8X.
Poletti, M., Cavallo, M., & Adenzato, M. (2017). Detecting dysexecutive syndrome in neurodegenerative diseases: Are we using an appropriate approach and effective diagnostic tools? *Journal of Neurology, Neurosurgery and Psychiatry, 88*(3), 195. https://doi.org/10.1136/jnnp-2016-314744.
Raz, N., & Daugherty, A. M. (2018). Pathways to brain aging and their modifiers: Free-radical-induced energetic and neural decline in senescence (FRIENDS) model-A mini-review. *Gerontology, 64*(1), 49–57.
Regard, M., Strauss, E., & Knapp, P. (1982). Children's production on verbal and non-verbal fluency tasks. *Perceptual and Motor Skills, 55,* 839–844. https://doi.org/10.2466/pms.1982.55.3.839.
Reitan, R., & Wolfson, D. (1993). *The Halstead-Reitan neuropsychological test battery: Theory and clinical interpretation*. Tucson, AZ: Neuropsychology Press.
Ridderinkhof, K. R., Span, M. M., & Van Der Molen, M. W. (2002). Perseverative behavior and adaptive control in older adults: Performance monitoring, rule induction, and set shifting. *Brain and Cognition, 49*(3), 382–401.

Rodríguez-Aranda, C., & Martinussen, M. (2006). Age-related differences in performance of phonemic verbal fluency measured by Controlled Oral Word Association Task (COWAT): A meta-analytic study. *Developmental Neuropsychology, 30*(2), 697–717.

Rodríguez-Aranda, C., & Sundet, K. (2006). The frontal hypothesis of cognitive aging: Factor structure and age effects on four frontal tests among healthy individuals. *The Journal of Genetic Psychology, 167*(3), 269–287.

Rönnlund, M., Lövdén, M., & Nilsson, L. G. (2001). Adult age differences in Tower of Hanoi performance: Influence from demographic and cognitive variables. *Aging, Neuropsychology, and Cognition, 8*(4), 269–283.

Rönnlund, M., Lövdén, M., & Nilsson, L. G. (2007). Cross-sectional versus longitudinal age gradients of Tower of Hanoi performance: The role of practice effects and cohort differences in education. *Aging, Neuropsychology, and Cognition, 15*(1), 40–67.

Rosselli, M., & Jurado, M. B. (2013). Las funciones ejecutivas y el lóbulo frontal en el envejecimiento típico y atípico. In J. Tirapu Ustárroz, A. García-Molina, M. Ríos Lago (Eds.), *Neuropsicología del córtex prefrontal y de las funciones ejecutivas*. Barcelona, España: Viguera Editores.

Rosselli, M., Tappen, R., Williams, C., Salvatierra, J., & Zoller, Y. (2009). Level of education and category fluency task among Spanish speaking elders: number of words, clustering, and switching strategies. *Aging, Neuropsychology, and Cognition, 16*(6), 721–744.

Roussel, M., Lhommée, E., Narme, P., Czernecki, V., Gall, D. L., Krystkowiak, P., … & GREFEX study group. (2017). Dysexecutive syndrome in Parkinson's disease: the GREFEX study. *Neuropsychology, Development, and Cognition. Section B, Aging, Neuropsychology and Cognition, 24*(5), 496–507. https://doi.org/10.1080/13825585.2016.1226248.

Sachdev, P. S., Chen, X., Brodaty, H., Thompson, C., Altendorf, A., & Wen, W. (2009). The determinants and longitudinal course of post-stroke mild cognitive impairment. *Journal of the International Neuropsychological Society: JINS, 15*(6), 915–923. https://doi.org/10.1017/S1355617709990579.

Salat, D. H. (2014). Diffusion tensor imaging in the study of aging and age-associated neural disease. In *Diffusion MRI* (pp. 257–281). Academic Press.

Salthouse, T. A. (1996). The processing-speed theory of adult age differences in cognition. *Psychological Review, 103*(3), 403–428.

Shallice, T., & Evans, M. E. (1978). The involvement of the frontal lobes in cognitive estimation. *Cortex, 14*(2), 294–303.

Slagter, H. A., Weissman, D. H., Giesbrecht, B., Kenemans, J. L., Mangun, G. R., Kok, A., et al. (2006). Brain regions activated by endogenous preparatory set shifting as revealed by fMRI. *Cognitive, Affective, & Behavioral Neuroscience, 6*(3), 175–189. https://doi.org/10.3758/CABN.6.3.175.

Sorel, O., & Pennequin, V. (2008). Aging of the planning process: The role of executive functioning. *Brain and Cognition, 66*(2), 196–201.

Stroop, J. R. (1935). Studies of interference in serial verbal reactions. *Journal of Experimental Psychology, 18*(6), 643.

Sudo, F. K., Alves, C. E. O., Alves, G. S., Ericeira-Valente, L., Tiel, C., Moreira, D. M., … Engelhardt, E. (2012). Dysexecutive syndrome and cerebrovascular disease in non-amnestic mild cognitive impairment: A systematic review of the literature. *Dementia & Neuropsychologia, 6*(3), 145–151. https://doi.org/10.1590/s1980-57642012dn06030006.

Sullivan, E. V., Rohlfing, T., & Pfefferbaum, A. (2010). Quantitative fiber tracking of lateral and interhemispheric white matter systems in normal aging: Relations to timed performance. *Neurobiology of Aging, 31*(3), 464–481.

Tas, A. C., Luck, S. J., & Hollingworth, A. (2016). The relationship between visual attention and visual working memory encoding: A dissociation between covert and overt orienting. *Journal of Experimental Psychology. Human Perception and Performance, 42*(8), 1121–1138. https://doi.org/10.1037/xhp0000212.

Thomson, D. R., & Hasher, L. (2017). On the preservation of vigilant attention to semantic information in healthy aging. *Experimental Brain Research, 235*(7), 2287–2300. https://doi.org/10.1007/s00221-017-4969-5.

Torralva, T., Roca, M., Gleichgerrcht, E., Bekinschtein, T., & Manes, F. (2009). A neuropsychological battery to detect specific executive and social cognitive impairments in early frontotemporal dementia. *Brain: A Journal of Neurology, 132*(Pt 5), 1299–1309. https://doi.org/10.1093/brain/awp041.

Van der Elst, W., Van Boxtel, M. P., Van Breukelen, G. J., & Jolles, J. (2006). The Stroop color-word test: Influence of age, sex, and education; and normative data for a large sample across the adult age range. *Assessment, 13*(1), 62–79.

van Reekum, C. M., Schaefer, S. M., Lapate, R. C., Norris, C. J., Tun, P. A., Lachman, M. E., ... Davidson, R. J. (2018). Aging is associated with a prefrontal lateral-medial shift during picture-induced negative affect. *Social Cognitive and Affective Neuroscience, 13*(2), 156–163. https://doi.org/10.1093/scan/nsx144.

West, R., & Alain, C. (2000). Age-related decline in inhibitory control contributes to the increased Stroop effect observed in older adults. *Psychophysiology, 37*(2), 179–189.

West, R. L. (1996). An application of prefrontal cortex function theory to cognitive aging. *Psychological Bulletin, 120,* 272–292.

West, R., & Baylis, G. C. (1998). Effects of increased response dominance and contextual disintegration on the Stroop interference effect in older adults. *Psychology and Aging, 13*(2), 206–217. https://doi.org/10.1037/0882-7974.13.2.206.

Williams, L. M., Kemp, A. H., Felmingham, K., Barton, M., Olivieri, G., Peduto, A., ... Bryant, R. A. (2006). Trauma modulates amygdala and medial prefrontal responses to consciously attended fear. *NeuroImage, 29*(2), 347–357. https://doi.org/10.1016/j.neuroimage.2005.03.047.

Williams-Gray, C. H., Foltynie, T., Brayne, C. E. G., Robbins, T. W., & Barker, R. A. (2007). Evolution of cognitive dysfunction in an incident Parkinson's disease cohort. *Brain: A Journal of Neurology*, *130*(Pt 7), 1787–1798. https://doi.org/10.1093/brain/awm111.

Wong, S., Strudwick, J., Devenney, E., Hodges, J. R., Piguet, O., & Kumfor, F. (2019). Frontal variant of Alzheimer's disease masquerading as behavioural-variant frontotemporal dementia: A case study comparison. *Neurocase*, 1–11.

Zook, N., Welsh, M. C., & Ewing, V. (2006). Performance of healthy, older adults on the Tower of London revised: Associations with verbal and nonverbal abilities. *Aging, Neuropsychology, and Cognition, 13*(1), 1–19.

[illegible]

Chapter 9
Executive Dysfunctions Associated with the Use of Information Technology

Mónica Rosselli and Deven M. Christopher

9.1 Introduction

Technology is used as a tool to perform goals in everyday life; however, for some, it can also be an agent of diverse negative consequences (Brand, Young, & Laier, 2014). Although Young (1998) used the term Internet addiction (IA) to define an Internet-related impulse control disorder, only Internet gaming disorder has been included in the appendix of the DSM-5. The term problematic Internet use (PIU) has been applied to address deficits in dimensions of executive functioning (Clemmons, 2017). Features of PIU include impairments in executive functioning related to overuse of the Internet such as decreased impulse control. Although there have been differences regarding the appropriate choice of term, in general there has been consensus that negative consequences or deficits due to Internet use are characterized by impaired impulse control, which accompanies a range of executive dysfunctions that negatively impact an individual's ability to function (Clemmons, 2017). Even for individuals who have not been diagnosed with a disorder, it is important to consider the potential drawbacks of technology use, such as the difficulty to maintain control over goal-directed or stimulus-driven attention in the midst of the many interruptions that can arrive while an individual is connected to the Internet.

How we adapt to technological advances and leverage them to our advantage by deciding what information we attend to at any moment in time has substantial implications on our ability to remain valuable and productive in our respective academic and economic domains. Information technology (IT) communicates and directs information via computers, networks, and other physical devices (e.g., smartphones and tablets) to create, process, and exchange electronic data (Khan, 2013). IT research

M. Rosselli (✉) · D. M. Christopher
Department of Psychology, Florida Atlantic University, Davie, FL, USA
e-mail: mrossell@fau.edu

D. M. Christopher
e-mail: dcchristopher2014@fau.edu

A. Ardila et al. (eds.), *Dysexecutive Syndromes*,
https://doi.org/10.1007/978-3-030-25077-5_9

defines information as data that is meaningful to the recipient and is of value in current or potential actions or decisions (Davis & Olson, 1984). IT enables the continuous connectivity often necessary to achieve goals by providing a means through which we accrue valuable information needed to accomplish our work. However, our computers and smartphones also induce attentional switching by facilitating a multitude of interruptions in the form of emails, text messages, app notifications, RSS feeds, and social networks, making it increasingly difficult to maintain directed attention toward a primary task.

Individuals progressively depend on IT and Internet access for every aspect of daily life. Today, it is used not only for business and education, but also to make basic or non-essential purchases, keep track of fitness and finances, and stay abreast socially with friends and family through text messaging, social networks, and file sharing (e.g., photos and videos). Further, computers and smartphones represent only two of the digital means used by individuals each day to remain informed and stay connected. There are many other physical devices from which to choose from such as tablets, television, watches, bracelets, and eyewear. The pervasiveness of information technology use and attentional switching between multiple forms of media have come to the forefront of society and have also produced scientific research to begin to study its effects on behavior, cognition, and brain structure and function in youth and adults (Uncapher et al., 2017).

The main purpose of this chapter is to review some of the current knowledge surrounding the influence of IT use on cognitive processes particularly on those abilities involving executive functions, and to present the clinical description of newly defined psychological disorders associated with the use of IT. An overview of the executive function subcomponents individuals are involved with during the complex interaction with IT is included as well as the characterization of clinical disorders in its overuse. A description of the assessment tools used in the diagnosis of these disorders is presented. The proposed neural substrates of the executive system underlying the use of IT are examined.

9.2 Information Technology and Executive Functions

The term executive function (EF) is a construct encompassing several cognitive abilities that permit holding information in working memory to inhibit highly automatic responses and to shift the focus of attention between different components of a specific task or problem. EF includes attentional and inhibitory control, planning, and set-shifting (Jurado & Rosselli, 2007). These cognitive control abilities allow us to focus attention strategically, to organize our thoughts in the face of distraction and complexity, and are useful when information technology is used.

The appropriate use of IT involves several of these EFs. First, the development of digital technology has required people to perform multiple tasks at the same time in an attempt to make their lives more productive. By definition, multi-tasking entails juggling different work activities and shifting attention from one task to another; this shifting in attention involves inhibitory control and decision-making. The executive control process involved in multi-tasking while using computers and smartphones induce attentional switching by facilitating a multitude of interruptions in the form of emails, text messages, app notifications, RSS feeds, and social networks, making it increasingly difficult to maintain directed attention toward a primary task. Informational intrusions are processed at the cognitive level (Wickens, 2002). They are one-way informational elements (e.g. email; instant messaging; pop-up displays) or task-irrelevant events (e.g. general reminders; announcements; status updates; notifications). Actionable intrusions draw attentional resources at the behavioral response level by requiring action (e.g. conducting online discussions; responding to information requests). They lead to task switching or simultaneous interactions (Barley, Meyerson, & Grodal, 2011), often require additional decision-making effort (Speier, Vessey, & Valacich, 2003), and are typically more demanding than those that only provide information (Kahneman, 1973). Dabbish, Kraut, Fussell, and Kiesler (2005) estimate one out of every three messages workers receive contain requests for action, which result in attentional switching.

Not only in the USA, but across many other countries (Kononova, 2013), youth spend more time with information technology, or media, than any other activity. The term "media" suggests all methods of mediated communication of information or data (Uncapher et al., 2017). Half of children (age range: 5–8) switch between several forms of media, for approximately two hours per day (Common Sense Media, 2013). Young children are particularly susceptible to novel stimuli; consequently, their attention can be enticed toward the rapidly changing appearance of digital media (such as animation and sounds) especially because they have the ability to direct their interaction by tapping and swiping (Chassiakos, Radesky, Christakis, Moreno, & Cross, 2016; Rothbart & Posner, 2015). Although there has been research that questions the effects of such features (i.e., rapid stimuli) on attention (Goodrich, Pempek, & Calvert, 2009), the long-term effects of rapid and repeated shifts in attention between multiple forms of digital media on children's attention span have not yet been reported (Chassiakos et al., 2016). Any detrimental effects from frequent attentional switching are important to investigate, especially for younger generations who find themselves growing increasingly more comfortable with switching attention between multiple technologies. On average, young people spend over seven hours per day with almost 30% of those hours spent switching their attention between more than one media stream (Rideout, Foehr, & Roberts, 2010). Ophir, Nass, and Wagner (2009) designed a series of experiments to study distinctions between the information processing styles of heavy media multitaskers (HMMs) and light media multitaskers (LMMs). Results showed HMMs performed worse on a test of task-switching ability. To identify HMMs, a questionnaire-based media multitasking index was developed to determine the mean number of media a person simultaneously consumed (HMMs were one standard deviation or more above the mean on this index). The authors examined the HMMs' abilities regarding the allocation of attention to environmental stimuli and their entry into working memory, the holding and manipulation of stimulus and task set representations in working memory, as well as the control of responses to stimuli and tasks. HMMs showed a reduced ability to filter out interference from irrelevant stimuli and irrelevant task sets (task-switching). The authors suggest attentional switching facilitated through technology, a growing social trend, places new demands on cognitive processing, in particular attention allocation, further stating HMMs use a "breadth-biased profile of cognitive control" necessary to manage multiple input streams (Ophir et al., 2009).

Although attentional switching between technology devices is commonplace [some individuals average more than four switches per minute (Brasel & Gips, 2011)], many adults aim to implement strategies in order to limit the amount of media streams they consume at any one time. However, that may not be the case for younger generations (and for the future, as youth continue to mature). Analyses of responses from 1,319 Americans from three generations revealed a clear generational effect; recent generations, identified as "Net Geners," switch their attention due to technology more than older generations. Net Geners find attentional switching to be easier (Carrier, Cheever, Rosen, Benitez, & Chang, 2009) and claim they switch their attention between tasks more efficiently than past generations. Notwithstanding, research thus far does not support this claim; during complex tasks, task switching eliminates cues needed to effectively perform the task (Gupta, Li, & Sharda, 2013) leading to performance degradation.

If, as the results Ophir et al. (2009) indicate, there is a growing trend to information technology processing, and that trend is rapid switching between tasks, it is important to investigate any consequences to performance, including subsequent volitional acts. Because a reduced ability to filter out interference from irrelevant stimuli (Ophir et al., 2009) due to attentional conflict impairs complex task performance (Gupta et al., 2013), resolving the conflict between attentional switching and goal performance seems essential for all individuals, from office workers to students and teachers. Future studies should investigate whether or not today's Net Gen college students (who have grown up with widespread access to technology) are developing a greater digital literacy (Oblinger & Oblinger, 2005) than have older generations, and if this has enriched them with an ability to switch their attention more efficiently.

The question of accrued executive dysfunction due to IT attentional switching remains important, not only for future generations, but for the current one as well. To better understand the potential negative consequences associated with the use of information technology (such as goal interference), it is important to investigate research which had defined the attention networks associated with it. It is equally valuable to consider the experiments that were designed and conducted with the purpose of simplifying the issues appropriately so that the underlying anatomy could be revealed. In addition, another area of research, resource depletion, may provide insight into any adverse effects from the use of information technology on subsequent acts of volition.

9.3 Attention Networks Associated with the Use of Information Technology

Rothbart & Posner (2015) describe specialized attention networks in the human brain as they relate to attentional switching that perform different but interrelated functions (i.e., alerting, orienting, and executive). First, they define alerting as attaining and maintaining a state of elevated sensitivity to arriving stimuli that involves preparation for identifying and reacting to an anticipated signal (Petersen & Posner, 2012). Orienting, they suggest, is the prioritization of information from sensory input by the selection of a modality. Finally, the authors state that executive attention includes means for monitoring and conflict resolution associated with thoughts, feelings, and behavior. Previous research has used the attention network test (ANT) and the data collected by using this task have been corroborated with data from neuroimaging studies to suggest that the three networks involve discrete brain mechanisms and are functionally independent (Fan, McCandliss, Sommer, Raz, & Posner, 2002; Rothbart & Posner, 2015).

9.3.1 Alerting

A function of the alerting network is to develop and maintain a vigilant state capable of detecting behaviorally relevant stimuli in the environment (Corbetta, & Shulman, 2002). One approach to the study of alerting is to use a warning signal prior to a target event to produce a phasic change in alertness (Petersen & Posner, 2012). In an alert state (that involves preparation for perceiving and reacting to an anticipated signal), an interruption can easily engage the mechanisms that produce detection (Posner & Petersen, 1990), and many people who work on devices with Internet access feel as if they are consistently placed in a state of vigilance. John Herrman, an editor at FEW, a tech site on BuzzFeed posted, “I’m never not looking sideways at what I’m doing, never not pulled to look at something else, never not reacting to whatever I’ve paused on” (Wortham, 2012). The alerting network has been associated with the right cerebral hemisphere (Posner & Petersen, 1990) and in particular the locus coeruleus (a nucleus of the brainstem and the primary source of noradrenaline to the brain), cingulate, frontal, and parietal regions (Rothbart & Posner, 2015). Noradrenergic modulation is an important component to change an individual from a default brain state (activity in the locus coeruleus accompanies a warning signal) to a state which expects an event (such as the arrival of a stimulus at the beginning of an experimental trial) (Rothbart & Posner, 2015).

9.3.2 Orienting

To switch attention between multiple sources of media such as computer, a smart phone, or tablet involves orienting to and prioritizing sensory input from the chosen device which is communicating (or is expected to communicate) information. An executive function essential for goal attainment involves an individual's ability to effectively decide where to direct attention at any moment in time. Attention can be subdivided into directed or involuntary, the former being when an individual attends to stimuli relevant to goal attainment (Kahneman, 1973). In contrast, involuntary attention is more automatically activated (Kaplan & Berman, 2010). Interruptions, characteristic to information technology use, can disrupt goal-directed orienting. When activating the orienting network, an individual may be engaged in overt (moving their head or eyes) or covert attention (e.g., shifting their attention to an alert from smartphone while maintaining fixation on a computer screen) (Petersen & Posner, 2012). Anatomically, a functional distinction has been made between two orienting systems, one to detect and another to alert (Corbetta & Shulman, 2002; Petersen & Posner, 2012). The first system is involved in goal-directed selection of sensory information and responses (directed attention) and is centered on the dorsal posterior parietal and frontal cortex (Corbetta & Shulman, 2002). Specifically, this cognitive (endogenous or top-down) system includes the frontal eye fields (FEF) and superior parietal lobe (Rothbart & Posner, 2015). A second sensory (exogenous or bottom-up) system is thought to involve a more ventral region including the parietal-temporal junction. This system is largely lateralized to the right hemisphere and involves automatic orienting induced by a cue. The separation of voluntary mechanisms from automatic ones may provide a foundation for understanding how directed attention can be involved in resistance to goal interference due to conscious and effortful choices on the part of the individual about where to orient and maintain attention.

9.3.3 Executive Attention

An individual activates the executive network when switching attention between media and while maintaining directed attention in the midst of IT interruptions. It is important for voluntary control of inhibition, excitation of emotions, thoughts and behavior (Bush, Luu, & Posner, 2000; Sheth et al., 2012), and a necessary mechanism for the ability to pursue goal-directed behavior through the control of directed and involuntary attention. Self-report temperament questionnaires are useful to assess executive attention in adults and older children (Rothbart & Posner, 2015; Rueda, 2012), while parent-report questionnaires can be utilized for younger children (Rothbart, Ahadi, Hershey, & Fisher, 2001). Tasks used to study the executive network include the go/no-go, the Stroop task, and flanker tasks. Areas involved in executive attention include midline frontal structures, the anterior cingulate cortex, the anterior insula, and the striatum. In addition, executive attention involves the regulation of other brain networks, such as the limbic system, related to emotion and detection of reward (Bush et al., 2000).

9.3.4 Attentional Switching

Attentional switching, defined as switching back and forth between more than one task or goal within a limited period, is the foundation for a type of goal interference: interruptions (Gazzaley & Rosen, 2016). Goals are plans that guide actions; they aid individuals in deciding how to respond to incoming external events (Gazzaley & Rosen, 2016). Goal interference can be defined as an externally generated event that uses cognitive resources to process information that is not directly related to a primary task or goal (Kraushaar & Novak, 2010). An interruption is an externally generated event which is engaged in as a simultaneous, secondary goal or task. The particular type of goal interference that interruptions present (in the context of attentional switching) could have negative effects on an individual which may even extend beyond their immediate circumstances (e.g., to subsequent tasks or goals that require inhibitory control). An aspect in which attentional switching can be observed is with the ubiquitous use of technology.

IT induced attention is highly complex; therefore, research seeks to simplify the issues accurately so that the underlying anatomy can be revealed. Simple tasks are used, such as those which only require switching from a resting state to performing a task, as well as a variety of auditory and visual tasks that required a high degree of vigilance in order to detect a critical target (Sridharan, Levitin, & Menon, 2008). Such tasks have revealed brain circuits that include the anterior insula, anterior cingulate, and connections to the underlying striatum. Specifically, the right insula cortex has been identified as being key in carrying out the switch from resting state to the state of directed attention needed for stimulus detection. Research is essential, not only to reveal the attention networks associated with the use of information technology, but also to investigate if IT use has negative consequences on subsequent acts (i.e., beyond the task at hand). Perhaps executive dysfunction associated with the use of information technology should be added to the well-established area of research concerning resource depletion.

9.3.4.1 Attentional Switching and Depletion

The particular type of goal interference that interruptions present (in the context of attentional switching) could have negative effects on an individual which may even extend beyond their immediate circumstances (e.g., to subsequent tasks or goals that require inhibitory control). The effort expended by attentional switching induced by interruptions may uniquely deplete an individual's resources. Although there is an acknowledgement of resource depletion, the field lacks a general framework for identifying the resource and understanding why a range of seemingly unrelated acts draw from this common resource (i.e., why one act of volition depletes volitional power for a second unrelated act) (Kaplan & Berman, 2010; Inzlicht & Gutsell, 2007). What is clear is that when an individual performs a task that requires directed attention, performance on the task immediately following is impaired due to fewer available resources (Baumeister, Bratslavsky, Muraven, & Tice, 1998; Tice, Baumeister, Shmueli, & Muraven, 2007; Vohs, Baumeister, & Ciarocco, 2005; Webb & Sheeran, 2003). Resources susceptible to depletion are shared between executive functioning and self-regulation (Vohs et al., 2008), and studies identify a range of behaviors affected as a result of resource depletion (Gailliot et al., 2007; Inzlicht & Gutsell, 2007; Kaplan & Berman, 2010).

If attentional switching induced by interruptions results in a greater depletion of resources, it is important to investigate the potential ramifications of performance on subsequent volitional acts, including inhibition. There are several explanations as to why IT interruptions may uniquely deplete an individual's resources. Research has shown interruptions manipulate and often divert attention involuntarily. IT interruptions are often unplanned, as well as the process they activate, and may involve an unseen cost in the form of anxiety. Finally, IT interruptions require additional decisions to be made by the individual.

9.3.4.2 IT Interruptions Divide Attention

Engaging in more than one task at a time may result in a more rapid depletion of resources. An individual who receives an IT interruption while working on a primary task is required to divide their attention between the task at hand and the incoming interruption. According to attention allocation perspective, attention is a limited, divisible resource, which comes from a limited pool of attentional capacity (Kahneman, 1973). Wickens (2002) uses the term "resources" to connote something that is limited and can be allocated. To "invest capacity," to "pay attention," and to "exert effort" are all expressions used interchangeably with "resources" concerning an implicit underlying reservoir (Hagger, Wood, Stiff, & Chatzisarantis, 2010) of limited availability that facilitates goal performance (Wickens, 1980; Kahneman, 1973). Therefore, if individuals choose to divide their attention between working on a primary task and an incoming IT interruption, they may inadvertently exert a higher degree of effort and deplete their resources more quickly than if they had maintained directed attention on their primary task.

9.3.4.3 IT Interruptions Are Unplanned

Because task demands are increased by interruptive external events (Addas & Pinsonneault, 2015; Kahneman, 1973), an individual may experience a greater depletion of resources if their attention is diverted involuntarily by way of an IT interruption. As stated, Kahneman (1973) subdivides attention into directed and involuntary. Involuntary attention, related to level of arousal, is more automatic, mostly stimulus-driven and less goal-directed (Kaplan & Berman, 2010). Surprising stimuli, which automatically attract attention, necessitate a greater effort of processing than do familiar stimuli (Falkinger, 2008; Kahneman, 1973). O'Conaill and Frohlich (1995) define interruptions as unscheduled. Therefore, externally generated events, such as interruptions which arrive and are unplanned or surprising, may also require more significant effort than maintaining directed attention on a primary task.

9.3.4.4 IT Interruptions Activate a Process

González and Mark (2004) maintain that it is not interruptions, but the entire process of frequent attentional switching (such as an alert of an email while working) that may result in a depletion of resources. After attending to an email, an individual may become aware (through the message content) of a number of additional tasks that need to be performed (Siu, Iverson, & Tang, 2006; Thomas et al., 2006; Tyler & Tang, 2003; Whittaker & Sidner, 1996; Whittaker, Bellotti, & Gwizdka, 2006; Whittaker, Bellotti, & Cwizdka, 2007). In addition, many emails cannot be discarded in a single session, but require multiple actions, as well as input or decisions from others (Thomas et al., 2006), further increasing task demands. Heavy demands such as these, which are often placed on an individual due to repeated IT interruptions, can deplete resources (Kaplan & Berman, 2010). Further, the effort an individual expends is not only on the interruption, but after the interruption has been attended to, the process of reorienting to the primary task once it has been revisited. The additional time it takes to reorient back to the primary task after the interruption is classified as a disruption cost (Mark, Gudith, & Klocke, 2008). Mark, González, and Harris (2005) report that after an interruption, it took individuals approximately 25 min to return to the original task. Jackson, Dawson, and Wilson (2003) report that email caused 96 interruptions in an eight hour day with an added hour and a half of recovery time per day.

9.3.4.5 IT Interruptions May Lead to Anxiety

IT interruptions can produce anxiety in several circumstances: if an individual works faster to compensate for time lost due to being interrupted; if an individual becomes aware that even if they work faster, they will not have enough time left to complete their primary task; or if, when their time to complete the task ends, the task is still incomplete. Bailey, Konstan, and Carlis (2001) investigated the effects of interruptions on anxiety by designing an experiment in which an interruption was a peripheral task presented to a user while performing a primary task. One of the key findings of their work was that a user experiences a greater increase in anxiety when a peripheral task interrupts their primary task than when it does not. The authors also found that when they interrupted a user during a document-editing task, the user completed the task faster than when they performed the same task without interruption. Additional studies have confirmed this finding and have also shown, as intrusions accumulate throughout the day, individuals do not necessarily exhibit decrements in performance; however working faster (Mark et al., 2008) in order to avoid productivity loss (tasks left incomplete) may be accompanied by feelings of anxiety. Glass, Singer, and Friedman (1969) concluded that adapting to unpredictable stress (such as an inability to complete tasks) involves a "psychic cost," suggesting a depletion of resources (Baumeister et al., 1998). Even if an individual shifts efficiently between a primary task and an IT interruption, they may not resume a suspended primary task in enough time to complete it (Iqbal & Horvitz, 2007). One study reports 41% of interruptions resulted in the discontinuation of the interrupted work entirely (O'Conaill & Frohlich, 1995). As the literature shows (Bailey et al., 2001; Baumeister et al., 1998; Glass et al., 1969; Iqbal & Horvitz, 2007; Mark et al., 2008; O'Conaill & Frohlich, 1995), anticipated productivity loss may contribute to anxiety felt by individuals who experience repeated IT interruptions.

9.3.4.6 IT Interruptions Generate Additional Decision-Making

Extensive active decision making has been shown to reduce self-control and result in poorer performance on subsequent acts of inhibition (Speier et al., 2003). Choosing is more depleting than merely establishing preferences (Vohs et al., 2008), and this may be another key in the literature as to why IT-induced attentional switching may uniquely deplete resources. If one-third of interruptions contain requests for action, with each of these requiring an assessment of whether and when the message content should be attended to (right away, at a later moment, or not at all) (Siu et al., 2006), an individual who continues to manage an increasing accumulation of minor decisions may be inadvertently lowering their threshold for self-control (Goleman, 2015). The greater demands on their attention could leave them susceptible to poorer decision making if, when faced with a truly significant decision toward the end of a day, they are not able to control impulsive actions because they have not retained enough energy to inhibit distractions or lower reflexive behaviors (Hartman & Miguel, 2017).

Christopher and Rosselli (2019) investigated if attentional switching due to information technology interruptions would deplete resources in a unique way and impair performance on a response inhibition task. The following were considered when investigating the costs of IT-induced attentional switching: (1) the expenditure of attentional resources and how these resources may be depleted more rapidly when attention is diverted involuntarily from a primary task to engage in one or more secondary tasks, and (2) how the process of IT-induced attentional switching and consequent resource depletion may have consequences that extend beyond the primary task. The study aimed to achieve ecological validity by simulating a typical working environment, applicable to either a business or academic setting, and help close the gap in the existing knowledge in this field by investigating whether attentional switching between two or more tasks due to IT interruptions would result in the depletion of resources of limited capacity, and due to depletion, would impair performance on an ostensibly unrelated task that measures response inhibition.

Three groups were compared on the Simon task after participants either did or did not receive interruptions during a self-regulation task. Participants who were interrupted with IT (in the form of informational and actionable intrusions) while performing a self-regulation task were expected to have poorer performance (a larger Simon effect) on the Simon task than participants who were not interrupted. Unexpectedly, poorer performance was found for participants who did not receive interruptions. These results (which conform to previous evidence which suggest sustained directed attention results in depletion and diminished performance on subsequent acts of inhibition) did not support predictions, but may provide a basis for further research, particularly because younger generations are developing in a more connected world than preceding generations and may therefore switch attention due to technology more efficiently than past generations.

9.4 Dysexecutive Related Disorders and the Information Technology Overuse

The use of IT is characterized by a dual nature in terms of its consequences. It can have benefits and positive aspects; for example, it facilitates exchange of information and communication, it allows people to have access to all types of resources overcoming geographical boundaries, to maximize the number of people to whom communication takes place with, and to be engaged in a variety of interactions and contexts. The use of these new technologies presents the user with a cognitive challenge since it requires not just the cognitive capabilities to adequate data processing, but the willingness to change and accept new devices. Also, IT users need some traits of personality such as technology enthusiasm and readiness (Bragazzi & Del Puente, 2014).

Interestingly, some research suggests that playing video games, even for a relatively short period of time, improves performance on visual and attentional tasks (Green & Bavelier, 2003). Boot, Kramer, Simons, Fabiani, & Gratton (2008) found that expert video gamers could track objects moving at greater speeds, were better in detecting changes to objects previously stored in visual short-term memory, switched faster from one task to another, and mentally rotated objects more efficiently, compared to non-gamers. In addition, Internet gaming may improve multitasking skills. Chen and Hsieh (2018) demonstrated that frequent Internet gaming individuals performed better than infrequent gaming experience individuals in tests that mimic everyday multitasking activities in a virtual environment (i.e., Edinburgh Virtual Errands Test); however, no differences were observed by these authors in conventional laboratory multitasks, such as the dual task and task switching. The authors concluded that playing Internet games are more related to higher-order executive functions such as reasoning, problem-solving, and planning rather than more basic executive functions such as inhibitory control, working memory, and cognitive flexibility.

Parallel to these positive challenges, the use of new technologies (such as smartphones) could result in negative consequences of social isolation and overuse. In some cases, the overuse may become an addition particularly to the abuse of specific social network sites (SNS) such as Facebook or Instagram (Donnelly & Kuss, 2016; Kuss & Griffiths, 2017). It has been suggested that excessive SNS use may lead to symptoms such as tolerance, withdrawal, and relapse traditionally associated with substance-related addictions (Kuss & Griffiths, 2017). Researchers have explored whether individuals become addicted to technology or to what technology allows them to do (Kuss & Griffiths, 2012). Technology seems to be the tool that allows individuals to engage in particular behaviors, such as social networking and gaming, rather than being addictive to the technology per se (Boyd, 2012). Kuss and Griffiths (2017) conclude that the addiction is not to the technology, but to connecting with people, and the good feelings that "likes" and positive comments of appreciation can produce. Therefore, it appears to be a "social networking addiction." In this section, we describe two of the most common disorders associated with IT excess: Nomophobia and Internet gaming disorder.

9.4.1 Nomophobia

Nomophobia (No Mobile Phone) refers to the reported uncontrollable fear of being without the mobile phone device or not having direct contact with it. This disorder has shown to share similar neuropsychological processes with drug addictions and pathologic gambling. In a 2012 survey conducted in the UK, it was found that 53% of smartphone users fear losing or being without their mobile phones (Elmore, 2014) particularly among young people between 18 ± 24 years old, followed by those between 25 ± 34 years (reported by Aguilera-Manrique et al., 2018). Data from studies in the USA indicate that sixty-six percent of the adults using mobile phones met the criteria for nomophobia (Elmore, 2014). Farooqui, Pore, and Gothankar (2018) found in a sample of 150 medical students in India who met the criteria for nomophobia, that 17.9% of the students had mild nomophobia, whereas 60% had moderate and 22.1% had severe nomophobia.

The disorder includes an obsession of using the phone, anxiety, stress, and even feelings of panic if the phone is not reachable for use (Adawi et al., 2019); it is as if smartphones actually have become an extension of themselves (Kuss & Griffiths, 2017). In some cases, there is mobile phone dependence defined as a loss of control on phone use that interferes with other activities, whereas in the actual case of nomophobia there is pathologic and irrational fear as it is found in the cases of specific phobias (anxiety disorder). This means that although nomophobia is related to abusive mobile phone and Internet use and dependence, it is a specific anxiety disorder that includes feeling anxious at the thought of being unable to use the phone due to lack of network coverage or flattened battery, trying to avoid places and situations in which the use of the device is prohibited (theaters, cinemas, etc.), and continuously looking at the phone's screen to see whether messages or calls have been or can be received (Bragazzi & Del Puente, 2014).

Nomophobia is fundamentally related to a fear of not being able to engage in social connections, and a preference for online social interaction (which is the key usage motivation for SNSs) (Kuss & Griffiths, 2011), and has been linked to problematic Internet use and negative consequences of technology use (Caplan, 2003), further pointing to a strong association between nomophobia and SNS addiction symptoms. To explain the high engagement in social networking such as Facebook, researchers have described the "fear of missing out" (FOMO) (Buglass, Binder, Betts, & Underwood, 2017; Oberst, Wegmann, Stodt, Brand, & Chamarro, 2017). FOMO has been defined as "a pervasive apprehension that others might be having rewarding experiences from which one is absent" and correlates with time invested in social networking (Przybylski, Murayama, DeHaan, & Gladwell, 2013). Moreover, FOMO predicts negative consequences of maladaptive SNS use (Buglass et al., 2017).

There is a growing usage of smartphone apps that track the time spent on the phone navigating the diverse apps, allowing the user to set use limits or to restrict its use, which suggests that there is a concern among online users of the Internet-related distractibility or other psychological problems (Aboujaoude, 2010).

A number of tools have been developed to assess behavioral problems related to IT disorders, including the Cellular Phone Dependence Questionnaire (CPDQ) (Toda, Monden, Kubo, & Morimoto, 2006), the Mobile Phone Dependence Inventory (MPDI) (Ezoe, Iida, Inoue, & Toda, 2016), or the Mobile Phone Problem Use Scale (MPPUS) (Bianchi & Phillips, 2005), the Facebook Dependence Questionnaire (FDQ) (Wolniczak et al., 2013), the Internet Addiction Test (Young, 1998), the Social Networking Addiction Scale (SNWAS) (Turel & Serenko, 2012), and the Bergen Social Media Addiction Scale (Andreassen, Pallesen, & Griffiths, 2017). For a review of these assessment tools and other ways of assessing social media overuse, see Kuss and Griffiths (2017).

A specific tool has been developed to evaluate the presence of nomophobia (using a self-reported questionnaire). The Nomophobia Questionnaire (NMP-Q), originally developed in English (Yildirim & Correia, 2015), has been adapted to other languages such as Italian (Adawi et al., 2018) and Spanish (González-Cabrera, León-Mejía, Pérez-Sancho, & Calvete, 2017).

Another assessment tool is the Nomophobia Questionnaire to assess nomophobia (QANIP; Olivencia-Carrión, Ferri-García, del Mar Rueda, Jiménez-Torres, & López-Torrecillas, 2018).

Studies have investigated the characteristic of young individuals who develop addiction disorders and have found that high impulsivity and low self-control are key risk factors in addiction (Lee et al., 2012; Reynolds, Ortengren, Richards, & de Wit, 2006). It has been found, for example, that self-control is negatively correlated with the use of tobacco, alcohol, and cannabis, along with problematic gambling and computer gaming. Mobile phone abuse is related to high impulsivity, and it has been identified as one of the risk factors for addiction to social networking sites among individuals who suffer from mobile phone abuse (Kim et al., 2017; Wu, Cheung, Ku,

& Hung, 2013). Also, individuals who score high in reward dependence are at higher risk to develop nomophobia (Olivencia-Carrión et al., 2018).

In summary, nomophobia is a common anxiety disorder related to mobile phone dependence and a fear of not being able to access it continually with high prevalence in young adults; like any other abuse problems, it is related to deficits in inhibitory control and the need to receive the reward that generates social media communications.

9.4.2 Internet Gaming Disorder

The Internet gaming disorder (IGD) is the inability to control excessive Internet game playing; it presents similar psychological and neuropsychological characteristics to drug addictions and pathologic gambling despite the fact that no chemical intake is needed. Individuals with IGD have a behavioral addiction with difficulties in controlling the desire to play online games despite significant negative consequences (King & Delfabbro, 2014). Although IGD has not yet been officially codified in the mental health disorders manual, it was included in Sect. 3 of the DSM-5, a part of the manual containing conditions warranting additional research (American Psychiatric Association, 2013; Petry et al., 2014). There are inconsistencies on the diagnostic criteria of IGD and some researchers have suggested that like other addictive behaviors including substance use and gambling, IGD should be classified as a reward deficiency syndrome (RDS), a condition characterized by an abnormal dopaminergic function in the nucleus accumbens (King & Delfabbro, 2014).

Comparable to individuals with substance addictions, persons with IGD show decreases in executive functions manifested by high levels of impulsivity (Ko et al., 2014; Lee et al., 2012; Zhou, Zhu, Li, & Wang, 2014) and problems with cognitive flexibility (Zhou et al., 2014).

9.5 Internet Addiction and Executive Dysfunction

Researchers have studied whether addiction to the Internet is associated with higher or lower executive functions (EFs). Findings suggest that individuals presenting this type of addiction have an EF profile like those suffering from other addiction disorders. For example, Lee et al. (2012) demonstrated that individuals with Internet addiction show increased levels of trait impulsivity as measured by the Barratt Impulsiveness Scale-11 (BIS-11) (Barratt, 1985), similar to those observed in patients with pathological gambling. Moreover, the severity of Internet addiction was positively correlated with the level of trait impulsivity in patients diagnosed with Internet addiction. By the same token, Zhou et al. (2014) showed that Internet addiction disorder (IAD), similar to alcohol-dependence, was associated with perseverative errors and failure to maintain set in the Wisconsin Card Sorting Test.

Dong, Lin, Zhou, & Lu (2014) studied performance in the Stroop test, while fMRI measures were used in a group of individuals diagnosed with IAD and another group of normal control. The authors created switching conditions between easy (congruent) to difficult (incongruent) trials or vice versa and compared them with no switching conditions (congruent-congruent; incongruent-incongruent). Although they found no significant behavioral group differences in the Stroop task, results showed higher superior temporal gyrus activations in the IAD group than in healthy controls during the switching conditions (easy to difficult; difficult to easy) than in the repeating trials. In addition, in the difficult-to-easy switching, IAD subjects showed higher brain activation in bilateral insula than healthy controls; in easy-to-difficult condition, IAD subjects show higher brain activation in bilateral precuneus than healthy controls. The authors concluded that the brains of individuals diagnosed with IAD present more effort in attentional shifting during the switching process compared to healthy controls.

More recently, Dong et al. (2018) analyzed white matter integrity between individuals with a more specific disorder: Internet gaming disorder (IGD); this group was compared to recreational Internet game use (RGU) individuals who spend similar amounts of time as the IGD individuals playing online games without developing the disorder. Whole-brain comparisons showed that IGD subjects demonstrated increased fractional anisotropy (FA; the higher the index, the higher the integrity of the tracks) in the bilateral anterior thalamic radiation, anterior limb of the internal capsule, bilateral corticospinal tract, bilateral inferior fronto-occipital fasciculus, corpus callosum, and bilateral inferior longitudinal fasciculus. In addition, Internet-addiction severity was positively correlated with FA values. The authors concluded that IGD is associated with measures of increased white-matter integrity in tracts linking reward circuitry and sensory and motor control systems. Ko et al. (2014) used fMRI to study response inhibition measures by an event-related designed Go/No-go task in individuals with IGD and normal controls. The severity of the Internet addiction, the lack of self-control, and the impulsivity was tested using the Chinese Internet Addiction Scale (CIAS) (Chen, Weng, Su, Wu, & Yang, 2003), the Barratt Impulsivity Scale 11(BIS-11) (Barratt, 1985), and Dickman's Impulsivity Scale (Dickman, 1990), respectively. Although the groups did not differ on the Go/No-go task, higher impulsivity and poorer self-control were observed in the IGD group compared to controls. When processing response inhibition, the IGD group exhibited higher brain activation in the left orbital frontal lobe and bilateral caudate nucleus than the control group. The authors suggest that the IGD individuals need higher activation of the fronto-striatal network to maintain inhibitory responses.

In conclusion, individuals suffering from Internet overuse disorders have a behavioral profile characterized by increased level of impulsivity and difficulties of cognitive control with poor cognitive flexibility corresponding to a dysexecutive syndrome. The behavioral addiction that these individuals present is kept in most cases by the reward generated by social media. In other words, different from substance additions, in Internet addiction, the "drug" seems to come from the content of social media. As described above, studies using functional neuroimaging techniques have shown that the brains of individuals diagnosed with this behavioral addiction have hyperactivation in the areas involved in the reward brain system—specifically the fronto-striatal circuitry—compared to healthy controls. Moreover, structural hyper-connectivity between the reward brain system and sensory and motor brain areas have also been described in Internet addicts.

Ardila (2013) suggested the distinction of two basic executive function systems; one involving metacognitive abilities (cool EFs) and the other one related to "Emotional/motivational behaviors" (hot EFs). Under the metacognitive abilities, problem-solving, abstracting, planning, anticipating the consequences of behavior, strategy development and implementation, and working memory are included, whereas the EFs included under the emotional/motivational EF are those abilities required to fulfill basic impulses following socially acceptable strategies in which inhibitory control plays a major role. Although many of the studies analyzing the EFs in Internet addicts are preliminary, and some suffer from methodological limitations (such as small samples), they seem to suggest that this addiction (like addictions to chemicals) involves mainly the emotional and motivational executive functions. The impact of IT on affect behavior, cognition, and brain function will be a topic of interest for researchers in the years to come.

References

Aboujaoude, E. (2010). Problematic internet use: An overview. *World Psychiatry, 9*(2), 85–90.

Addas, S., & Pinsonneault, A. (2015). The many faces of information technology interruptions: A taxonomy and preliminary investigation of their performance effects. *Information Systems Journal, 25*(3), 231–273.

Adawi, M., Bragazzi, N. L., Argumosa-Villar, L., Boada-Grau, J., Vigil-Colet, A., Yildirim, C., ... & Watad, A. (2018). Translation and validation of the Nomophobia questionnaire in the Italian language: exploratory factor analysis. *JMIR mHealth and uHealth, 6*(1), e24.

Adawi, M., Zerbetto, R., Re, T. S., Bisharat, B., Mahamid, M., Amital, H., ... & Bragazzi, N. L. (2019). Psychometric properties of the Brief Symptom Inventory in nomophobic subjects: insights from preliminary confirmatory factor, exploratory factor, and clustering analyses in a sample of healthy Italian volunteers. *Psychology Research and Behavior Management, 12*, 145.

Aguilera-Manrique, G., Márquez-Hernández, V. V., Alcaraz-Córdoba, T., Granados-Gámez, G., Gutiérrez-Puertas, V., & Gutiérrez-Puertas, L. (2018). The relationship between nomophobia and the distraction associated with smartphone use among nursing students in their clinical practicum. *PLoS ONE, 13*(8), e0202953.

American Psychiatric Association. (2013). *Diagnostic and statistical manual of mental disorders* (DSM-5®). American Psychiatric Pub.

Andreassen, C. S., Pallesen, S., & Griffiths, M. D. (2017). The relationship between addictive use of social media, narcissism, and self-esteem: Findings from a large national survey. *Addictive Behaviors, 64*, 287–293.

Ardila, A. (2013). There are two different dysexecutive syndromes. *Journal of Neurological Disorders, 1*(1), 1–4.

Bailey, B. P., Konstan, J. A., & Carlis, J. V. (2001). The effects of interruptions on task performance, annoyance, and anxiety in the user interface. In *Interact* (Vol. 1, pp. 593–601).

Barley, S. R., Meyerson, D. E., & Grodal, S. (2011). E-mail as a source and symbol of stress. *Organization Science, 22*(4), 887–906.

Barratt, E. S. (1985). Impulsiveness subtraits: Arousal and information processing. In J. T. Spence & C. E. Izard (Eds.), *Motivation, emotion and personality* (pp. 137–146). Elsevier Science: North Holland.

Baumeister, R. F., Bratslavsky, E., Muraven, M., & Tice, D. M. (1998). Ego depletion: Is the active self a limited resource? *Journal of Personality and Social Psychology, 74*(5), 1252.

Bianchi, A., & Phillips, J. G. (2005). Psychological predictors of problem mobile phone use. *CyberPsychology & Behavior, 8*(1), 39–51.

Boot, W. R., Kramer, A. F., Simons, D. J., Fabiani, M., & Gratton, G. (2008). The effects of video game playing on attention, memory, and executive control. *Acta Psychologica, 129*(3), 387–398.

Boyd, D. (2012). Participating in the always-on lifestyle. In M. Mandiberg (Ed.), *The Social Media Reader* (pp. 71–76). New York: New York University.

Bragazzi, N. L., & Del Puente, G. (2014). A proposal for including nomophobia in the new DSM-V. *Psychology Research and Behavior Management, 7,* 155.

Brand, M., Young, K. S., & Laier, C. (2014). Prefrontal control and Internet addiction: A theoretical model and review of neuropsychological and neuroimaging findings. *Frontiers in Human Neuroscience, 8,* 375.

Brasel, S. A., & Gips, J. (2011). Media multitasking behavior: Concurrent television and computer usage. *Cyberpsychology, Behavior, and Social Networking, 14*(9), 527–534.

Buglass, S. L., Binder, J. F., Betts, L. R., & Underwood, J. D. (2017). Motivators of online vulnerability: The impact of social network site use and FOMO. *Computers in Human Behavior, 66,* 248–255.

Bush, G., Luu, P., & Posner, M. I. (2000). Cognitive and emotional influences in anterior cingulate cortex. *Trends in cognitive sciences, 4*(6), 215–222.

Caplan, S. E. (2003). Preference for online social interaction: A theory of problematic Internet use and psychosocial well-being. *Communication Research, 30*(6), 625–648.

Carrier, L. M., Cheever, N. A., Rosen, L. D., Benitez, S., & Chang, J. (2009). Multitasking across generations: Multitasking choices and difficulty ratings in three generations of Americans. *Computers in Human Behavior, 25*(2), 483–489.

Chassiakos, Y. L. R., Radesky, J., Christakis, D., Moreno, M. A., & Cross, C. (2016). Children and adolescents and digital media. *Pediatrics, 138*(5), e20162593.

Chen, S. H., Weng, L. J., Su, Y. J., Wu, H. M., & Yang, P. F. (2003). Development of a Chinese internet addiction scale and its psychometric study. *Chinese Journal of Psychology*.

Chen, Y. Q., & Hsieh, S. (2018). The relationship between internet-gaming experience and executive functions measured by virtual environment compared with conventional laboratory multitasks. *PLoS ONE, 13*(6), e0198339.

Christopher, D. M. & Rosselli, M. (2019). Information technology induced attentional switching effects on inhibitory control. *Applied Neuropsychology: Adult*. https://doi.org/10.1080/23279095.2019.1633535.

Clemmons, D. (2017). *Parental perceptions of children and adolescent internet use, executive functioning, and parenting style*. Doctoral dissertation, Middle Tennessee State University.

Common Sense Media. (2013). *Zero to eight: Children's media use in America 2013*.

Corbetta, M., & Shulman, G. L. (2002). Control of goal-directed and stimulus-driven attention in the brain. *Nature Reviews Neuroscience, 3*(3), 201.

Dabbish, L. A., Kraut, R. E., Fussell, S., & Kiesler, S. (2005, April). Understanding email use: Predicting action on a message. In *Proceedings of the SIGCHI Conference on Human Factors in Computing Systems* (pp. 691–700). ACM.

Davis, G. B., & Olson, M. H. (1984). *Management information systems: Conceptual foundations, structure, and development.* McGraw-Hill, Inc.

Dickman, S. J. (1990). Functional and dysfunctional impulsivity: Personality and cognitive correlates. *Journal of Personality and Social Psychology, 58*(1), 95.

Dong, G., Lin, X., Zhou, H., & Lu, Q. (2014). Cognitive flexibility in internet addicts: fMRI evidence from difficult-to-easy and easy-to-difficult switching situations. *Addictive Behaviors, 39*(3), 677–683.

Dong, G., Wu, L., Wang, Z., Wang, Y., Du, X., & Potenza, M. N. (2018). Diffusion-weighted MRI measures suggest increased white-matter integrity in Internet gaming disorder: Evidence from the comparison with recreational Internet game users. *Addictive Behaviors, 81,* 32–38.

Donnelly, E., & Kuss, D. J. (2016). Depression among users of social networking sites (SNSs): The role of SNS addiction and increased usage. *Journal of Addiction and Preventive Medicine, 1*(2), 107.

Elmore, T. (2014). Nomophobia: A rising trend in students. *Psychology Today*. Available from: https://www.psychologytoday.com/blog/artificial-maturity/201409/nomophobia-rising-trend-in-students. Last accessed April 17, 2019.

Ezoe, S., Iida, T., Inoue, K., & Toda, M. (2016). Development of Japanese version of smartphone dependence scale. *Open Journal of Preventive Medicine, 6*(07), 179.

Falkinger, J. (2008). Limited attention as a scarce resource in information-rich economies. *The Economic Journal, 118*(532), 1596–1620.

Fan, J., McCandliss, B. D., Sommer, T., Raz, A., & Posner, M. I. (2002). Testing the efficiency and independence of attentional networks. *Journal of Cognitive Neuroscience, 14*(3), 340–347.

Farooqui, I. A., Pore, P., & Gothankar, J. (2018). Nomophobia: An emerging issue in medical institutions? *Journal of Mental Health, 27*(5), 438–441.

Gailliot, M. T., Baumeister, R. F., DeWall, C. N., Maner, J. K., Plant, E. A., Tice, D. M., ... & Schmeichel, B. J. (2007). Self-control relies on glucose as a limited energy source: Willpower is more than a metaphor. *Journal of Personality and Social Psychology*, 92(2), 325.

Gazzaley, A., & Rosen, L. D. (2016). *The distracted mind: Ancient brains in a high-tech world.* Mit Press.

Glass, D. C., Singer, J. E., & Friedman, L. N. (1969). Psychic cost of adaptation to an environmental stressor. *Journal of Personality and Social Psychology, 12*(3), 200.

Goleman, D. (2015). *Focus: The hidden driver of excellence*. New York: Harper.

González-Cabrera, J., León-Mejía, A., Pérez-Sancho, C., & Calvete, E. (2017). Adaptation of the Nomophobia Questionnaire (NMP-Q) to Spanish in a sample of adolescents. *Actas Españolas de Psiquiatria, 45*(4), 137–144.

González, V. M., & Mark, G. (2004, April). Constant, constant, multi-tasking craziness: Managing multiple working spheres. In In *Proceedings of the SIGCHI conference on Human factors in computing systems* (pp. 113–120). ACM.

Goodrich, S. A., Pempek, T. A., & Calvert, S. L. (2009). Formal production features of infant and toddler DVDs. *Archives of Pediatrics and Adolescent Medicine, 163*(12), 1151–1156.

Green, C. S., & Bavelier, D. (2003). Action video game modifies visual selective attention. *Nature, 423*(6939), 534.

Gupta, A., Li, H., & Sharda, R. (2013). Should I send this message? Understanding the impact of interruptions, social hierarchy and perceived task complexity on user performance and perceived workload. *Decision Support Systems, 55*(1), 135–145.

Hagger, M. S., Wood, C., Stiff, C., & Chatzisarantis, N. L. (2010). Ego depletion and the strength model of self-control: A meta-analysis. *Psychological Bulletin, 136*(4), 495.

Hartman, B., & Miguel, S. F. S. (2017). Optimizing client and student learning from the brain's perspective. *Journal of the American Veterinary Medical Association, 251*(1), 33–35.

Inzlicht, M., & Gutsell, J. N. (2007). Running on empty: Neural signals for self-control failure. *Psychological Science, 18*(11), 933–937.

Iqbal, S. T., & Horvitz, E. (2007, April). Disruption and recovery of computing tasks: Field study, analysis, and directions. In *Proceedings of the SIGCHI Conference on Human Factors in Computing Systems* (pp. 677–686). ACM.

Jackson, T., Dawson, R., & Wilson, D. (2003). Reducing the effect of email interruptions on employees. *International Journal of Information Management, 23*(1), 55–65.

Jurado, M. B., & Rosselli, M. (2007). The elusive nature of executive functions: A review of our current understanding. *Neuropsychology Review, 17*(3), 213–233.

Kahneman, D. (1973). *Attention and effort* (Vol. 1063). Englewood Cliffs, NJ: Prentice-Hall.

Kaplan, S., & Berman, M. G. (2010). Directed attention as a common resource for executive functioning and self-regulation. *Perspectives on Psychological Science, 5*(1), 43–57.

Khan, J. (2013, October 19). *Information technology definition and examples*. Retrieved from http://www.byte-notes.com/information-technology-definition-and-examples.

Kim, Y. J., Lim, J. A., Lee, J. Y., Oh, S., Kim, S. N., Kim, D. J., … & Choi, J. S. (2017). Impulsivity and compulsivity in Internet gaming disorder: A comparison with obsessive–compulsive disorder and alcohol use disorder. *Journal of Behavioral Addictions*, *6*(4), 545–553.

King, D. L., & Delfabbro, P. H. (2014). The cognitive psychology of Internet gaming disorder. *Clinical Psychology Review, 34,* 298–308.

Ko, C. H., Hsieh, T. J., Chen, C. Y., Yen, C. F., Chen, C. S., Yen, J. Y., … & Liu, G. C. (2014). Altered brain activation during response inhibition and error processing in subjects with Internet gaming disorder: a functional magnetic imaging study. *European Archives of Psychiatry and Clinical Neuroscience*, *264*(8), 661–672.

Kononova, A. (2013). Multitasking across borders: A cross-national study of media multitasking behaviors, its antecedents, and outcomes. *International Journal of Communication, 7,* 23.

Kraushaar, J. M., & Novak, D. C. (2010). Examining the affects of student multitasking with laptops during the lecture. *Journal of Information Systems Education, 21*(2), 241.

Kuss, D. J., & Griffiths, M. D. (2011). Online social networking and addiction—A review of the psychological literature. *International Journal of Environmental Research and Public Health, 8*(9), 3528–3552.

Kuss, D. J., & Griffiths, M. D. (2012). Internet gaming addiction: A systematic review of empirical research. *International Journal of Mental Health and Addiction, 10*(2), 278–296.

Kuss, D., & Griffiths, M. (2017). Social networking sites and addiction: Ten lessons learned. *International Journal of Environmental Research and Public Health, 14*(3), 311.

Lee, H. W., Choi, J. S., Shin, Y. C., Lee, J. Y., Jung, H. Y., & Kwon, J. S. (2012). Impulsivity in internet addiction: A comparison with pathological gambling. *Cyberpsychology, Behavior, and Social Networking, 15*(7), 373–377.

Mark, G., González, V. M., & Harris, J. (2005, April). No task left behind?: Examining the nature of fragmented work. In *Proceedings of the SIGCHI Conference on Human Factors in Computing Systems* (pp. 321–330). ACM.

Mark, G., Gudith, D., & Klocke, U. (2008, April). The cost of interrupted work: more speed and stress. In *Proceedings of the SIGCHI conference on Human Factors in Computing Systems* (pp. 107–110). ACM.

Oberst, U., Wegmann, E., Stodt, B., Brand, M., & Chamarro, A. (2017). Negative consequences from heavy social networking in adolescents: The mediating role of fear of missing out. *Journal of Adolescence, 55,* 51–60.

Oblinger, D., & Oblinger, J. (2005). Is it age or IT: First steps toward understanding the Net generation. *Educating the Net Generation, 2*(1–2), 20.

O'Conaill, B., & Frohlich, D. (1995, May). Timespace in the workplace: Dealing with interruptions. In *Conference Companion on Human Factors in Computing Systems* (pp. 262–263). ACM.

Olivencia-Carrión, M. A., Ferri-García, R., del Mar Rueda, M., Jiménez-Torres, M. G., & López-Torrecillas, F. (2018). Temperament and characteristics related to nomophobia. *Psychiatry Research, 266,* 5–10.

Ophir, E., Nass, C., & Wagner, A. D. (2009). Cognitive control in media multitaskers. *Proceedings of the National Academy of Sciences, 106*(37), 15583–15587.

Petersen, S. E., & Posner, M. I. (2012). The attention system of the human brain: 20 years after. *Annual Review of Neuroscience, 35,* 73–89.

Petry, N. M., Rehbein, F., Gentile, D. A., Lemmens, J. S., Rumpf, H. J., Mossle, T., … O'Brien, C. P. (2014). An international consensus for assessing internet gaming disorder using the new DSM-5 approach. *Addiction, 109,* 1399–1406.

Posner, M. I., & Petersen, S. E. (1990). The attention system of the human brain. *Annual Review of Neuroscience, 13*(1), 25–42.

Przybylski, A. K., Murayama, K., DeHaan, C. R., & Gladwell, V. (2013). Motivational, emotional, and behavioral correlates of fear of missing out. *Computers in Human Behavior, 29*(4), 1841–1848.

Reynolds, B., Ortengren, A., Richards, J. B., & de Wit, H. (2006). Dimensions of impulsive behavior: Personality and behavioral measures. *Personality and Individual Differences, 40*(2), 305–315.

Rideout, V. J., Foehr, U. G., & Roberts, D. F. (2010). Generation M 2: Media in the lives of 8- to 18-year-olds. *Henry J. Kaiser Family Foundation.*

Rothbart, M. K., Ahadi, S. A., Hershey, K. L., & Fisher, P. (2001). Investigations of temperament at three to seven years: The Children's behavior questionnaire. *Child Development, 72*(5), 1394–1408.

Rothbart, M. K., & Posner, M. I. (2015). The developing brain in a multitasking world. *Developmental Review, 35,* 42–63.

Rueda, M. R. (2012). Effortful control. *Handbook of Temperament*, 145–167.

Sheth, S. A., Mian, M. K., Patel, S. R., Asaad, W. F., Williams, Z. M., Dougherty, D. D., … & Eskandar, E. N. (2012). Human dorsal anterior cingulate cortex neurons mediate ongoing behavioural adaptation. *Nature, 488*(7410), 218.

Siu, N., Iverson, L., & Tang, A. (2006, November). Going with the flow: Email awareness and task management. In *Proceedings of the 2006 20th Anniversary Conference on Computer Supported Cooperative Work* (pp. 441–450). ACM.

Speier, C., Vessey, I., & Valacich, J. S. (2003). The effects of interruptions, task complexity, and information presentation on computer-supported decision-making performance. *Decision Sciences, 34*(4), 771–797.

Sridharan, D., Levitin, D. J., & Menon, V. (2008). A critical role for the right fronto-insular cortex in switching between central-executive and default-mode networks. *Proceedings of the National Academy of Sciences, 105*(34), 12569–12574.

Thomas, G. F., King, C. L., Baroni, B., Cook, L., Keitelman, M., Miller, S., et al. (2006). Reconceptualizing e-mail overload. *Journal of Business and Technical Communication, 20*(3), 252–287.

Tice, D. M., Baumeister, R. F., Shmueli, D., & Muraven, M. (2007). Restoring the self: Positive affect helps improve self-regulation following ego depletion. *Journal of Experimental Social Psychology, 43*(3), 379–384.

Toda, M., Monden, K., Kubo, K., & Morimoto, K. (2006). Mobile phone dependence and health-related lifestyle of university students. *Social Behavior and Personality: An International Journal, 34*(10), 1277–1284.

Turel, O., & Serenko, A. (2012). The benefits and dangers of enjoyment with social networking websites. *European Journal of Information Systems, 21*(5), 512–528.

Tyler, J. R., & Tang, J. C. (2003). When can I expect an email response? A study of rhythms in email usage. In *ECSCW 2003* (pp. 239–258). Dordrecht: Springer.

Uncapher, M. R., Lin, L., Rosen, L. D., Kirkorian, H. L., Baron, N. S., Bailey, K., … & Wagner, A. D. (2017). Media multitasking and cognitive, psychological, neural, and learning differences. *Pediatrics, 140*(Supplement 2), S62–S66.

Vohs, K. D., Baumeister, R. F., & Ciarocco, N. J. (2005). Self-regulation and self-presentation: Regulatory resource depletion impairs impression management and effortful self-presentation depletes regulatory resources. *Journal of Personality and Social Psychology, 88*(4), 632.

Vohs, K. D., Baumeister, R. F., Schmeichel, B. J., Twenge, J. M., Nelson, N. M., & Tice, D. M. (2008). Making choices impairs subsequent self-control: A limited-resource account of decision making, self-regulation, and active initiative. In *Self-regulation and self-control* (pp. 45–77). Routledge.

Webb, T. L., & Sheeran, P. (2003). Can implementation intentions help to overcome ego-depletion? *Journal of Experimental Social Psychology, 39*(3), 279–286.

Whittaker, S., & Sidner, C. (1996, April). Email overload: Exploring personal information management of email. In *Proceedings of the SIGCHI Conference on Human Factors in Computing Systems* (pp. 276–283). ACM.

Whittaker, S., Bellotti, V., & Gwizdka, J. (2006). Email in personal information management. *Communications of the ACM, 49*(1), 68–73.

Whittaker, S., Bellotti, V., & Cwizdka, J. (2007). CD everything through Email. *Personal Information Management*, 167.

Wickens, C. D. (1980). The structure of attentional resources. *Attention and Performance VIII, 8,* 239–257.

Wickens, C. D. (2002). Multiple resources and performance prediction. *Theoretical Issues in Ergonomics Science, 3*(2), 159–177.

Wolniczak, I., Cáceres-DelAguila, J. A., Palma-Ardiles, G., Arroyo, K. J., Solís-Visscher, R., Paredes-Yauri, S., … & Bernabe-Ortiz, A. (2013). Association between Facebook dependence and poor sleep quality: A study in a sample of undergraduate students in Peru. *PloS One*, *8*(3), e59087.

Wortham, J. (2012, June 30). When internet distractions make us more efficient. Retrieved from https://www.nytimes.com/2012/07/01/technology/when-internet-distractions-make-us-more-efficient.html.

Wu, A. M., Cheung, V. I., Ku, L., & Hung, E. P. (2013). Psychological risk factors of addiction to social networking sites among Chinese smartphone users. *Journal of Behavioral Addictions, 2*(3), 160–166.

Yildirim, C., & Correia, A. P. (2015). Exploring the dimensions of nomophobia: Development and validation of a self-reported questionnaire. *Computers in Human Behavior, 49,* 130–137.

Young, K. S. (1998). Internet addiction: The emergence of a new clinical disorder. *Cyberpsychology & Behavior, 1*(3), 237–244.

Zhou, Z., Zhu, H., Li, C., & Wang, J. (2014). Internet addictive individuals share impulsivity and executive dysfunction with alcohol-dependent patients. *Frontiers in Behavioral Neuroscience, 8,* 288.

Part IV
Executive Dysfunction and Personality Disorders

Chapter 10
Executive Dysfunction in Violent and Criminal Behavior

Feggy Ostrosky Shejet and Karla Ximena Díaz Galván

10.1 Introduction

Human behavior and its neural causes is still not understood completely, especially in most complex behavior that involves volitional and moral facts, where stimuli, memories, beliefs, and other factors exert their effects. To identify the cause associated with a specific behavior has been a hopeless attempt; however, it has provided valuable facts that help us understand the complicated neural basis of human behavior. Some authors have described specific lesion in neural circuitry associated to specific behaviors. For example, in the case of criminal behavior, a number of rare cases have now been described in whom a focal lesion caused criminality; these are neither very consistent (the lesions occur in several different anatomical locations) nor at all reliable (only a small fraction of patients, for any lesion location, show criminal behavior) (Adolphs, Gläscher, & Tranel, 2018). Maybe, this is due to the complexity of neural mechanisms that interact with genetics, neurochemistry, and cognitive processes that build a human being. Additionally, the nature of these interactions has shown that most neural, functional, or anatomical patterns overlap, and then they are not unique to a pathology nor a specific personality disorder.

Darby, Horn, Cushman, and Fox (2018) probe this issue by examining the overlap of these core criminality-associated regions with brain regions inferred from functional imaging data to subserve processes that might well come into play during criminal behavior. Overlap was found with brain regions known to be important for theory of mind and value-based decision-making, a finding also consistent with prior studies showing deficits in these abilities in patients whose lesions. How much this partial decomposition begins to explain criminality, however, seems still very much open to question because, again, the vast majority of patients with impairments in

F. Ostrosky Shejet (✉) · K. X. Díaz Galván
Laboratorio de Psicofisiología y Neuropsicología, Facultad de Psicología, Universidad Nacional Autonoma de Mexico, Av. Universidad 3004 Copilco-Universidad, Facultad de Psicología, Edificio D Cubículo 211, 04510 Mexico City, Mexico
e-mail: feggy@unam.mx

A. Ardila et al. (eds.), *Dysexecutive Syndromes*,
https://doi.org/10.1007/978-3-030-25077-5_10

theory of mind or value-based decision-making are not criminals. In a way, this is good news for folk psychology and jurisprudence: our concepts of moral responsibility and free will are not challenged by these data, since neither the brain lesions nor the lesion network maps explain criminality.

One of the most frequently associated traits of criminal behavior is violence.

10.2 Violence Versus Aggression

In contemporary literature, there is not a clear difference between violence and aggression, and it is continually misused and referenced as synonyms. However, it is of great importance to understand its differences.

Aggression is defined as a basic primitive behavior in every living being. From the very evolutionary point of view, aggression is considered as the behavioral manifestation in which its aim is to cause physical damage to an individual in order to maintain the species (Alcázar, Verdejo, Bouso, & Bezos, 2010; Ostrosky & Ardila, 2018).

On the other hand, violence is defined by the World Health Organization as "the intentional use of physical force or power, threatened or actual, against oneself, another person, or against a group or community, which either results in or has a high likelihood of resulting in injury, death, psychological harm, maldevelopment, or deprivation," although the group acknowledges that the inclusion of "the use of power" in its definition expands on the conventional understanding of the word.

Violence definition is not included in aggression characteristics. This means that an aggressive behavior may be legitimate, legal, and could be used to defend itself from an external attack; it has the characteristics that justifies it appearance. Hence, violence does include aggression, but not every aggressive act can be considered as violent (Anderson & Bushman, 2002). Since ethologists have identified aggression in different animal species is a term more often used in animal behavior context, whereas violent behavior is exclusive to the human race (Carrasco & González, 2006).

10.3 Components of Violence

The violence definition above allows to delimit a very clear behavioral pattern, which represents an advantage from the scientific research point of view, because it allows us to study the associated traits to these behaviors and does not only focus on the aggression–violence relationship. Researchers have reported these traits associated with violent behavior, starting from the premise that violent conduct is composed of 3 basic components:

1. Affective (anger-rage)
2. Cognitive or temperamental (impulsivity, hostility)
3. Behavioral, that represents the act itself

Rage is an emotional state that includes a wide range of feelings that includes from irritability, annoyance, anger, and so on up to intense rage that emerge from unpleasant experiences that are not goal directed. Besides, it also occurs in the conscience of physiological changes that are associated withviolent behavior like motor responses, thoughts, and memories linked to such unpleasant events. These anger characteristics arc known as "slate anger" that is generally matched with an autonomous activation of the nervous system. Another anger characteristic that is considered as a "trait" and its related to low reactivity threshold in which the anger feelings are triggered by certain stimulus relatively innocuous or very specific stimulus related to rejection or injustice. In general, anger may be considered as a personality trait in terms of the experience of anger and to be ready for an angry response (Carrasco & González, 2006; Ramírez & Andreu, 2005).

In a study that investigated proneness to anger, both emotion and preparation to the action, a positive correlation between the experience of anger and the preparation to express it was found, which indicates that those who experience anger with frequency have an increased probability of expressing it behaviorally (Ramírez, Santisteban, Fujihara, & Van Goozen, 2002).

Within the cognitive component of violence is the hostility that can be defined as the set of attitudes that lead to the negative assessment of people or things that is often accompanied by a desire to damage objects or people by aggressive behaviors aimed at a goal (Carrasco & González, 2006; Ostrosky, 2011; Ramírez & Andreu, 2005).

The hostility is composed of attitudes of resentment and mistrust that can be expressed through verbal and physical violence. The cognitive phenomenon of hostility consists of beliefs and negative attitudes toward others, including cynicism and denigration. The hostility is usually accompanied by feelings of anger, both showing similar physiological effects that predispose to violent behavior aimed at the destruction of objects, insults, or to inflict harm (Ramírez & Andreu, 2005). Some hostility components have been studied the influence of biological maturation on the levels of irritability and resentment (components of hostility). They have reported that these variables although they decrease with the passage of time shows stability. High levels of irritability were also associated with high levels of physical and verbal aggression, while high levels of resentment were associated with high levels of violent behavior. Another interesting finding was a correlation between irritability and resentment that increased with the passage of time (Caprara, Paciello, Gerbino, & Cugini, 2007).

Another component of violence is impulsivity. Impulsivity is a multidimensional concept that refers to the tendency to act quickly without thinking. There is a difference between an impulsive act and the psychological process underlying it, which is why impulsivity can be considered as behavior and as a cognitive process—the latter refers to a feature of stable personality that is related to the control of the thoughts and behaviors (Ramírez & Andreu, 2005).

Another concept related to violence is empathy, which has a cognitive and an affective-emotional component. Empathy is generally defined as the ability to share another person's emotional state that includes the ability to identify and understand the perspective of another person (cognitive component), while the emotional component is characterized by the tendency to experience feelings of concern or sympathy toward others. The empathic response usually causes an individual to moderate his aggressive behavior, i.e. people highly empathic are able to anticipate the consequences of their own behavior toward another person emotionally. Some studies have suggested that the relationship between empathy and violence can be explained by the affective component, since low levels of emotional empathy is associated with an increased frequency of violence (Jolliffe & Farrington, 2006). On the other hand, other studies have suggested that cognitive empathy is preserved in psychopathic individuals since they use this advantage of understanding others feelings to manipulate their prey and reach their personal goals engaging in frequent deceit and pathological lying (Díaz-Galván, Ostrosky-Shejet, & Romero-Rebollar, 2015).

Finally, the behavioral field includes the type of aggression used during the violent act. In literature, the aggressive and violent behavior has been classified into 2 subtypes: one reactive, affective, and impulsive, and another proactive, premeditated, or predatory (Stanford et al., 2003). The use of these subtypes of violence allows to distinguish biological, psychological, and social correlates as well as general characteristics that underlie them (Andreu, 2009).

Reactive aggression refers to acts whose main purpose would be to harm another individual, and it has been associated with failures in behavioral inhibition, high levels of impulsivity, and hostility. It is considered that this type of aggression occurs in reaction to any provocation, characterized by defensive reactions, fear, irritability, hostility and provocation, in addition to disturbances in social information processing. Also deemed that the reactions of this type of aggression are disproportionate and exaggerated. The evolutionary basis of reactive aggression is self-protection (Andreu, 2009; Meloy, 2006). Physiologically reactive aggression is associated with a sympathetic hyperactivity, and neurobiological and cognitive characteristics as a lower intellectual capacity, as well as poor verbal skills and a decreased performance of the executive functions (Andreu, 2009).

On the other hand, the proactive aggression is a behavior that occurs in the absence of provocation or anger, is intentional, and is intended to dominate or intimidate. This subtype of aggression is based on the idea that aggression is a way to achieve a particular purpose. Neuropsychologically speaking, proactive aggression is associated with normal executive performance and physiologically with a low arousal of the autonomic nervous system (Andreu, 2009; Meloy, 2006; Merk, Orobio de Castro, Koops, & Matthys, 2005).

10.4 Psychopathy

Psychopathy is not a component of violence, but it is a frequently associated variable. Psychopathy is one of the variables with the greatest predictive power of violent conduct; when the defining traits of this disorder are revised features like insensitivity, impulsivity, self-centeredness, lack of empathy, among others, it is proposed that a psychopath is more likely to violate rules and laws (Hare, 1999).

From the development and use of the Hare psychopathy scale-revised (PCL-R, Hare, 2003) the evaluation of this disorder has been improved. Psychopathy, measured by the PCL-R and its derivatives, is related to interpersonal and affective dimensions of personality as manipulation, pathological lies, and absence of remorse and guilt, grouped in the Factor 1 (F1); on the other hand, antisocial tendencies like irresponsibility, impulsivity, and criminal conduct are grouped in the Factor 2 (F2) (Hare & Neumann, 2008). Several studies have attempted to identify what traits of psychopathy are more associated with violent behavior. Two meta-analysis results have shown that the F2 has better predictive efficacy with an effect size that varies between 0.4 and 0.6, compared to the F1 ranging between 0.1 and 0.2, which means that the predictive utility of the F2 does not depend on the measured traits by the F1 (Kennealy, Skeem, Walters, & Camp, 2010; Yang, Wong, & Coid, 2010). In another study, which evaluated the combination of these two factors predictive ability, they found similar results (Walsh & Kosson, 2008).

Neuropsychological Findings Related to Violent Behavior
Literature has suggested that the origin of aggression is the existence of cognitive deficits in aggressive, mostly in executive functions, attention, memory, and language (Elliot & Mirsky, 2002). However, current literature about violent behavior is heterogeneous and includes samples from institutionalized populations that committed murder to violent personality traits in general population participants; as mentioned before, violence can be manifested by a wide range of behaviors. Hence, this chapter aims to integrate results in all these populations for a better understanding of the neuropsychological mechanisms that underlies violence, but first we will make a short review of the main findings separately.

10.5 Studies in Institutionalized Populations

The study of aggression has been carried out mostly in institutionalized populations (psychiatric and prison participants). These studies have focused on the psychiatric diagnosis of conduct disorders, which has been reported to be more prevalent in men than in women (Connor, Aderson, & Melloni, 2002). In this regard, several authors have studied murderers, as Barratt, Stanford, Kent, and Felthous (1997). They used two groups of inmates, divided based on the type of aggression of the crime they had committed, compared to a non-institutionalized control group. They reported lower performance in functions of the orbitofrontal cortex, as inhibitory control and decision-making in tasks where the emotional response and task processing of reward/punishment are evaluated. They also found dorsolateral alterations and argue that they can predispose the perseveration of a response (anti-social behavior throughout life despite repeated punishment), and poor planning and organization bringing as consequences of occupational and social dysfunctional life style.

However, results have not been consistent. It appears that the way the sample is divided has a big impact on the results of the study in violent behavior. Regarding this matter, Arias and Ostrosky (2008) did an investigation using two different violent subjects ratings: (1) impulsive (reactive) against premeditated (proactive) and (2) psychopaths against non-psychopaths. Fifty inmates were assessed at state prisons and 25 external controls matched on age and education. They measured their neuropsychological performance through two batteries: the NEUROPSI attention and memory (Ostrosky-Solís et al., 2007) that measures different types of attention and memory, and a battery of frontal and executive functions (BANFE) (Flores, Ostrosky, & Lozano, 2008) that provides three total scores: orbitomedial, dorsolateral, and anterior prefrontal. The results of the study indicated that violent populations regardless of their classification can be differentiated from non-violent population. However, no significant differences in neuropsychological assessments was found with the classification of impulsive and premeditated violence, while the results among non-psychopaths and psychopaths show significant differences between the control group and the non-psychopath. The authors conclude that their results support other studies where there are alterations in the executive functions of violent people, and they find differences in tasks related to both the orbitomedial and the dorsolateral prefrontal cortex, in addition to alterations in attention and memory, emphasizing the importance of the classification used for his study, where the criterion of psychopathy seems to be more sensitive to differentiate violent individuals by their cognitive performance.

10.6 Studies in Psychopathic Population

The relationship between psychopathic personality and executive functions has been made repeatedly over the years in the field of study of violent behavior. Several authors (Gorenstein, 1982; Ostrosky, 2017; Raine, 1997) have postulated that the alterations in the executive functions are an important risk factor for the development of antisocial and violent behavior. This hypothesis of prefrontal substrates in antisocial subjects is shown in a study by Gorenstein (1982) where they presented a greater number of perseverations on the Wisconsin Card Sorting Test, related to the functioning of the dorsolateral prefrontal cortex. Dolan and Park (2002) show that antisocial subjects showed irregularities in tasks of planning and set-shifting, as well as deficits in tasks of inhibition of behavior using GO/NO GO test.

In a study carried out by Díaz, Ostrosky, Romero, and Pérez (2013) aiming to assess cognitive performance in orbito-medial-related tasks in psychopaths evaluated 63 adult men (20–59 years of age) divided into 2 groups: inmate psychopaths ($n =$

30) and a control group from general population ($n = 33$) using the psychopathy checklist of Hare (PCL-R). They found that psychopaths obtained lower orbito-medial performance, committing a greater number of errors in the stroop task. They also found a positive correlation between the number of maintenance errors in WCST and psychopathy scores in factor 1, as well as a positive correlation between the percentage of risk cards in an adaptation of the IGT (Iowa Gambling Task) and the factor 2 of psychopathy. The authors suggest that the neuropsychological profile of psychopaths was significantly lower compared with the controls, especially in tasks that involve inhibition and decision-making processes support the hypothesis of the damage in orbito-medial regions in this population.

10.7 Studies in General Population

Studies carried out on members of the community are even scarcer since the traits of violence are more difficult to identify. However, the findings indicate the great need to increase these investigations to be able to distinguish them from institutionalized populations. In this regard, some authors have tried to characterize the types of violence and associate them with a specific cognitive pattern, as it is the case of the study of Stanford, Greve, and Gerstle (1997) whose objective was to assess the impulsive aggression in subjects considered socially as normal (college students). Twelve subjects participated (6 women and 6 men) classified as aggressive impulsive according to four criteria as attacks of anger in the last 6 months, 2 or more episodes of aggression, episodes of violence against objects or physical, high score (8 points) in the subscale of irritability of the Buss-Durkee hostility scale, compared with a control group control. The groups were different in the performance of the WCST, Word Association test, and the percentage of perseverations in a verbal fluency test. These results suggest that in impulsive aggression there is a flaw to control internal trends and issue a response and that there is a difficulty in verbal strategic processing. These results are consistent with those reported in impulsive aggressive inmates, which suggests the existence of a specific behavioral syndrome characterized by a poor impulse control and an altered verbal processing, which is associated with spontaneous aggressive attacks.

However, up to date, neuropsychological evaluation has only been done using isolated tasks, and this may have misleading results. In this regard, Díaz, Ostrosky, and Camarena (2012) assessed 60 subjects from the general population classified as violent (30) and controls (30) through his score on the scale of Reactive-Proactive-Aggression Questionnaire (RPQ) with the objective to evaluate the cognitive functioning of the CPF using a neuropsychological battery providing 3 indexes: dorsolateral, orbito-medial, and anterior pre-fontal performance. The results they found were similar to those reported before in institutionalized samples; differences were found only in the orbito-medial index, showing the violent group's lower performance. Nevertheless, the authors discussed the role that could play the component of antisocial personality in violent behavior and the neuropsychological performance since there was no difference in performance dorsolateral and anterior prefrontal, where these preserved functions may have an important role to compensate the orbito-medial flaws, hence keeping them from antisocial behavior.

Other authors have suggested that bad temper, just like patients with acquired prefrontal damage traits as cognitive inflexibility, emotional dysregulation, and impulsiveness (including impulsive aggression) is very common. Indicating that executive functions play an important role in the regulation of impulsive aggression, suggesting that it is the executive functions that play an important role in mediating the relationship between temper and aggression in men (Giancola, Roth, & Parrott, 2006). Hence, executive dysfunction found in aggressive impulsive people interferes with the ability to generate long-term goals, control, and monitor your own behavior (Villemarette-Pittman, Stanford, & Greve, 2002).

10.8 A Study Considering Violence as a Continuum

As previously mentioned, violent behavior has been associated with orbital functioning; however, other studies have reported fails related to dorsolateral functioning, probably related to antisocial components in violent behavior. To probe if findings reported in institutionalized samples are generalizable to non-institutionalized violent people, Díaz and Ostrosky (in press) evaluated a sample of 123 men, divided into non-violent controls (29 subjects) with low levels of aggression, hostility, anger, impulsiveness and traits of psychopathy from a community sample, a group of 30 violent individuals (not institutionalized), characterized by high levels of aggression, hostility, anger, impulsiveness, and psychopathy; and a group of 64 criminals that were identified as violent according to the offence such as homicide, injury, or attempted murder, kidnapping, or that exerted violence to the time of the crime (p. e. armed robbery). The results showed that there was an effect of the grouping variable (control, violent inmate, or violent from the community) in orbital ($F = 7.03$, $p = 0.002$) and dorsolateral ($F = 4.93$, $p = 0.010$) scores. Additionally, the control group had better orbitofrontal scores compared to both violent groups and only the violent inmate group had dorsolateral deficiencies (being the group with highest psychopathy scores) and suggesting a relationship between violence, psychopathy antisocial traits and low dorsolateral performance.

10.9 The Prefrontal Cortex and the Cognitive Mediation of Violent Behavior

The development of the prefrontal cortex has helped humans navigate a social system in which emphasizes cooperation, reciprocal altruism, and group living, which requires an efficient system that regulates violence (Raine, 2002). Since Phineas

Gage's case, it has been hypothesized that impairment in cognitive functions related to damage in the prefrontal cortex may lead to impulsiveness, poor planning, mental inflexibility, low verbal IQ, and deficiencies in attention, and predispose individuals to have feelings of frustration and anxiety, difficulty in emotional regulation and finally to an increase risk for violent behavior (Elliot & Mirsky, 2002). It has been proposed that functionally the orbitofrontal cortex and a region of the medial prefrontal cortex and anterior cingulate are part of the same system, since both regions are fundamental in the inhibition and the regulation of emotional states as well as in the regulation of aggression and violence (Kringelbach & Rolls, 2004; Ongür & Price, 2000). This network receives input from all sensory modalities and, on the other hand, outputs of processing systems that reacts to primary reinforces, also essential for learning the by association of stimuli reinforcer. The orbital cortex also receives projections with visceral information coming from various nuclei of the amygdala, anterior cingulate, and hippocampus (Kringelbach & Rolls, 2004).

On the other hand, psychopathy that is an additional factor frequently associated, but not equivalent to violence, has been neuropsychological described depending on the traits of this personality disorder. A study carried out in our laboratory pointed out (Díaz et al., 2013) that in criminal psychopaths there is a positive correlation between the number of maintenance errors from the WCST and the interpersonal factor of psychopathy (F1). Maintenance errors have been linked initially to problems of working memory (and short-term memory), as well as difficulties in the maintenance of attention. Tasks that require the use of working memory have been linked primarily with dorsolateral areas, while the maintenance of attention has been associated with superior medial areas (Fuster, 2008). Studies in psychopathic individuals suggest that the standard tests used to measure executive functions may not be sensitive enough to detect the ventral or orbital disorders relevant to aggression (Brower & Price, 2001).

Stuss and Alexander (2000) suggest that maintenance errors are related to a failure in the automatic processing and maintenance of attention. Factor 1 of psychopathy reflects interpersonal and affective components of the disorder which include callousness, inability to establish strong emotional bonds, lack of empathy, no guilt or remorse. These interpersonal and affective traits of psychopathy are more closely related to the functioning of the orbito-medial cortex, which could explain the relationship found between the number of maintenance errors and features interpersonal and affective of psychopathy, suggesting that these behavioral manifestations could be due to deficiencies in functioning of the orbito-medial cortex.

Dorsolateral failures in violent inmates have been reported less regularly in the literature as it is the case of the study previously cited Díaz et al. (2013) where psychopaths get lower scores in the dorsolateral performance-related tasks and also found a positive correlation between the percentage of high risk scores in the IGT and the factor 2 of psychopathy (antisocial traits). Decision-making based on emotional states has been previously reported in patients who have ventromedial damage (Bechara, Damasio, Tranel, & Damasio, 1997) expressing problems in risk-benefit processing, thus choosing a greater amount of high risk cards where preference is given to the immediate reward rather than delay it to get more benefits. The factor 2 of psychopathy that includes features such as the need for constant stimulation, the tendency to boredom, a parasitic lifestyle, unrealistic goals, impulsivity, irresponsibility, including a tendency to ignore or violating the conventions and social norms. A failure in risk-benefit processing could explain some of the features present in the factor 2 of psychopathy as irresponsibility and impulsiveness, presenting an increased risk of committing crimes, breaking social conventions without properly evaluating the possible consequences of their acts. The dorsolateral prefrontal cortex also participates in the mental representation of emotions and the regulation of these (Barrett, Mesquita, Ochsner, & Gross, 2007); the variation of its activation has been associated with this processing depending on the approach or avoidance that can cause the emotion (Harmon-Jones, 2003). During decision-making, category elements are brought to the "working memory," maintaining an active representation of memory over a period of delay that involves the dorsolateral prefrontal cortex area.

It has been reported that subjects with pre-frontal lesions and patients with Korsakoff's syndrome have difficulties in abstract categorization suggesting that failures in behavioral regulation contribute to the alteration in the resolution of problems in these patients (Delis, Squire, Bihrle, & Massman, 1992). Additionally, other authors have suggested that language deficiencies are related to impulsivity (Villemarette-Pittman et al., 2002). Taken this altogether, it is possible that the lack of a conceptual organization reflects executive problems associated with the functioning of the dorsolateral regions of the prefrontal cortex and not only to the deficiencies from the orbito-medial (Ostrosky, 2011, 2017; Romero, 2014). The deficit of the dorsolateral prefrontal cortex has been most frequently linked to antisocial disorder, where its malfunction can lead to impulsivity committing recidivism and breaking social conventions, often found in criminal populations (Raine & Yang, 2006).

In resume, it appears that neuropsychological deficiencies associated with orbito-medial functioning are a common characteristic in violent behavior samples and that the executive functioning linked to dorsolateral performance mediate the risk for violent acts. The difference between the violent sample from general population and the violent inmate sample seems to be the relative preservation of this executive "cold" control. Individuals from the community sample may have difficulties for regulating and inhibiting their own emotions but the executive supra-ordinate control related to dorsolateral regions could be compensating the orbital deficiencies, giving them enough cognitive strategies and resources for not breaking social rules and conventions. Recent studies have suggested the existence of a hierarchical control of the behavior where the rostral regions of the prefrontal cortex play an important role in the regulation of more caudal regions (Badre & Nee, 2018).

In future research, it would be important to implement a different strategy to explore the effect of these two factors on violent behavior, one of these strategies is the measurement of anti-social traits independently, since due to the high correlation between the scores obtained by the PCL-R it could mask the real effects of the factors of psychopathy on neuropsychological performance associated with violent behavior traits.

Funding This work was partially supported by PAPIIT UNAM (IN302016).

References

Adolphs, R., Gläscher, J., & Tranel, D. (2018). Searching for the neural causes of criminal behavior. *Proceedings of the National Academy of Sciences, 115*, 451–452. https://doi.org/10.1073/pnas.1720442115.

Alcázar, M., Verdejo, A., Bouso, J. C., & Bezos, L. (2010). Neuropsicología de la agresión impulsiva. *Revista de Neurología, 50*(5), 291–299.

Anderson, C., & Bushman, B. J. (2002). Human aggression. *Annual Review of Psychology, 53*, 27–51.

Andreu, J. M. (2009). Propuesta de un modelo integrador de la agresividad impulsiva y premeditada en función de sus bases motivacionales y socio-cognitivas. *Psicopatología Clínica Legal y Forense, 9*, 85–98.

Arias, N., & Ostrosky, F. (2008). Neuropsicología de la Violencia y sus Clasificaciones. *Revista Neuropsicología, Neuropsiquiatría y Neurociencias, 8*(1), 95–114.

Badre, D., & Nee, D. E. (2018). Frontal cortex and the hierarchical control of behavior. *Trends in Cognitive Sciences, 22*(2), 170–188. https://doi.org/10.1016/j.tics.2017.11.005.

Barratt, E., Stanford, M., Kent, T., & Felthous, A. (1997). Neuropsychological and cognitive psychophysiological substrates of impulsive aggression. *Biological Psychiatry, 41*(10), 1045–1061.

Barrett, B., Mesquita, K. N., Ochsner, J. J., & Gross, J. (2007). The experience of emotion. *Annual Review of Psychology, 58*, 373–403.

Bechara, A., Damasio, H., Tranel, D., & Damasio, A. (1997). Deciding advantageously before knowing the advantageous strategy. *Science, 257*, 1293–1295.

Brower, M. C., & Price, B. H. (2001). Neuropsychiatry of frontal lobe dysfunction in violent and criminal behavior: A critical review. *Journal of Neurology, Neurosurgery and Psychiatry, 71*, 720–726.

Caprara, G., Paciello, M., Gerbino, M., & Cugini, C. (2007). Individual differences conducive to aggression and violence: Trajectories and correlates of irritability and hostile rumination through adolescence. *Aggressive Behavior, 33*, 359–374.

Carrasco, M. A., & González, M. J. (2006). Aspectos conceptuales de la agresión: definición y modelos explicativos. *Acción Psicológica, 4*(2), 7–38.

Connor, D. F., Aderson, J. J., & Melloni, R. (2002). Gender differences in reactive and proactive aggression. *Child Psychiatry and Human Development, 33*(4), 279–294.

Darby, R., Horn, A., Cushman, F., & Fox, M. (2018). Lesion network localization of criminal behavior. *Proceedings of the National Academy of Sciences, 115*(3), 601–606. https://doi.org/10.1073/pnas.1706587115.

Delis, D. C., Squire, L. R., Bihrle, A., & Massman, P. (1992). Componential analysis of problem-solving ability: Performance of patients with frontal lobe damage and amnesic patients on a new sorting test. *Neuropsychologia, 30*(8), 683–697.

Díaz, K., & Ostrosky, F. (En prensa). Caracterización de la conducta violenta: un estudio de individuos violentos dentro y fuera de reclusorios.

Díaz, K. X., Ostrosky, F., & Camarena, B. (2012). Desempeño Neuropsicológico Prefrontal en Sujetos Violentos de la Población General. *Acta de Investigación Psicológica, 2*(1), 555–567.

Díaz, K. X., Ostrosky, F., Romero, C., & Pérez, M. (2013). Desempeño Neuropsicologico Orbitomedial en Psicópatas. *Neuropsicología, Neuropsiquiatría y Neurociencias, 13*(1), 43–58.

Díaz-Galván, K. X., Ostrosky-Shejet, F., & Romero-Rebollar, C. (2015). Cognitive and affective empathy: The role in violent behavior and psychopathy. *Revista Médica del Hospital General de México, 78*, 27–35.

Dolan, M., & Park, I. (2002). The neuropsychology of antisocial personality disorder. *Psychological Medicine, 32*(3), 417–427.

Elliot, A. K., & Mirsky, A. F. (2002). Cognitive antecedents of violence and aggression. *The Neurobiology of Criminal Behavior, 8*(3), 111–136.

Flores, J. C., Ostrosky, F., & Lozano, A. (2008). Batería de Funciones Frontales y Ejecutivas: Presentación. *Revista Neuropsicología, Neuropsiquiatría y Neurociencias, 8*(1), 141–158.

Fuster, J. M. (2008). *The prefrontal cortex* (4th ed.). London: Academic Press.
Giancola, P. R., Roth, R. M., & Parrott, D. J. (2006). The mediating role of executive functioning in the relation between difficult temperament and physical aggression. *Journal of Psychopathology and Behavioral Assessment, 28*(4), 211–221.
Gorenstein, E. E. (1982). Frontal lobe functions in psychopaths. *Journal of Abnormal Psychology, 91*(5), 368.
Hare, R. D. (1999). Psychopathy as a risk factor for violence. *The Psychiatric Quarterly, 70*(3), 181–197.
Hare, R. D. (2003). *Manual for the revised psychopathy checklist* (2nd ed.). Toronto, ON: Multi-Health Systems.
Hare, R. D., & Neumann, C. S. (2008). Psychopathy as a clinical and empirical construct. *Annual Review of Clinical Psychology, 4,* 217–246.
Harmon-Jones, E. (2003). Clarifying the emotive functions of asymmetrical frontal cortical activity. *Psychophysiology, 40,* 838–848.
Jolliffe, D., & Farrington, D. P. (2006). Examining the relationship between low empathy and bullying. *Aggressive Behavior, 32,* 540–550.
Kennealy, P. J., Skeem, J., Walters, G. D., & Camp, J. (2010). Do core interpersonal and affective traits of PCL-R psychopathy interact with antisocial behavior and disinhibition to predict violence? *Psychological Assessment, 22*(3), 569–580.
Kringelbach, M. L., & Rolls, E. T. (2004). The functional neuroanatomy of the human orbitofrontal cortex: Evidence from neuroimaging and neuropsychology. *Progress in Neurobiology, 72*(5), 341–372.
Meloy, J. R. (2006). Empirical basis and forensic application of affective and predatory violence. *The Australian and New Zealand Journal of Psychiatry, 40*(6–7), 539–547.
Merk, W., Orobio de Castro, B., Koops, W., & Matthys, W. (2005). The distinction between reactive and proactive aggression: Utility for theory, diagnosis and treatment? *European Journal of Developmental Psychology, 2*(2), 197–220.
Ongür, D., & Price, J. L. (2000). The organization of networks within the orbital and medial prefrontal cortex of rats, monkeys and humans. *Cerebral Cortex, 10*(3), 206–219.
Ostrosky, F. (2011). *Mentes Asesinas. La violencia en tu Cerebro*. ISBN 97860795535-2-4. Ed.Quinto Sol.2 edición.
Ostrosky, F. (2017). Conducta Violenta y sus Bases Biológicas: Neuroimagen, Neuropsicología, Electrofisiología y Genética. In E. García-López (Ed.), *Psicopatología Forense. Comportamiento Humano y Tribunales de Justicia.* México: Manual Moderno.
Ostrosky, F., & Ardila, A. (2018). *Neuropsychology of criminal behavior* (142 pp.). New York: Routledge, Taylor & Francis Group. ISBN 9781138092112.
Ostrosky-Solís, F., Esther Gómez-Pérez, M., Matute, E., Rosselli, M., Ardila, A., & Pineda, D. (2007). Neuropsi attention and memory: A neuropsychological test battery in Spanish with norms by age and educational level. *Applied Neuropsychology, 14*(3), 156–170.
Raine, A. (1997). *The psychopathology of crime: Criminal behavior as a clinical disorder*. New York: Academic press.
Raine, A. (2002). Psicopatía, violencia y neuroimagen. In A. Raine & J. Sanmartín (Comps.), *Violencia y psicopatía* (pp. 59–88). España: Ariel.
Raine, A., & Yang, Y. (2006). Neural foundations to moral reasoning and antisocial behavior. *Social cognitive and Affective Neuroscience, 1*(3), 203–213.
Ramírez, J. M., & Andreu, J. M. (2005). Aggression, and some related psychological constructs (anger, hostility, and impulsivity); some comments from a research project. *Neuroscience and Biobehavioral Reviews, 30*(3), 276–291.
Ramírez, J. M., Santisteban, C., Fujihara, T., & Van Goozen, S. (2002). Differences between experience of anger and readiness to angry action: A study of Japanese and Spanish students. *Aggressive Behavior, 28*(6), 429–438.
Romero. (2014). *Desempeño Neuropsicológico y Genes Asociados a la Conducta Violenta (Tesis Doctoral)*. Universidad Nacional Autónoma de México, Ciudad de México, México.

Stanford, M. S., Greve, K. W., & Gerstle, J. E. (1997). Neuropsychological correlates of self-reported impulsive aggression in a college sample. *Personality and Individual Differences, 23*(6), 961–965.

Stanford, M. S., Houston, R. J., Mathias, C. W., Villemarette-Pittman, N. R., Helfritz, L. E., & Conklin, S. M. (2003). Characterizing aggressive behavior. *Assessment, 10*(2), 183–190.

Stuss, D. T., & Alexander, M. P. (2000). Executive functions and the frontal lobes: A conceptual view. *Psychology Research, 63*(3), 289–298.

Villemarette-Pittman, N. R., Stanford, M. S., & Greve, K. W. (2002). Language and executive function in self-reported impulsive aggression. *Personality and Individual Differences, 34,* 1533–1544.

Walsh, Z., & Kosson, D. S. (2008). Psychopathy and violence: The importance of factor level interactions. *Psychological Assessment, 20*(2), 114–120.

Yang, M., Wong, S., & Coid, J. (2010). The efficacy of violence prediction: A meta-analytic comparison of nine risk assessment tools. *Psychological Bulletin, 136*(5), 740–767.

Chapter 11
Executive Control Guided by Context in Colombian Ex-Combatants

Carlos Tobón and David Pineda

11.1 Introduction

Cognitive neuroscience theories have been built around cognitive psychology models of information computational analogy of boxes and arrows and neuroimages related to controlled cognitive tasks which are administered in different experimental conditions, while electrical–magnetic brain signals are registered using advanced functional neuroimaging techniques (Forstmann, Ratcliff, & Wagenmakers, 2016; Forstmann, Wagenmakers, Eichele, Brown, & Serences, 2011; Sebastian, Forstmann, & Matzke, 2018). The different models for explaining the diversity of cognitive functions would include (1) the classical neurocognitive model that would hypothesize mind- and brain-linked functioning as some complex sets of encapsulated information processors (semantic, visual perception, phonologic loop, executive control, immediate memory, etc.) and (2) the functional connectionist model that would assume the relation between cognition and brain as several complex systems of interconnected nodules of basic information processing, such as priming, binding, sequencing, integrating, analyzing, synthetizing, coupling and deleting. These theoretical models recently have begun to focus on searching for explanation models related to brain processes involved in the social interaction, and the adaptation of individuals to different social environments, in peaceful and violent situations (Decety & Cowell, 2015; Forbes & Grafman, 2013; Yoder & Decety, 2018). In this way, when cognitive neuroscience models were constructed, the assumption of a restrictive intrinsic mechanism of internal (self) control over cognition and emotion would lead to the statement of a metaphysic circular metaphor of an inner causal entity: the

C. Tobón
Grupo Neuropsicología y Conducta—GRUNECO, Facultad de Medicina, Universidad de Antioquia UdeA, Calle 70 No. 52-21, Medellín, Colombia

D. Pineda (✉)
Grupo Neuropsicología y Conducta—GRUNECO, Facultad de Psicología, Universidad de San Buenaventura, Carrera 56 C # 51-90 Of 302B, Medellín, Colombia
e-mail: dpineda51@une.net.co

A. Ardila et al. (eds.), *Dysexecutive Syndromes*,
https://doi.org/10.1007/978-3-030-25077-5_11

central executive device. To break this tautological hypothesis, some interactive limited resources of internal (neurophysiological) and external (contextual) mechanisms should be admitted, which must compete for perceptual attention and programming control of actions, to get the adequate solving problem processes (Fernandez-Duque & Johnson, 2002).

Armed conflicts are special scenarios where human behavior could generate psychological and biological adaptations and display emotional exacerbation of violent behaviors, oriented to handle highly stressful conditions of this chaotic environment (Gallaway, Fink, Millikan, & Bell, 2012; Jakupcak et al., 2007; Taft et al., 2007). Exposure to multiple or chronic traumatic events can influence several domains, such as affect regulation and cognition, generating specific biases (Williams, 2006). Individuals exposed to traumatic events may exhibit different emotion recognitions (Marsh et al., 2008), novelty seeking behaviors, regardless of the consequences (Brazil et al., 2011) and a higher frequency of hard cognitive preconceptions (Heilbrun, 1982; Nelson & Trainor, 2007; Paschall, 2002).

Context and emotional processing may influence over the executive mechanisms, and then, over the interpretation of social perceptions and memory about the experiences, which would produce biased actions, with variations according the physical conditions (Fernandez-Duque & Johnson, 2002; Ibanez, Melloni, et al., 2012). These factors, in turn, are shaped by learned rules, social conventions and interactions typically identified as social cognition (Decety & Cowell, 2015; Eslinger, Moore, Anderson, & Grossman, 2011). To engage in such flexible behavior, our cerebral active circuitries must access the available contextual information to predict social meanings (e.g., others' intentions, feelings and behavior), based on previous experiences and their relevance for the situation (Melloni, Lopez, & Ibanez, 2014). Complex social skills would emerge from the complex interaction between the emotional processes and the executive controlling mechanisms that would regulate intricate actions, by competition for the available neurophysiological resources (Eslinger, 1998; Fernandez-Duque & Johnson, 2002; Grossmann, 2010). Contextual modulation of empathy may represent an adaptive advantage, making behavior more sensitive to different environmental conditions. Experiences acquired in a specific context, as armed conflict, could modify implicit and explicit emotional processes, favoring inadequate responses to a peaceful social context with probably unfair executive planning on the actions, which could be related the accessible neurophysiological resources of the orbitofrontal circuitries (OFC) (Forbes & Grafman, 2013).

Different social factors are involved in the Colombian armed conflict, including territorial conflicts, socioeconomic inequities, forced displacement and even cultural factors that have normalized violent behaviors. Across more than 50 years of army conflict, Colombia has nearly 7,265,072 victims of forced displacement and 11,140 victims of antipersonnel mines (Amnesty International Report 2017/18, 2018). This includes 363,374 victims of threats, 22,915 victims of sexual offenses, 167,809 victims of enforced disappearance. Violence in Colombia has been exerted by drug cartels, Marxist–Leninist guerrillas (e.g., FARC and ELN), paramilitary armies and national army forces, among other actors. The Colombian conflict is a great example of the inherent complexity of the sources, actors and effects of violence (Baez, Santamaría-García, & Ibáñez, 2019).

In this chapter, the main neurophysiological mechanisms involved in the identification of the contextual characteristics of the environment and its interaction with emotional information processes and executive controlling activities will be addressed. Likewise, the changes in processing of information related to participation in armed conflicts will be reviewed, focusing on neurophysiological executive control resources. Finally, the cognitive and behavioral changes generated in response to physiological adaptations under the war environment will be discussed.

11.2 Context Identification, Emotional Processing and Executive Control

One of the main characteristics of the human brain would lies in selecting and processing sensitive (input) information. These inputs that enter through each of the sensory pathways (visual, auditory, olfactory, gustatory and somatic sensation) must be (mandatory) processed. Once the input reaches the central nervous system, classification mechanisms are used to identify the relevance of the stimulus to assign enough attentional resources to this recognition process (Seeley et al., 2007). The inputs with high emotional content—either faces or affective images—would produce a greater activation of the cerebral areas involved in recognition and association processes, evidencing a higher level of appropriation of attentional resources; then, it is supposed that these kinds of information are prioritized at this first level of processing (Bayle & Taylor, 2010; Herrmann et al., 2008).

From the first approach, following the feedback theory, the response to an emotional stimulus generates an activation of cortical and subcortical structures, which have an important role in the generation of behavioral responses. There are enough evidences that the structures involve in this processing are the diencephalon, the neocortex, the thalamus, the hippocampus, the hypothalamus and cingulate gyrus (LeDoux, 2003; Phelps, 2006). Subsequently, the amygdala and the OFC have been added to this cataloged as visceral brain. According to this neurophysiological model, the cortical path obtains sensory information from the thalamus, which lets it to be processed by sensory neocortex circuitries, and later, the perceptual representation reaches the cingulate gyrus. On the other hand, another subcortical parallel way (sensations path) takes the information from the thalamus, interacts with the mammillary bodies of the hypothalamus and then, is projected to the cingulate gyrus through the anterior thalamus. This subcortical circuit is closed by the cingulate neurons that are projected to the hypothalamus through the hippocampus, using the fornix connections (Papez, 1995). Then, the emotionally charged stimulus is responsible for obtaining the available attentional resources, which would produce the perceptual process, to generate the conscious sensation and the related autonomic physiological response.

The recent neurophysiological data, based on studies of functional magnetic resonance images (fMRI), event-related potentials (ERPs) and magnetoencephalography (MEG), have let to determine those structures involved in the temporal course, the correlation between the emotional and recognition phases and other cognitive processes (Adolphs, 2002; Ibanez, Melloni, et al., 2012). Using these advanced neuroimages techniques, it has been identified that emotional information provides neurophysiological cues to cortical systems to construe some specific contexts, which are involved in the decision-making processes. Under stressful situations, the processing of emotional information could change the relevance of the stimuli, generating modulations in the interpretation of the scenarios, facilitating or not secondary adaptive decision making. These intentional actions also are modified by physical general conditions (exertion, exhaustion, sleep deprivation, illness, etc.) (Weippert et al., 2018).

11.2.1 Faces Recognition

In social interactions, an important amount of emotional information comes from the faces, so at the brain level there are two parallel specialized processes: (1) to identify the characteristics of identity (more related to the semantic component) and (2) to recognize facial expression (emotional recognition).

In the first step, the occipital cortex and the posterior temporal cortex are responsible for the perceptual processing of the stimuli. At the perceptual level, a greater activation of the visual cortex is observed in the presentation of faces with emotional expressions in comparison with the neutral ones. This pattern of activation occurs at both the level of the visual cortex in the occipital lobe (early processing) and the fusiform gyrus and inferior temporal sulcus (delayed processing) (Haxby, Hoffman, & Gobbini, 2000; Pessoa, 2010). Subsequently, the fusiform gyrus participates in the decoding of the identity of the face, and specifically it has seen the activation of an area of the cortex around this gyrus, which is activated more by the presentation of faces than objects, so it has been called the fusiform area of the faces (Kanwisher, McDermott, & Chun, 1997; Patterson, Nestor, & Rogers, 2007). For the recognition of personal identity and its semantic associations, such as the name and biographical information of the face, connections with structures of the anterior temporal lobe are required. In parallel, the superior temporal gyrus would be in charge of recognizing the changing characteristics of the faces, such as the kind of the gazes, the facial expressions, the movement of the lips, among others (Calder & Young, 2005). Finally, the OFC participates in the explicit identification of facial expression. This cortex shows greater activation when the subject is instructed in the specific identification of facial expression (Ghashghaei, Hilgetag, & Barbas, 2007).

The processing of emotional information in faces serves as a stage for the demonstration of how the brain, through the competition for neurophysiological attentional resources, filters the perceived information to prioritize the process with relevant information, which will be crucial in the organization of the intentional behaviors. In the processes of social interaction, this facilitation in the recognition of the faces allows the individual to identify facial expressions that indicate the friendliness of the other in front of the information that is being shared. Under more complex situations such as the war environment, these facial features could help in the recognition of the enemy, or the identification of threat signals in the other, leading to the modulation of behavioral responses depending on the signal identified. Modulations in identifying faces emotional characteristics observed in individuals with disorders such as autism, schizophrenia and psychopathy have been linked to abnormalities in social interaction of these individuals, helping to elucidate the role of this recognition in such interactions.

When multifaceted social interactions constitute the scenario, both people and multiple meaning environmental elements are presented together; then, another level of neurophysiological processing for these complex scenarios is required. As the neurophysiological resources are limited for all brain circuitries involved in the processing of social information, these complex situations should be edited by our brain as one scope image, and the final affective value depends on the interactions among all its elements (Weippert et al., 2018).

11.2.2 Affective Images Processing

In the processing of affective images, after basic characteristic identification in the primary sensory and associative areas, sensory information can follow two parallel routes for analysis, the subcortical or the cortical pathways. At the subcortical level, the sensory information is driven to the limbic structures where the valence of the stimuli is recognized (Purves et al., 2008). The amygdala has been implicated in the associative learning of inputs, using reward and punishment feedback, and the amygdala activation has been connected with experiments of induced fear (Davidson, Putnam, & Larson, 2000). This structure has a great connectivity pattern with the visual cortex, which facilitates the detection of stimuli with emotional relevance; Likewise, it presents afferent projections to the ventral visual pathway, which allows to enhance or decrease the response to the neural stimulus and thus exert a feedback effect (Swanson, 2003; Young, Scannell, Burns, & Blakemore, 1994). Additionally, some structures such as the hypothalamus, the basal ganglia and the nucleus basalis of Meynert produce intricate networks with the amygdala to associate the input recognitions with reward and punishment feedback, as well as with the autonomic responses, which function as bottom-up processes toward the prefrontal cortex, acting as behavior regulators (Passamonti et al., 2008; Phelps, 2006).

This cerebral mechanism for selecting information can be considered one of the processes that would explain how the affective information generates a limbic activation. In faces, facilitation toward specific facial expressions has been reported, mainly with negative valence, which would suggest that executive control guided by emotional modulations would occur even in early perceptual stages (Adolph, Meister, & Pause, 2013). The amygdala receives information from the pulvinar nucleus of the thalamus and the superior colliculus, and it is mainly activated by the emotional recognition, especially fear expressions (LeDoux, 2003). A similar phenomenon has been detected using stimuli that represent threats, which activate the same circuitries; thus, these evidences would reflect that negative valence of face recognition would facilitate the affective information process and the executive control of the responses (Coccaro, McCloskey, Fitzgerald, & Phan, 2007; LeDoux, 2012; McGaugh, 2004). An increase in this activation has been described in individuals with post-traumatic stress disorder (PTSD), which has been correlated with failures in cognition (attention, memory and executive control) and in social interactions (to avoid people, diminished participation in social activities, low emotional expression), evidencing how alterations in the perceptual recognition of emotional processes can be related to some cognitive and behavioral symptoms (Morey et al., 2012).

Then, during the information recognition, the limbic structures would generate responses of "emotional activation," which would trigger neurophysiological mechanism of frontal and insular structures related to the executive control of behavioral responses. Three mechanisms of interaction between the amygdala and the OFC have been described, which could contribute to the activation, recognition and modulation of emotional inputs, and then to the executive control of behaviors. The first mechanism would be a feedback path, which would modulate the perceptual representation, and it would participate in the tuning of attention to dispose resources on a specific characteristic of stimuli; a second mechanism allows the evocation of the conceptual knowledge of emotion through the stimulation of the hippocampal networks. Finally, the system would produce emotional controlled responses through connections with motor circuitries, including the basal nuclei and efferent visceral structures, among which hypothalamus/OFC networks would contribute to the identification and imitation of the emotional states of the other persons (Adolphs, 2002). These three mechanisms would represent an interconnected system of complex interactions among structures related to the different processes of emotional information, some of them related to social cognition and others involved in emotionally regulated responses.

11.2.3 Integration of Perceptual and Emotional Elements in the Generation of Contexts

In the cortical path of emotional processing, the driven information has the purpose of associating the elements of the facts in a general contextual frame (Adolphs, Damasio, Tranel, Cooper, & Damasio, 2000). In this process, the integration of sensory and spatial–temporal elements allows to delimit the interaction of the individual with his social environment. The anterior cortex of the cingulum (Medalla & Barbas, 2010), the insula (Singer, Critchley, & Preuschoff, 2009) and the prefrontal cortex (Ghashghaei et al., 2007) are the main structures involved in this step. The insula and the cortex of the cingulum are in charge of the constant updating of sensory information, integrating the conceptual elements with their episodic components, also coupling them with the active products of the subcortical pathway. Consequently, the cortex of the cingulate presents a large number of projections toward inhibitory structures such as the lateral hypothalamus, the gray periaqueductal substance and the parabrachial nuclei, possibly involved in the regulation of autonomic responses (Passamonti et al., 2008; Pessoa, 2010). This network would modulate affective, sensorimotor and cognitive components of the empathic process. In bottom-up processing, it would underlie components automatically elicited by affective arousal, emotional responses and basic understanding; during top-down processing, it would prompt executive controlled mechanisms in which the perceiver's motivation, memories, intentions and attitudes influence the extent of an empathic experience (Melloni et al., 2014).

Once the context interpretation is generated, the following step is integration of this information with other specific sensorial information, to actualize the scenario and determine the relevance of each information under the social contextual frame guidance. This idea is part of one of the most traditional psychological approaches, which assumed that some complex psychological phenomena are perceived as whole. For this step, the insula assumed the main role to integrate the interoceptive and exteroceptive stimuli now associated with the conjunction of the current context as a complete scope of work. Then, in the context model, the social complex environment is interpreted as a unified gestalt; then, in some social chaotic contexts, the social inputs would be proprietarily processed as threats, which would be related to the disposition of emotional resources for planed aggressive, defensive–evading responses. While, very organized, predictable and peaceful social context would be related to different emotional cognition with consequent probably well organized and refined behaviors in most of the people (Couto et al., 2012). The insula has multiples connections with frontal and temporal lobes, which would regulate the representational processes about others, especially those related to the feelings, which would confer a very important role inside of this entire social context model.

The prefrontal cortex would be responsible for integrating the social contextual information with the circuitries that would activate the programs and plans for the intentional and purposeful behaviors, providing the available neurophysiological pool of resources, a process known as a top-down executive control (Criaud, Wardak, Ben Hamed, Ballanger, & Boulinguez, 2012). Reversal learning experiments, in which emotional stimuli are nonpredictably shifted, according to the subject changes of responses to reward or punishment feedback, serve to exemplify the involvement of these structures in emotional processing and behavioral regulation. The mechanism underlying the modulation of the emotion and behavior is related to connections of inhibitory control from regions of the prefrontal cortex (especially the OFC) to the amygdala (Couto et al., 2012). In this sense, the structures involved in the generation of the context would use the emotional signals coming from the limbic system to modulate the interpretation of the complete situation. In cases of violent environments, the feelings and intentions of others are evaluated and biased as part of the threatening context. Then, the emotional signal is sorted by the cognition as part of an extreme dichotomy: friends and enemies/cares and threats, creating a social cognition without nuances. In these conditions, the emotional process is included rapidly by the context biases as part of the complete environment, following the principle of the cognitive economy (Tobón et al., 2015).

11.2.4 Emotional Regulation and Executive Control

The efficiency on the competition for executive control and emotional resources would derive in the construction of social perceptions, actions and experiences stores (Baez et al., 2013; Melloni et al., 2014). These factors in turn are bound by learned rules, social conventions and interaction, typically identified as social cognition (Eslinger et al., 2011).

Interacting with the process of emotional regulation, the executive control mechanisms would have a vital role. The neurophysiological resources are related to the activities of the intrinsic and bidirectional connections among the OFC, the medial prefrontal cortex (MPFC) and the frontal dorsolateral cortex (FDLC), which are mixed with subcortical limbic structures. The emotional information processed is obtained by the OFC to be integrated with cognitive information and context perception, to organize a controlled response according to the demands of the environment (Dougherty et al., 2004). In this step, the reciprocal communication between the anterior cortex of the cingulum, the insula and the OFC allows the processing of cognitive and sensory information and influences the motor inhibitory control, mainly to negative stimuli (Singer et al., 2009). Likewise, the anterior cortex of the cingulate provides a regulation on the hypothalamus, adapting the autonomic response, according to the input of cognitive and contextual information. A final information, mediated by the reward system, through GABAergic neurons of the basalis nucleus of Meynert, would guide the OFC neurophysiological resources to attach to the efficient and adequate response and rapidly to block the inadequate ones, according to the context (Barkley, 2001; Goldstein, Naglieri, Princiotta, & Otero, 2014; Rueda, Posner, & Rothbart, 2004). Then, executive control is assumed by contextual model as a pool of limited neurophysiological resources that allows one to adapt from situation to situation, depending upon the subject goals in each recognized context (Checa, Rodríguez-Bailón, & Rueda, 2008).

Frontal regions (OFC, MPFC and FDLC) are involved in the prediction of the meaning of actions based on the integration of contextual information with the coding and evocation of episodic learning. The prefrontal neurons present a fast adaptation to the context-dependent information with behavioral significance. The contextual modulation of the frontotemporal regions could influence and at the same time be influenced by the insula (Goldstein et al., 2014; Ibañez & Manes, 2012; Melloni et al., 2014). Because of its modulating role in affective activation and emotional response, as well as its interaction for emotional regulation, the social contextual network can affect the different affective, cognitive and behavioral components of individuals.

The anatomical structures related to the contextual social network are the same that allow the individuals to understand the differences between the diverse environmental conditions, triggering the correct processes to performance according to social demands. The processes occurs by activation of the orbital superior sulcus, which predicts and anticipates grounded on the perceived information, and guided by the contextual structure. During this activity, connections with temporal lobe, especially the hippocampus, amygdala and perirhinal cortex, let the generation of complex cognitive associations and categorizations, representing and generalizing the contextual information (Bar, 2004). Moreover, the para-hippocampal cortex generates processes of detection to distinguish familiar (previous experienced information) from unfamiliar data inside of the entire context (Checa et al., 2008).

The war environment would generate a modulated state of the activation of the perceptual structures before the recognition of the emotional information. In the relationship between the visual and emotional system, through communication between the superior colliculus and amygdala via the thalamus pulvinar, this modulation initially facilitates the identification of the characteristics of the visual stimuli, which is especially more effective in detecting emotional stimuli (e.g., negative valence), generating a greater relevance of this information on associative structures such as the insula and the anterior cortex of the cingulum. Likewise, through the amygdala and the associative areas, the prefrontal cortex would be activated for the construction of the behavioral response. The greater activation of the perceptual and associative areas, reflected in the greater relevance of the stimulus, produces biases in the behavioral response reflected in states of hypervigilance and poor cognitive control to regulate the affective areas.

11.3 Adaptive Responses Associated with the War's Context

As it was discussed previously, for social relationships, especially for social cognition representations, the contextual cues guide the cognitive predictions, which allow selecting the more adaptive responses to each community (Ibañez & Manes, 2012). These keys help each person to concentrate on the current information in order to choose rapidly the best adaptive behavior. In war environments, contextual elements can be modulated by emotional processing, leading to physiological adaptations of behavioral responses to stressful situations. Associated with these physiological changes have been described processes involved in both the generation of violent behaviors and pathological processes in ex-combatants such as anxiety, depression or PTSD, such as the adaptation to the war environment.

Some authors have discussed the role of cognitive biases that could contribute to aggressive behavior in ex-combatants. Through the description of the "survival model," these researchers have explained the activation of context-inappropriate cognitive processes in ex-combatants with PTSD. The authors exemplified how this population, by virtue of its previous threat exposure, could more easily recognize aversive (threatening) stimuli, even in the absence of real threatening stimuli. The characteristics of hypervigilance and sustained physiological reactivity before the stimuli would facilitate the production of the cognitive biases that lead to the aggressive behaviors (Chemtob, Novaco, Hamada, & Gross, 1997; Taft et al., 2015).

In Colombian ex-combatants, different cognitive and neurophysiological studies have been developed. In this population, chronic exposure to the war environment could reshape the emotional processing system so as to become more efficient for socially relevant cue. Two kinds of modulations could be expected in the war context; first, it could facilitate the identification of the adverse stimuli oriented toward the recognition of threatening situations. Also, modulations could be observed in the process of perceptual identification of neutral stimuli, attributing valences to them, as a compensatory mechanism aimed at reducing failures in recognition of aversive stimuli under conditions of ambiguity (Tobón et al., 2015; Trujillo, Valencia, et al. 2017).

In everyday social cognition contexts, facial emotional expressions involve an automatic, rapid shortcut to representation of the essential features of interpersonal communication and for understanding, acting and predicting social outcomes. ERP research has demonstrated early, automatic and unacquainted processing of emotion in faces, words and pictures (Ibanez, Urquina, et al., 2012). The N170 is a negative peak around 170 ms in the temporal–occipital regions (Bentin, Allison, Puce, Perez, & McCarthy, 1996), sourced in the superior temporal sulcus and the fusiform gyrus (two neural areas associated with face processing) (Deffke et al., 2007). Its amplitude is greater for human faces compared to objects or words. The N170 component has shown amplitude/latency modulation based on emotional variables (Escobar et al., 2013; Petroni et al., 2011). Thus, the N170 represents adequate neurocognitive marker of face recognition and valence processing, which has been also associated with social cognition and executive functions.

A research in our group, oriented to assess ERPs responses to emotional stimuli in Colombian ex-combatants with different empathy profiles (Normal and Low) and their relation to emotional and executive processing, using a modified version of the dual valence task (DVT), showed the expected N170 modulation for stimulus type in all groups, but modulation in ERP waveforms underlay face valence discrimination only in control (never combatant) but not in both normal empathy and low empathy ex-combatant groups (see Fig. 11.1), indicating that ex-combatants are impaired in cortical emotional processing, regardless of their dispositional empathy profiles (unpublished data yet).

Several studies have reported a stimulus type effect in the N170 amplitude (e.g., face > word) (Frühholz, Jellinghaus, & Herrmann, 2011; Holmes, Vuilleumier, & Eimer, 2003; Ibanez, Urquina, et al., 2012). However, against our predictions, we did not find significant statistical differences between group on faces and words discrimination (see Fig. 11.2). The implication of a preserved facial processing in ex-combatants is not entirely surprising; however, in a war environment, combatants need to promptly identify risky situations and alterations in facial discrimination would imply disadvantages for survival (Anaki, Brezniak, & Shalom, 2012; Miller & Litz, 2004). In the same vein, a previous report of our group (Tobón et al. 2015) with the same population had also shown unimpaired basic cortical responses to

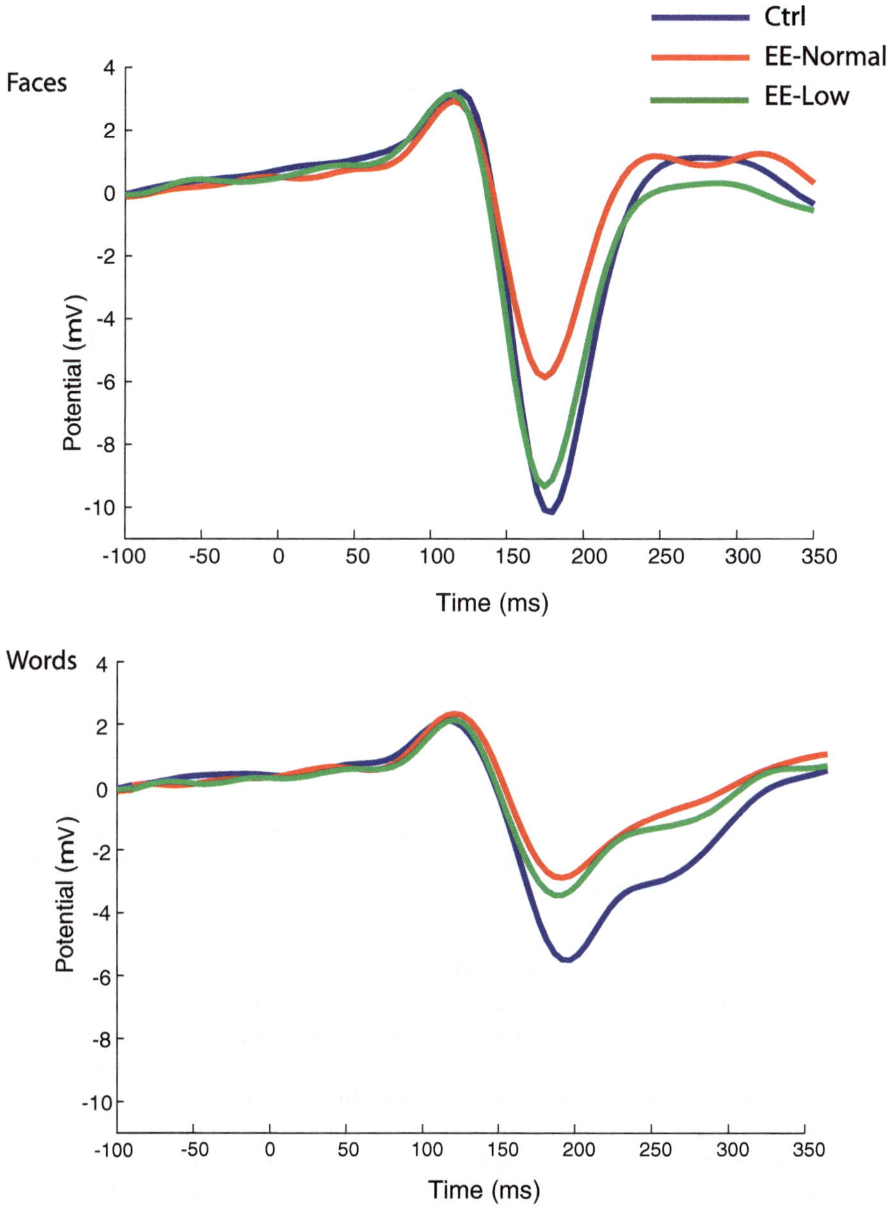

Fig. 11.1 Stimulus type (words and faces). Average waveforms in the right (P4) electrode for each group (normal-empathy ex-combatants EE-Normal, low-empathy ex-combatants EE-Low and Ctrl). Average waveforms were generated by taking the mean of each participant's waveform for each category (words and faces)

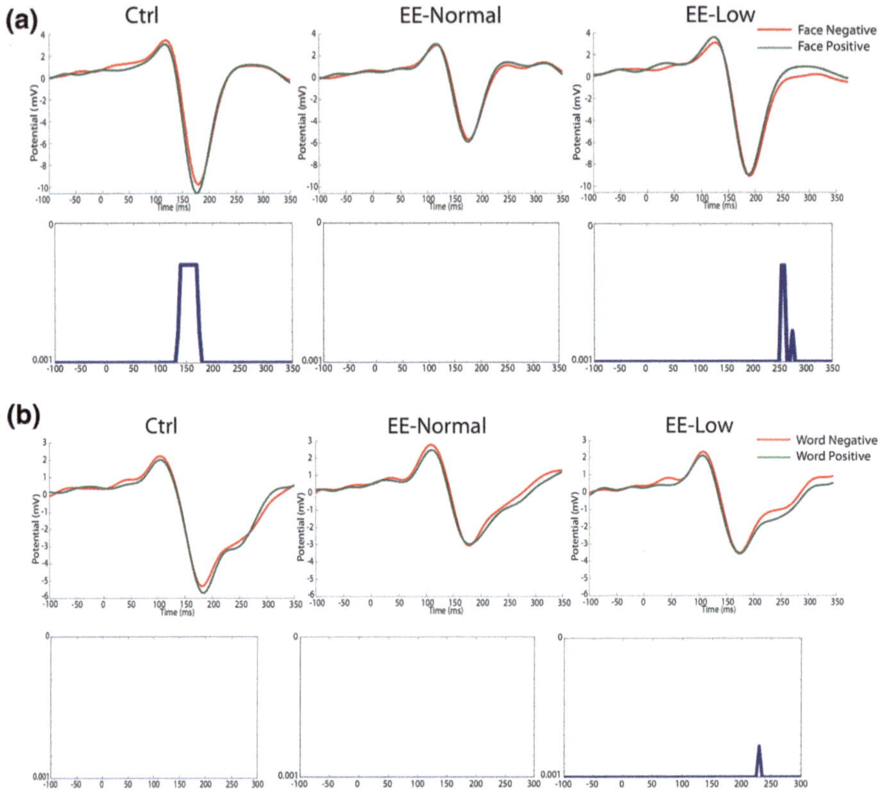

Fig. 11.2 Word and face valence. **a** and **b** display results for facial and lexical stimuli, respectively. The upper row in each one shows the mean amplitude of each valence (positive and negative) among groups. The bottom row shows the permutation results

other stimuli (scenarios), suggesting that preserved rapid stimulus processing in ex-combatants could represent an adaptation to violent environments.

In this study, cognitive, electrophysiological and correlational results suggest different neurocognitive profiles for each group (see Fig. 11.3). Dimensional and group correlations are consistent with previous findings, suggesting that self-reported empathy goes along with enhanced processing of emotion in social stimuli (Kanske, Schönfelder, & Wessa, 2013). Normal empathy ex-combatants showed impairments in executive control that were associated with N170 modulations to face valence. Such executive dysfunctions could be reflected in nonplanning actions, poor consequence evaluation and emotional oriented behavior (Criaud et al., 2012). Conversely, low-empathy ex-combatants could understand the pain and feelings of others but failed to identify with them. In other words, they exhibited normal cognitive empathy and abnormal emotional empathy (Pineda et al., 2013). Moreover, affective empathy in this group was associated with a specific pattern of abnormal N170 modulations to face valence. Populations with instrumental aggression exhibit similar patterns

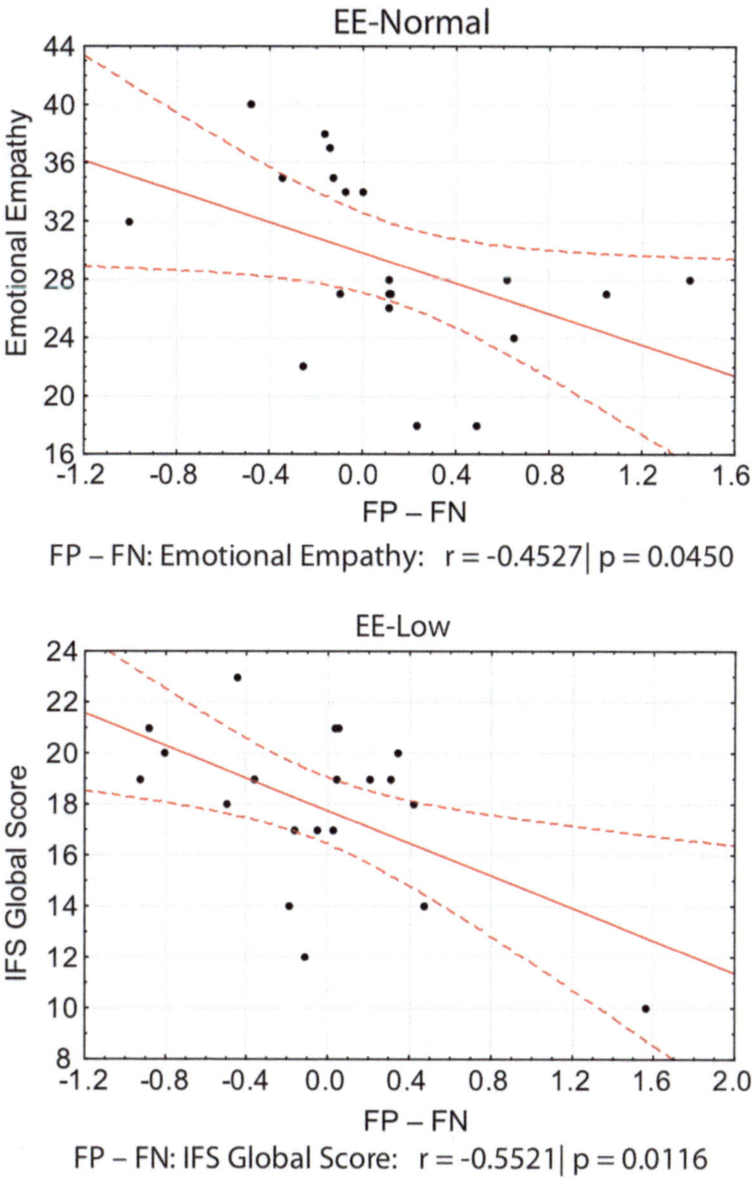

Fig. 11.3 Groups correlations. For each of the ex-combatant groups, the scatterplot graph shows significant effects between cortical measures of face valence and individual cognitive profiles (emotional empathy and executive functions)

of poor or normal executive functions but low personal distress (Barratt, Stanford, Dowdy, Liebman, & Kent, 1999). By the same token, absent N170 valence modulation in low-empathy ex-combatants could reflect a subtle involvement of dispositional affective empathy. In brief, normal-empathy ex-combatants may exhibit poor executive functioning and abnormal N170 modulation as a possible consequence of general lenient impairments in frontal functions. In turn, low-empathy ex-combatants would be characterized by empathy abnormalities and absent neural differentiation of emotional processing.

Emotional inference of facial clues is one of the most important steps in the development of social cognition behaviors. Successful social interaction depends on the ability to infer other people's emotions, beliefs and intentions based on their emotional facial and bodily language (de Gelder et al., 2010). Moreover, empathy, emotional inference and social cognition intertwine during social cognition processes. Consistent with these observations, in this study N170 modulations to face valence were inversely correlated with emotional empathy: Impairments in cortical markers of face valence were associated with poor emotional empathy profile. Similarly, other studies have found N170 valence modulations associated with affective empathy traits (Soria Bauser, Thoma, & Suchan, 2012). Brain–behavior associations among different affective processes show a convergent pattern along the individuals.

Studies in different populations suggest that facial processing is required for several high-level social executive skills. In healthy participants, the cognitive and affective dimensions of theory of mind (as well as executive performance) were predicted by the N170 valence discrimination (positive/negative), suggesting that basic social cognition processes are supported, at least in part, by early brain activity that is sensitive to facial emotional valence (Petroni et al., 2011). Similar results are observed in clinical populations with bipolar disorder, ADHD and schizophrenia families (Ibáñez et al., 2014). Here, we suggest that failures in cortical markers of N170 emotional modulation can be associated with poor empathic response and executive dysfunctions in ex-combatants. This model could serve as a theoretical basis to explain the observed correlation between facial valence N170 modulations and emotional empathy.

Semantic recognition refers to the ability to assign and use the meanings of words and other stimuli. This capacity relies on both stored semantic knowledge (semantic representations) and executive control mechanisms that shape semantic activation in line with current goals and constraints (semantic control). In this line, inverse correlations between cortical activity for words and executive function (the more negative the N170, the better the executive performance) could reflect the important role of frontal lobe in semantic processing. Impairments in executive control have direct effects on different components of semantic recognition (Whitney, Kirk, O'Sullivan, Ralph, & Jefferies, 2012) and on cortical responses to semantic emotional stimuli (Ibáñez et al., 2014).

Consistent with previous reports (Eder, 2011; Hartley, Jonides, & Sylvester, 2011; Ibanez, Urquina, et al., 2012; Petroni et al., 2011), we found N170 emotional modulations in never-combatant controls but not in ex-combatants. Emotional facial expressions play a crucial role in social interaction. For instance, angry faces activate the human fear system and modulate human behavior (Mühlberger et al., 2009). Impairments in this domain have been associated with abnormal behaviors, such as poor social adaptation (Criaud et al., 2012). An ERP study examined the neural and personality correlates of processing infant facial expressions in mothers with substantiated neglect (Rodrigo et al., 2011). As opposed to control mothers, neglectful mothers did not exhibit increased N170 amplitude at temporal leads for crying than for laughing and neutral. Similar absent neural markers of emotional processing (N170 face valence effect) are observed in subjects with attachment problems (Escobar et al., 2013). In this population, brain failures in valence discrimination could be correlated with social anhedonia (Rodrigo et al., 2011). In special conditions, changes in valence recognition could be reflected in both top-down and bottom-up regulation processes. In physicians, not modulation of early N110 between pain and no-pain stimuli (over the frontal area or late P3 over the centroparietal regions) was observed. Those results could indicate that emotion regulation in physicians inhibited bottom-up processing of the perception of pain in others. Down-regulation of negative arousal in response to the pain of others may have many beneficial consequences, including the release of cognitive resources necessary for being of assistance (Decety, 2010).

We speculate that changes in cortical valence processing may be necessary to deal with salient emotional stimuli during combat. Stress conditions in war environments could induce adaptations in emotional processing and modulate the identification and reactivity against facial valence. Thus, different levels of cortical emotional processing (for faces vs. scenarios) seem to be affected in ex-combatants regardless of their level of dispositional empathy. Nevertheless, individual differences in both empathy levels and executive functions seem to be related to these cortical abnormalities.

In a similar population, a study explored the relationship between emotional processing modulation and social cognition and behavior patterns using an ERPs design with an emotional recognition task for faces and words (Trujillo, Valencia, et al. 2017). In this paper, ex-combatants presented higher assertion skills and showed more salient brain responses to faces than controls and no bias toward anger was observed in ex-combatants. Again, the relationship between emotional processing and the social cognition and behavior components of ex-combatants shows patterns of adaptation associated with the war environment.

Besides, the identification of the perceptual characteristics of the emotional stimuli also in the subsequent processes associated with this recognition could present significant differences between never combatant and ex-combatant groups. The relevance given to emotional information by the control mechanisms is another possible target for modulation of the war environment in the individual.

Using an ERPs experiment, an adequate discrimination of the emotional stimuli in the subjects, in relation to their valence, was evidenced, both in the behavioral data and in the modulation of the amplitude of the EPN-evoked potential; then, changes in the networks involved in the identification of the valence of the stimuli were not demonstrated. However, differences were found in the relevance that these stimuli had on the generation of contexts and associated behavioral responses, a phenomenon evaluated through the differences in the amplitude of the ERP named late posterior potential (LPP). (Tobón et al., 2015). Similar effects have been described in war veterans with and without posttraumatic stress disorder (PTSD) who present an attentional bias reflected in an attenuated frontal P3 response to neutral target and increased response to trauma-relevant combat stimuli (Stanford, Vasterling, Mathias, Constans, & Houston, 2001); also an enhanced P3 and N1 amplitudes in the PTSD patients in nontarget combat-related pictures and prolonged P3 latencies have been reported (Attias, Bleich, Furman, & Zinger, 1996). In this sense, although speculative, combat environment could produce a high reactivity to emotional salience, for all positive, negative and neutral valences, which would result from a perceptual bias in processing information. This bias would be the result of biological adaptations to deal with the stressing conditions of war environment. Also, high reactivity could facilitate changes in responses to social situations, affecting empathy processes.

In Colombia, an important characteristic of the armed conflict was a very lack of empathy for the enemy, led by social/ideological/political biases, which could explain why the combatants committed acts of extreme violence, brutality and cruelty, like enforced disappearances, murders, massacres, quarters and tortures (Maguen et al., 2009). These characteristics on the social representations associated with the war environment could not only generate changes in the emotional processing system, but also in the different cognitive and behavioral processes of the ex-combatants (Anaki et al., 2012).

11.4 Cognitive and Behavioral Profile in Colombian Ex-Combatants

Contextual modulation of empathy may represent an adaptive advantage, making behavior more sensitive to different environmental conditions. To perform this flexible behavior, our brain must access the available contextual information to predict the social meaning (e.g., others' intentions, feelings and behavior) based on previous experiences and the relevance of the specific situation (Melloni et al., 2014). Complex social skills are dependent of emotional and executive control processes (Eslinger, 1998; Grossmann, 2010). Changes in sociocultural environments related to extremely brutal armed conflicts would be reflected in a different process of social information and emotional recognition, favoring inadequate responses to a peaceful social context, which would be determined by contextual learned biases. Thus, cognitive strategies and executive control would be strongly associated with both emotional processing and social cognition.

Individuals involved in an armed conflict would tend to generate biological and psychological adaptations aimed at dealing with the adverse conditions of the war environment. These environments would generate situations of chronic stress resulting from the hostile environment, in which the rapid identification of the stimuli, as well as the response generated before processing, is necessary to produce their coupling to the environment. The complex effect, caused by the exposition to these multiples and chronic adverse traumatic events, could affect several domains such as affect regulation, behavioral control and cognition (Williams, 2006). Deficits in recognizing emotional expressions (Marsh et al., 2008; Petroni et al., 2011), the propensity to seek rewarding stimuli with little or none concern over the consequences (Brazil et al., 2011) and a high frequency of cognitive deficits especially at inhibitory control, complex ideational reasoning and working memory (Heilbrun, 1982; Nelson & Trainor, 2007; Paschall, 2002) have been reported. In ex-combatants of the Colombian armed conflict, worse performance in executive control and low scores in the personal distress component in the empathic domain, compared to a control group, were described. This low performance in executive resources could reflect patterns of poor inhibitory control, as well as difficulties in planning, motor programming and complex ideological reasoning (Tobón et al., 2016).

The modulations in the empathic components could be more related to the generation of strategies to face the actions that should be taken in the combat environment. An exploration of the different empathy dimensions of Colombian ex-combatants, through the Interpersonal Reactivity Index (IRI), showed changes in these subjects in relation to controls (Tobón et al., 2016). The described IRI's profile shows a reduction in the component of personal distress, with a preservation of the other domains (fantasy, empathic concern and perspective taking). This profile could mean that the subjects would have the ability to understand the point of view, the pain and the affective state of the other, but with a low impact of these elements in the social decision making, which would involve the relationship with the other and could explain the alteration in the prosocial behaviors of these individuals, probably related to their irregular military training and combat experiences. This poor emphatic feature could be an enabling factor of the violent behaviors, developed in the war environment, a phenomenon known as callous unemotional traits syndrome (Marsh et al., 2008).

The cognitive effect of the perceptual bias produced by modulation in emotional processing (explained above), associated with a low sociocultural level and poor performance on the executive control tasks, becomes a risk factor for the generation of behaviors with a high propensity to search for dangerous novelty, manifesting behaviors such as substance abuse/dependence (SAD) and violent criminal behavior. In Colombian ex-combatant population, these deviated comportments were frequently found using rating scales and structured psychiatric interviews (Ramos et al., 2018).

For psychiatric profile, these contextual associations are related to neurophysiological changes in the cortical networks involved in social interaction. This network would affect the different affective, sensitive-motor and cognitive components of the empathic process at bottom-up (components automatically elicited by affective arousal, emotional responses and basic understanding) and top-down (controlled processes in which the perceiver's motivation, memories, intentions and attitudes influence the extent of an empathic experience) information processing. In a study oriented to assess the effect of PTSD on volumetric changes in the amygdala and hippocampus, and the contribution of illness duration, trauma load and depressive symptoms, comparing a group of veterans with posttraumatic stress disorder (PTSD) versus a control group, significant statistical structural differences were found in the amygdala volumes (Brown & Morey, 2012; Morey, Petty, Cooper, Labar, & McCarthy, 2008). In this study, the lack of correlation between trauma load and amygdala volumes suggests that changes in amygdala volumes could be implied in impairments in social interactions associated with war environment exposition. Another study in a similar population showed that scores in Clinician-Administered PTSD Scale scores were inversely correlated with volumes of the subgenual cingulate, caudate, hypothalamus, insula and left middle temporal gyrus (Herringa, Phillips, Almeida, Insana, & Germain, 2012). Similarly, impairments in salience network have been associated with postwar exposition conditions in veterans and it was associated with patterns of PTSD (Sripada et al., 2012). Since PTSD is one of the main disorders observed in veterans, alteration of structures involved in the contextual network suggests that these possible changes may also be involved in emotional processing deficits in ex-combatants.

Another possible effect of modulation in contextual context networks would be related to the expression of violent behaviors and antisocial personality disorder (ASPD). In a sample of Colombian ex-combatants with ASPD and a control group, the cortical activity patterns were evaluated through the quantitative electroencephalogram (qEEG) (Ramos et al., 2018). In this work, a higher prevalence of ASPD (68.4%) and a greater spectral power of the alpha-2 and beta frequency bands were identified in the ex-combatants with ASPD than the controls. These different modulations in the brain electrical activity had a direct significant correlation with 16/20 items of the structured Psychopathy Checklist-Revised (PCL-R) interview, which would support the theory that the adaptative behaviors generated under war environments could have a physiological substratum over the networks of emotional processing and executive control (Ramos et al., 2018; Tobón et al., 2015).

11.5 Conclusions

Several raising set of evidences about the emotional processing and their impact on executive control mechanisms, to generate contextual perceptual biases, related to the production of adaptive responses in a war environment of the Colombian ex-combatant have been briefly summarized. These biases could represent strong determinant features of cognition and behavior of this specific population with executive and empathic dysregulations, which have been found associated with psychopathological problems, such as PTSD, depression, anxiety, SAD, ASPD and violent criminal behaviors.

The description of contextual modulations as a crucial mechanism of emotional processing and executive control opens a new frame for therapeutic approaches, focused on the intervention of social, cognitive and affective processes. That would let to integrate strategies to assess multilevel (social, cultural, political, biological and neurocognitive) perspectives (Baez et al., 2019).

The reviewed evidences would demonstrate that the modulations in the cognitive and emotional mechanisms are related to threatening context of the war environments. Given that social cognitive abilities allow individuals to process emotional information, interpret and predict the consequences of an action, and determine an appropriate response in different contexts of daily life, it is necessary to guarantee an adequate functioning of these skills to assure the return to the civilian life of the ex-combatants (Baez et al., 2019). Then, the interventions should consider the contextual conditions in which the violence has arisen for evaluating interpersonal and intrapersonal factors that could promote violent behavior. At this level, it would be reasonable that mental training treatments should be related to the different cognitive and social skills and promotion of personal abilities for emotional regulation and executive control (Baez et al., 2019; Tobón et al., 2016; Trujillo, Trujillo, et al. 2017; Trujillo, Valencia, et al. 2017).

References

Adolph, D., Meister, L., & Pause, B. M. (2013). Context counts! Social anxiety modulates the processing of fearful faces in the context of chemosensory anxiety signals. *Frontiers in Human Neuroscience, 7,* 283. https://doi.org/10.3389/fnhum.2013.00283.

Adolphs, R. (2002). Neural systems for recognizing emotion. *Current Opinion in Neurobiology, 12*(2), 169–177. https://doi.org/10.1016/S0959-4388(02)00301-X.

Adolphs, R., Damasio, H., Tranel, D., Cooper, G., & Damasio, A. R. (2000). A role for somatosensory cortices in the visual recognition of emotion as revealed by three-dimensional lesion mapping. *The Journal of Neuroscience: The Official Journal of the Society for Neuroscience, 20*(7), 2683–2690.

Anaki, D., Brezniak, T., & Shalom, L. (2012). Faces in the face of death: Effects of exposure to life-threatening events and mortality salience on facial expression recognition in combat and noncombat military veterans. *Emotion (Washington, D.C.), 12*(4), 860–867. https://doi.org/10.1037/a0029415.

Attias, J., Bleich, A., Furman, V., & Zinger, Y. (1996). Event-related potentials in post-traumatic stress disorder of combat origin. *Biological Psychiatry, 40*(5), 373–381. https://doi.org/10.1016/0006-3223(95)00419-X.

Baez, S., Herrera, E., Villarin, L., Theil, D., Gonzalez-Gadea, M. L., Gomez, P., … Ibañez, A. M. (2013). Contextual social cognition impairments in schizophrenia and bipolar disorder. *PloS One, 8*(3), e57664. https://doi.org/10.1371/journal.pone.0057664.

Baez, S., Santamaría-García, H., & Ibáñez, A. (2019). Disarming ex-combatants' minds: Toward situated reintegration process in post-conflict Colombia. *Frontiers in Psychology, 10,* 73. https://doi.org/10.3389/fpsyg.2019.00073.

Bar, M. (2004). Visual objects in context. *Nature Reviews Neuroscience, 5*(8), 617–629. https://doi.org/10.1038/nrn1476.

Barkley, R. A. (2001). The executive functions and self-regulation: An evolutionary neuropsychological perspective. *Neuropsychology Review, 11*(1), 1–29. https://doi.org/10.1023/A:1009085417776.

Barratt, E. S., Stanford, M. S., Dowdy, L., Liebman, M. J., & Kent, T. A. (1999). Impulsive and premeditated aggression: A factor analysis of self-reported acts. *Psychiatry Research, 86*(2), 163–173.

Bayle, D. J., & Taylor, M. J. (2010). Attention inhibition of early cortical activation to fearful faces. *Brain Research, 1313,* 113–123. https://doi.org/10.1016/j.brainres.2009.11.060.

Bentin, S., Allison, T., Puce, A., Perez, E., & McCarthy, G. (1996). Electrophysiological studies of face perception in humans. *Journal of Cognitive Neuroscience, 8*(6), 551–565. https://doi.org/10.1162/jocn.1996.8.6.551.

Brazil, I. A., Mars, R. B., Bulten, B. H., Buitelaar, J. K., Verkes, R. J., & De Bruijn, E. R. A. (2011). A neurophysiological dissociation between monitoring one's own and others' actions in psychopathy. *Biological Psychiatry, 69*(7), 693–699. https://doi.org/10.1016/j.biopsych.2010.11.013.

Brown, V. M., & Morey, R. A. (2012). Neural systems for cognitive and emotional processing in posttraumatic stress disorder. *Frontiers in Psychology, 3,* 449. https://doi.org/10.3389/fpsyg.2012.00449.

Calder, A. J., & Young, A. W. (2005). Understanding the recognition of facial identity and facial expression. *Nature Reviews Neuroscience, 6*(8), 641–651. https://doi.org/10.1038/nrn1724.

Checa, P., Rodríguez-Bailón, R., & Rueda, M. R. (2008). Neurocognitive and temperamental systems of self-regulation and early adolescents' social and academic outcomes. *Mind, Brain, and Education, 2*(4), 177–187. https://doi.org/10.1111/j.1751-228X.2008.00052.x.

Chemtob, C. M., Novaco, R. W., Hamada, R. S., & Gross, D. M. (1997). Cognitive-behavioral treatment for severe anger in posttraumatic stress disorder. *Journal of Consulting and Clinical Psychology, 65*(1), 184–189.

Coccaro, E. F., McCloskey, M. S., Fitzgerald, D. A., & Phan, K. L. (2007). Amygdala and orbitofrontal reactivity to social threat in individuals with impulsive aggression. *Biological Psychiatry, 62*(2), 168–178. https://doi.org/10.1016/j.biopsych.2006.08.024.

Couto, B., Sedeño, L., Sposato, L. A., Sigman, M., Riccio, P. M., Salles, A., … Ibanez, A. (2012). Insular networks for emotional processing and social cognition: Comparison of two case reports with either cortical or subcortical involvement. *Cortex; a Journal Devoted to the Study of the Nervous System and Behavior*. https://doi.org/10.1016/j.cortex.2012.08.006.

Criaud, M., Wardak, C., Ben Hamed, S., Ballanger, B., & Boulinguez, P. (2012). Proactive inhibitory control of response as the default state of executive control. *Frontiers in Psychology, 3*. https://doi.org/10.3389/fpsyg.2012.00059.

Davidson, R. J., Putnam, K. M., & Larson, C. L. (2000). Dysfunction in the neural circuitry of emotion regulation—A possible prelude to violence. *Science (New York, N.Y.), 289*(5479), 591–594.

de Gelder, B., Van den Stock, J., Meeren, H. K. M., Sinke, C. B. A., Kret, M. E., & Tamietto, M. (2010). Standing up for the body. Recent progress in uncovering the networks involved in the perception of bodies and bodily expressions. *Neuroscience and Biobehavioral Reviews, 34*(4), 513–527. https://doi.org/10.1016/j.neubiorev.2009.10.008.

Decety, J. (2010). The neurodevelopment of empathy in humans. *Developmental Neuroscience, 32*(4), 257–267. https://doi.org/10.1159/000317771.

Decety, J., & Cowell, J. M. (2015). Empathy, justice, and moral behavior. *AJOB Neuroscience, 6*(3), 3–14. https://doi.org/10.1080/21507740.2015.1047055.

Deffke, I., Sander, T., Heidenreich, J., Sommer, W., Curio, G., Trahms, L., et al. (2007). MEG/EEG sources of the 170-ms response to faces are co-localized in the fusiform gyrus. *NeuroImage, 35*(4), 1495–1501. https://doi.org/10.1016/j.neuroimage.2007.01.034.

Dougherty, D. D., Rauch, S. L., Deckersbach, T., Marci, C., Loh, R., Shin, L. M., … Fava, M. (2004). Ventromedial prefrontal cortex and amygdala dysfunction during an anger induction positron emission tomography study in patients with major depressive disorder with anger attacks. *Archives of General Psychiatry, 61*(8), 795–804. https://doi.org/10.1001/archpsyc.61.8.795.

Eder, A. B. (2011). Control of impulsive emotional behaviour through implementation intentions. *Cognition and Emotion, 25*(3), 478–489. https://doi.org/10.1080/02699931.2010.527493.

Escobar, M. J., Rivera-Rei, A., Decety, J., Huepe, D., Cardona, J. F., Canales-Johnson, A., … Ibañez, A. (2013). Attachment patterns trigger differential neural signature of emotional processing in adolescents. *PloS One, 8*(8), e70247. https://doi.org/10.1371/journal.pone.0070247.

Eslinger, P. J. (1998). Neurological and neuropsychological bases of empathy. *European Neurology, 39*(4), 193–199.

Eslinger, P. J., Moore, P., Anderson, C., & Grossman, M. (2011). Social cognition, executive functioning, and neuroimaging correlates of empathic deficits in frontotemporal dementia. *The Journal of Neuropsychiatry and Clinical Neurosciences, 23*(1), 74–82. https://doi.org/10.1176/appi.neuropsych.23.1.74.

Fernandez-Duque, D., & Johnson, M. L. (2002). Cause and effect theories of attention: The role of conceptual metaphors. *Review of General Psychology, 6*(2), 153–165. https://doi.org/10.1037/1089-2680.6.2.153.

Forbes, C. E., & Grafman, J. (2013). Social neuroscience: The second phase. *Frontiers in Human Neuroscience, 7*. https://doi.org/10.3389/fnhum.2013.00020.

Forstmann, B. U., Ratcliff, R., & Wagenmakers, E.-J. (2016). Sequential sampling models in cognitive neuroscience: Advantages, applications, and extensions. *Annual Review of Psychology, 67*, 641–666. https://doi.org/10.1146/annurev-psych-122414-033645.

Forstmann, B. U., Wagenmakers, E.-J., Eichele, T., Brown, S., & Serences, J. T. (2011). Reciprocal relations between cognitive neuroscience and formal cognitive models: Opposites attract? *Trends in Cognitive Sciences, 15*(6), 272–279. https://doi.org/10.1016/j.tics.2011.04.002.

Frühholz, S., Jellinghaus, A., & Herrmann, M. (2011). Time course of implicit processing and explicit processing of emotional faces and emotional words. *Biological Psychology, 87*(2), 265–274. https://doi.org/10.1016/j.biopsycho.2011.03.008.

Gallaway, M. S., Fink, D. S., Millikan, A. M., & Bell, M. R. (2012). Factors associated with physical aggression among US army soldiers. *Aggressive Behavior, 38*(5), 357–367. https://doi.org/10.1002/ab.21436.

Ghashghaei, H. T., Hilgetag, C. C., & Barbas, H. (2007). Sequence of information processing for emotions based on the anatomic dialogue between prefrontal cortex and amygdala. *NeuroImage, 34*(3), 905–923. https://doi.org/10.1016/j.neuroimage.2006.09.046.

Goldstein, S., Naglieri, J. A., Princiotta, D., & Otero, T. M. (2014). Introduction: A history of executive functioning as a theoretical and clinical construct. In S. Goldstein & J. A. Naglieri (Eds.), *Handbook of executive functioning* (pp. 3–12). New York, NY: Springer. https://doi.org/10.1007/978-1-4614-8106-5_1.

Grossmann, T. (2010). The development of emotion perception in face and voice during infancy. *Restorative Neurology and Neuroscience, 28*(2), 219–236. https://doi.org/10.3233/RNN-2010-0499.

Hartley, A. A., Jonides, J., & Sylvester, C.-Y. C. (2011). Dual-task processing in younger and older adults: Similarities and differences revealed by fMRI. *Brain and Cognition, 75*(3), 281–291. https://doi.org/10.1016/j.bandc.2011.01.004.

Haxby, Hoffman, & Gobbini. (2000). The distributed human neural system for face perception. *Trends in Cognitive Sciences, 4*(6), 223–233.

Heilbrun, A. B. (1982). Cognitive models of criminal violence based upon intelligence and psychopathy levels. *Journal of Consulting and Clinical Psychology, 50*(4), 546–557. https://doi.org/10.1037/0022-006X.50.4.546.

Herringa, R., Phillips, M., Almeida, J., Insana, S., & Germain, A. (2012). Post-traumatic stress symptoms correlate with smaller subgenual cingulate, caudate, and insula volumes in unmedicated combat veterans. *Psychiatry Research, 203*(2–3), 139–145. https://doi.org/10.1016/j.pscychresns.2012.02.005.

Herrmann, M. J., Huter, T., Plichta, M. M., Ehlis, A.-C., Alpers, G. W., Mühlberger, A., et al. (2008). Enhancement of activity of the primary visual cortex during processing of emotional stimuli as measured with event-related functional near-infrared spectroscopy and event-related potentials. *Human Brain Mapping, 29*(1), 28–35. https://doi.org/10.1002/hbm.20368.

Holmes, A., Vuilleumier, P., & Eimer, M. (2003). The processing of emotional facial expression is gated by spatial attention: Evidence from event-related brain potentials. *Cognitive Brain Research, 16*(2), 174–184. https://doi.org/10.1016/S0926-6410(02)00268-9.

Ibáñez, A., Aguado, J., Baez, S., Huepe, D., Lopez, V., Ortega, R., … Manes, F. (2014). From neural signatures of emotional modulation to social cognition: Individual differences in healthy volunteers and psychiatric participants. *Social Cognitive and Affective Neuroscience, 9*(7), 939–950. https://doi.org/10.1093/scan/nst067.

Ibañez, A., & Manes, F. (2012). Contextual social cognition and the behavioral variant of frontotemporal dementia. *Neurology, 78*(17), 1354–1362. https://doi.org/10.1212/WNL.0b013e3182518375.

Ibanez, A., Melloni, M., Huepe, D., Helgiu, E., Rivera-Rei, A., Canales-Johnson, A., … Moya, A. (2012). What event-related potentials (ERPs) bring to social neuroscience? *Social Neuroscience, 7*(6), 632–649. https://doi.org/10.1080/17470919.2012.691078.

Ibanez, A., Urquina, H., Petroni, A., Baez, S., Lopez, V., do Nascimento, M., … Manes, F. (2012). Neural processing of emotional facial and semantic expressions in euthymic bipolar disorder (BD) and its association with theory of mind (ToM). *PloS One, 7*(10), e46877. https://doi.org/10.1371/journal.pone.0046877.

Jakupcak, M., Conybeare, D., Phelps, L., Hunt, S., Holmes, H. A., Felker, B., … McFall, M. E. (2007). Anger, hostility, and aggression among Iraq and Afghanistan war veterans reporting PTSD and subthreshold PTSD. *Journal of Traumatic Stress, 20*(6), 945–954. https://doi.org/10.1002/jts.20258.

Kanske, P., Schönfelder, S., & Wessa, M. (2013). Emotional modulation of the attentional blink and the relation to interpersonal reactivity. *Frontiers in Human Neuroscience, 7,* 641. https://doi.org/10.3389/fnhum.2013.00641.

Kanwisher, N., McDermott, J., & Chun, M. M. (1997). The fusiform face area: A module in human extrastriate cortex specialized for face perception. *The Journal of Neuroscience: The Official Journal of the Society for Neuroscience, 17*(11), 4302–4311.

LeDoux, J. (2003). The emotional brain, fear, and the amygdala. *Cellular and Molecular Neurobiology, 23*(4–5), 727–738.

LeDoux, J. (2012). Rethinking the emotional brain. *Neuron, 73*(4), 653–676. https://doi.org/10.1016/j.neuron.2012.02.004.

Maguen, S., Metzler, T. J., Litz, B. T., Seal, K. H., Knight, S. J., & Marmar, C. R. (2009). The impact of killing in war on mental health symptoms and related functioning. *Journal of Traumatic Stress, 22*(5), 435–443. https://doi.org/10.1002/jts.20451.

Marsh, A. A., Finger, E. C., Mitchell, D. G. V., Reid, M. E., Sims, C., Kosson, D. S., … Blair, R. J. R. (2008). Reduced amygdala response to fearful expressions in children and adolescents with callous-unemotional traits and disruptive behavior disorders. *The American Journal of Psychiatry, 165*(6), 712–720. https://doi.org/10.1176/appi.ajp.2007.07071145.

McGaugh, J. L. (2004). The amygdala modulates the consolidation of memories of emotionally arousing experiences. *Annual Review of Neuroscience, 27,* 1–28. https://doi.org/10.1146/annurev.neuro.27.070203.144157.

Medalla, M., & Barbas, H. (2010). Anterior cingulate synapses in prefrontal areas 10 and 46 suggest differential influence in cognitive control. *The Journal of Neuroscience: The Official Journal of the Society for Neuroscience, 30*(48), 16068–16081. https://doi.org/10.1523/JNEUROSCI.1773-10.2010.

Melloni, M., Lopez, V., & Ibanez, A. (2014). Empathy and contextual social cognition. *Cognitive, Affective & Behavioral Neuroscience, 14*(1), 407–425. https://doi.org/10.3758/s13415-013-0205-3.

Miller, M. W., & Litz, B. T. (2004). Emotional-processing in posttraumatic stress disorder II: Startle reflex modulation during picture processing. *Journal of Abnormal Psychology, 113*(3), 451–463. https://doi.org/10.1037/0021-843X.113.3.451.

Morey, R. A., Gold, A. L., LaBar, K. S., Beall, S. K., Brown, V. M., Haswell, C. C., … McCarthy, G. (2012). Amygdala volume changes with posttraumatic stress disorder in a large case-controlled veteran group. *Archives of General Psychiatry, 69*(11), 1169–1178. https://doi.org/10.1001/archgenpsychiatry.2012.50.

Morey, R. A., Petty, C. M., Cooper, D. A., Labar, K. S., & McCarthy, G. (2008). Neural systems for executive and emotional processing are modulated by symptoms of posttraumatic stress disorder in Iraq war veterans. *Psychiatry Research, 162*(1), 59–72. https://doi.org/10.1016/j.pscychresns.2007.07.007.

Mühlberger, A., Wieser, M. J., Herrmann, M. J., Weyers, P., Tröger, C., & Pauli, P. (2009). Early cortical processing of natural and artificial emotional faces differs between lower and higher socially anxious persons. *Journal of Neural Transmission (Vienna, Austria: 1996), 116*(6), 735–746. https://doi.org/10.1007/s00702-008-0108-6.

Nelson, R. J., & Trainor, B. C. (2007). Neural mechanisms of aggression. *Nature Reviews Neuroscience, 8*(7), 536–546. https://doi.org/10.1038/nrn2174.

Papez, J. W. (1995). A proposed mechanism of emotion. 1937. *The Journal of Neuropsychiatry and Clinical Neurosciences, 7*(1), 103–112.

Paschall, M. (2002). Executive cognitive functioning and aggression: A public health perspective. *Aggression and Violent Behavior, 7*(3), 215–235. https://doi.org/10.1016/S1359-1789(00)00044-6.

Passamonti, L., Rowe, J. B., Ewbank, M., Hampshire, A., Keane, J., & Calder, A. J. (2008). Connectivity from the ventral anterior cingulate to the amygdala is modulated by appetitive motivation in response to facial signals of aggression. *NeuroImage, 43*(3), 562–570. https://doi.org/10.1016/j.neuroimage.2008.07.045.

Patterson, K., Nestor, P. J., & Rogers, T. T. (2007). Where do you know what you know? The representation of semantic knowledge in the human brain. *Nature Reviews Neuroscience, 8*(12), 976–987. https://doi.org/10.1038/nrn2277.

Pessoa, L. (2010). Emergent processes in cognitive-emotional interactions. *Dialogues in Clinical Neuroscience, 12*(4), 433–448.

Petroni, A., Canales-Johnson, A., Urquina, H., Guex, R., Hurtado, E., Blenkmann, A., … Ibañez, A. (2011). The cortical processing of facial emotional expression is associated with social cognition skills and executive functioning: A preliminary study. *Neuroscience Letters, 505*(1), 41–46. https://doi.org/10.1016/j.neulet.2011.09.062.

Phelps, E. A. (2006). Emotion and cognition: Insights from studies of the human amygdala. *Annual Review of Psychology, 57,* 27–53. https://doi.org/10.1146/annurev.psych.56.091103.070234.

Pineda, D. A., Aguirre-Acevedo, D. C., Trujillo, N., Valencia, A. M., Pareja, Á., Tobón, C., … Ibáñez, A. (2013). Dimensions of empathy in ex-combatants of the Colombian armed conflict using a standardized scale. *Revista Colombiana de Psiquiatría, 42*(1), 9–28.

Purves, D., Brannon, E. M., Cabeza, R., Huettel, S. A., LaBar, K. S., Platt, M. L., & Woldorff, M. G. (2008). *Principles of cognitive neuroscience*. USA: Sinauer Associates.

Ramos, C., Duque-Grajales, J., Rendón, J., Montoya-Betancur, A., Baena, A., Pineda, D., et al. (2018). Changes in resting EEG in Colombian ex-combatants ith antisocial personality disorder. *Revista Colombiana De Psiquiatria, 47*(2), 90–97. https://doi.org/10.1016/j.rcp.2017.02.001.

Rodrigo, M. J., León, I., Quiñones, I., Lage, A., Byrne, S., & Bobes, M. A. (2011). Brain and personality bases of insensitivity to infant cues in neglectful mothers: An event-related potential study. *Development and Psychopathology, 23*(1), 163–176. https://doi.org/10.1017/S0954579410000714.

Rueda, M. R., Posner, M. I., & Rothbart, M. K. (2004). Attentional control and self-regulation. *Handbook of self-regulation: Research, theory, and applications* (pp. 283–300). New York, NY, US: The Guilford Press.

Sebastian, A., Forstmann, B. U., & Matzke, D. (2018). Towards a model-based cognitive neuroscience of stopping—A neuroimaging perspective. *Neuroscience and Biobehavioral Reviews, 90,* 130–136. https://doi.org/10.1016/j.neubiorev.2018.04.011.

Seeley, W. W., Menon, V., Schatzberg, A. F., Keller, J., Glover, G. H., Kenna, H., … Greicius, M. D. (2007). Dissociable intrinsic connectivity networks for salience processing and executive control. *The Journal of Neuroscience: The Official Journal of the Society for Neuroscience, 27*(9), 2349–2356. https://doi.org/10.1523/JNEUROSCI.5587-06.2007.

Singer, T., Critchley, H. D., & Preuschoff, K. (2009). A common role of insula in feelings, empathy and uncertainty. *Trends in Cognitive Sciences, 13*(8), 334–340. https://doi.org/10.1016/j.tics.2009.05.001.

Soria Bauser, D., Thoma, P., & Suchan, B. (2012). Turn to me: Electrophysiological correlates of frontal vs. averted view face and body processing are associated with trait empathy. *Frontiers in Integrative Neuroscience, 6*. https://doi.org/10.3389/fnint.2012.00106.

Sripada, R. K., King, A. P., Welsh, R. C., Garfinkel, S. N., Wang, X., Sripada, C. S., et al. (2012). Neural dysregulation in posttraumatic stress disorder: Evidence for disrupted equilibrium between salience and default mode brain networks. *Psychosomatic Medicine, 74*(9), 904–911. https://doi.org/10.1097/PSY.0b013e318273bf33.

Stanford, M. S., Vasterling, J. J., Mathias, C. W., Constans, J. I., & Houston, R. J. (2001). Impact of threat relevance on P3 event-related potentials in combat-related post-traumatic stress disorder. *Psychiatry Research, 102*(2), 125–137.

Swanson, L. W. (2003). The amygdala and its place in the cerebral hemisphere. *Annals of the New York Academy of Sciences, 985,* 174–184.

Taft, C. T., Kaloupek, D. G., Schumm, J. A., Marshall, A. D., Panuzio, J., King, D. W., & Keane, T. M. (2007). Posttraumatic stress disorder symptoms, physiological reactivity, alcohol problems, and aggression among military veterans. *Journal of Abnormal Psychology, 116*(3), 498–507. https://doi.org/10.1037/0021-843X.116.3.498.

Taft, C. T., Weatherill, R. P., Scott, J. P., Thomas, S. A., Kang, H. K., & Eckhardt, C. I. (2015). Social information processing in anger expression and partner violence in returning U.S. veterans. *Journal of Traumatic Stress, 28*(4), 314–321. https://doi.org/10.1002/jts.22017.

Tobón, C., Aguirre-Acevedo, D. C., Velilla, L., Duque, J., Ramos, C. P., & Pineda, D. (2016). Psychiatric, cognitive and emotional profile in ex-combatants of illegal armed groups in Colombia. *Revista Colombiana De Psiquiatria, 45*(1), 28–36. https://doi.org/10.1016/j.rcp.2015.07.004.

Tobón, C., Ibañez, A., Velilla, L., Duque, J., Ochoa, J., Trujillo, N., … Pineda, D. (2015). Emotional processing in Colombian ex-combatants and its relationship with empathy and executive functions. *Social Neuroscience, 10*(2), 153–165. https://doi.org/10.1080/17470919.2014.969406.

Trujillo, S., Trujillo, N., Lopez, J. D., Gomez, D., Valencia, S., Rendon, J., … Parra, M. A. (2017). Social cognitive training improves emotional processing and reduces aggressive attitudes in ex-combatants. *Frontiers in Psychology, 8*, 510. https://doi.org/10.3389/fpsyg.2017.00510.

Trujillo, S. P., Valencia, S., Trujillo, N., Ugarriza, J. E., Rodríguez, M. V., Rendón, J., … Parra, M. A. (2017). Atypical modulations of N170 component during emotional processing and their links to social behaviors in ex-combatants. *Frontiers in Human Neuroscience, 11*, 244. https://doi.org/10.3389/fnhum.2017.00244.

Weippert, M., Rickler, M., Kluck, S., Behrens, K., Bastian, M., Mau-Moeller, A., … Lischke, A. (2018). It's harder to push, when I have to push hard—Physical exertion and fatigue changes reasoning and decision-making on hypothetical moral dilemmas in males. *Frontiers in Behavioral Neuroscience, 12*. https://doi.org/10.3389/fnbeh.2018.00268.

Whitney, C., Kirk, M., O'Sullivan, J., Ralph, M. A. L., & Jefferies, E. (2012). Executive semantic processing is underpinned by a large-scale neural network: Revealing the contribution of left prefrontal, posterior temporal, and parietal cortex to controlled retrieval and selection using TMS. *Journal of Cognitive Neuroscience, 24*(1), 133–147. https://doi.org/10.1162/jocn_a_00123.

Williams, R. (2006). The psychosocial consequences for children and young people who are exposed to terrorism, war, conflict and natural disasters. *Current Opinion in Psychiatry, 19*(4), 337–349. https://doi.org/10.1097/01.yco.0000228751.85828.c1.

Yoder, K. J., & Decety, J. (2018). The neuroscience of morality and social decision-making. *Psychology, Crime & Law, 24*(3), 279–295. https://doi.org/10.1080/1068316X.2017.1414817.

Young, M. P., Scannell, J. W., Burns, G. A., & Blakemore, C. (1994). Analysis of connectivity: Neural systems in the cerebral cortex. *Reviews in the Neurosciences, 5*(3), 227–250.

Part V
Executive Dysfunction in Neuropsychiatric Disorders

Chapter 12
Executive Dysfunction in Depressive Disorders

Mónica Rosselli, Merike Lang and Fernanda Arruda

12.1 Introduction

Depression is defined as a mood disorder associated with a persistent emotional state of sadness and loss of interest that affects thoughts and behavior, leading to physical and cognitive problems. Therefore, depression includes cognitive (i.e., memory deficits), behavioral (i.e., less daily activity), emotional (i.e., feeling misery), motivational (i.e., lack of initiative and despondency), and physical (i.e., disturbances in sleep and eating) symptoms (Comer, 2016). Some of the cognitive symptoms described in depression may include deficits in executive functions (EFs). Research has demonstrated that patients diagnosed with major depression had widespread cognitive impairment (Ravnkilde et al., 2002). However, not all depressed individuals have cognitive defects; the manifestation of depressive symptoms may be due to an interaction between motivation, emotional, and cognitive symptoms (Austin, Mitchell, & Goodwin, 2001).

EFs, a set of cognitive abilities that guide behavior toward the completion of a goal, are involved in the conscious control of thought and action (Kerr & Zelazo, 2004). EFs permit quick set-shifting and inhibition of inappropriate behaviors (Jurado & Rosselli, 2007). Lezak (1983) viewed EFs as the dimension of human behavior that deals with 'how' behavior is expressed. It is an umbrella term that includes a wide variety of components such as planning, set-shifting, updating, cognitive flexibility, working memory, inhibitory control, multitasking, and abstraction (Jurado

M. Rosselli (✉) · M. Lang · F. Arruda
Department of Psychology, Florida Atlantic University, Davie, FL, USA
e-mail: mrossell@fau.edu

M. Lang
e-mail: mlang2015@fau.edu

F. Arruda
e-mail: farruda2016@fau.edu

A. Ardila et al. (eds.), *Dysexecutive Syndromes*,
https://doi.org/10.1007/978-3-030-25077-5_12

& Rosselli, 2007; Miyake et al., 2000; Snyder, 2013). Moral and ethical behaviors also represent EFs (Ardila & Surloff, 2004).

An important distinction in the classification of EFs accounts for whether they are affective or cognitive processes. EFs that have an affective/emotional component are considered 'hot' EFs, while those that are relatively abstract and non-affective, relating to cognition (e.g., working memory and multitasking), are known as 'cool' or 'cold' EFs, although some authors argue that both should be viewed as multidimensional and in a dynamic continuum rather than in dichotomy (Kluwe-Schiavon, Viola, Sanvicente-Vieira, Malloy-Diniz, & Grassi-Oliveira, 2017). 'Cool' EFs include self-management skills with no involvement of emotion such as updating, inhibition, and set-shifting (Ho, Hsu, Lu, Gossop, & Chen, 2018). The 'hot' EFs include affective decision making for events with emotionally significant consequences (i.e., meaningful rewards and/or losses) (Kerr & Zelazo, 2004). Ardila (2013) suggested that cool EFs constitute a metacognitive group of cognitive abilities, whereas the hot EFs comprise emotional/motivational processes. The latter EFs include abilities required to fulfill basic impulses following socially accepted strategies in which inhibitory control plays a major role.

EFs rely heavily on the prefrontal cortex (PFC). Three main subdivisions of the PFC relevant to EFs are the dorsolateral prefrontal cortex (DLPFC), the orbitofrontal cortex (OFC), and the medial prefrontal cortex (MPFC) (Ochsner & Gross, 2007; Goldman-Rakic, 1995). Studies have demonstrated that the DLPFC plays a major role in metacognitive EFs, whereas the OFC and MPFC are relevant to the mediation of EFs in which emotions are involved (Ardila, 2013). More recently, an emphasis has been placed on the ventromedial frontal lobe (Farrar, Mian, Budson, Moss, & Killiany, 2018; Peters, Fellows, & Sheldon, 2017) and the ventrolateral prefrontal cortex (VLPFC) as relevant structures in the decision-making and regulatory processes of behavior (Light et al., 2011), respectively.

Some depressed individuals present deficits in EFs such as shifting, inhibition, working memory, and planning as part of their neuropsychological profiles (Zakzanis, Leach, & Kaplan, 1998; Lockwood, Alexopoulos, & van Gorp, 2002; Snyder, 2013). Since the PFC demonstrates changes in depressive symptoms, there is an overlap of the areas involved in depression and the neural mechanisms of EFs (Pizzagalli, 2011; Rogers et al., 2004). Therefore, the dysexecutive syndrome has been suggested for depressed individuals. This depression-dysexecutive syndrome has been considered a distinct type of depression characterized by psychomotor retardation and a reduced interest in activities, as well as reduced verbal fluency (Alexopoulos, 2001).

The main purpose of this chapter is to review the current knowledge surrounding the association between depression and cognitive processes, particularly those abilities involved in EFs. The first section will define the different depressive disorders and will be followed by a description of the proposed neural substrates of the executive system in depressed individuals across the lifespan.

12.1.1 Defining Depressive Disorders

Clinical depression can manifest with major depressive episodes (MDE) and major depressive disorder (MDD). An MDE is a period of two or more weeks marked by at least five symptoms of depression, which include sad mood and/or loss of pleasure. An MDE is considered recurrent when there is an interval of at least two consecutive months between separate episodes (DSM-5; American Psychiatric Association, 2013). People who experience recurrent MDEs without having any history of mania receive a diagnosis of MDD (APA, 2013). MDD is diagnosed when, for at least two weeks, a patient has experienced depressed mood or loss of interest or pleasure associated with other symptoms such as a change in appetite and body weight, sleep alteration, psychomotor agitation or retardation, fatigue, negative feelings about the self, decreased concentration, and suicidal ideation (APA, 2013). The International Statistical Classification of Diseases and Related Health Problems (ICD-10; World Health Organization, 2004) criteria distinguish three degrees of severity in depressive episodes: mild (few distressing symptoms and minor social/occupational impairment), moderate (greater intensity and number of symptoms with functional impairment), and severe (intense symptoms which are distressing/unmanageable and interfere with social/occupational functioning).

Persistent depressive disorder (dysthymia) is the consolidation of two diagnoses from the DSM-IV: chronic MDD and dysthymic disorder. This diagnosis refers to those who present depressed mood for most of the day for at least two years; children and adolescents can receive this diagnosis when symptoms are present for at least one year, and they may additionally experience irritable mood (APA, 2013). A third type of depressive disorder (DD) is premenstrual dysphoric disorder, a diagnosis given to women who repeatedly have clinically significant depressive and related symptoms, such as marked affective lability, irritability or anger, depressed mood, and anxiety, during the week before menstruation in the majority of menstrual cycles. These symptoms must cause significant distress and interfere with the patient's social and/or work life.

The DSM-5 divides mood disorders into two groups: bipolar and related disorders, and depressive disorders (APA, 2013; Tandon, 2015). The bipolar and related disorders section includes major depression in combination with episodes of mania and is placed between the section of the schizophrenia spectrum/other psychotic disorders and the section pertaining to depressive disorders. This change from the DSM-IV was made with the consideration that bipolar disorder shares both clinical features with unipolar depression and with schizophrenia (Tandon, 2015).

Table 12.1 includes a list of all depressive disorders according to the DSM-5. The common feature of all of these disorders is the presence of sadness, emptiness, or irritability in mood, accompanied by somatic and cognitive changes that significantly affect the individual's capacity to function. Duration, timing, or presumed etiology distinguishes them.

Disruptive mood dysregulation disorder, a childhood depressive disorder, is characterized by children and adolescents who have severe and recurrent temper outbursts

Table 12.1 Depressive disorders (DD) based on the DSM-5 (APA, 2013)

Disruptive mood dysregulation disorder
Major depressive disorder (including major depressive episode)
Persistent depressive disorder (dysthymia)
Premenstrual dysphoric disorder
Substance/medication-induced depressive disorder
Depressive disorder due to another medical condition
Other specified depressive disorder
Unspecified depressive disorder

that are out of proportion to the given situation and express a persistent irritable or angry mood (APA, 2013).

12.2 Executive Function and Depression

12.2.1 Child/Adolescent MDD and Executive Dysfunction

There is no consistency in the findings regarding the association between depression and EFs for children and adolescents. Some studies have shown that they score similarly to healthy controls on neuropsychological tasks measuring EFs. Favre et al. (2009) found that 39 children and adolescents (between the ages of 8–17 years) with a diagnosis of MDD had similar EF scores compared to healthy controls ($n = 24$) on the Wisconsin Card Sorting Test (WCST), Trail Making Test (TMT), Control Oral Word Association Test (COWAT) and the Stroop test. Only mental processing speed was significantly lower in those with MDD, as demonstrated by the processing speed index from the Wechsler Intelligence Scales (third edition; WISC-III and WAIS-III). The authors suggested that lower processing speed may be due to lower motivation and psychomotor retardation (a symptom of MDD), and not likely due to deficits in attention and concentration. In addition, this study included ten participants with comorbid ADHD, and this subgroup of ADHD and MDD performed worse on the WCST and TMT-B compared to depressed children without ADHD. The authors speculated that with a larger sample, these differences would have been detected.

Metanalytic reports have found significant impairments in some EFs for children and adolescents suffering from depression. Wagner, Müller, Helmreich, Huss, and Tadić (2015) analyzed 17 studies relating to intelligence, EFs, verbal memory, and attention in 447 patients (age range of 9–15.3 years) with an MDD diagnosis. These individuals were compared to 1347 healthy participants (ranging in age from 9–15.8 years). The EF measures included inhibition (Stroop Color-Word interference test), set-shifting (TMT-B, Cambridge Neuropsychological Test Automated Batteries [CANTAB], supervisory attention system [SAS] and shifting attention test [SAT]), working memory (digit span [Wechsler Intelligence Scale for Children—WISC], n-back, symbol digit encoding [Amsterdam Neuropsychological Tasks—ANT] and spatial working memory), planning (Tower of Hanoi and Stockings of Cambridge [CANTAB]), and verbal fluency (phonemic and semantic fluencies). Their results demonstrated significantly lower EF test performance in MDD, especially for inhibition capacity, semantic verbal fluency, sustained attention, verbal memory, and shifting/planning. In addition, healthy children and adolescents had higher full-scale IQ scores (on verbal and performance measures) compared to MDD patients. Günther and collaborators (2011) also reported difficulties in EF tasks of inhibitory control such as go/no-go and set-shifting tasks of 61 children with depressive disorders including MDD and dysthymic disorder (age range of 10–15) compared to healthy controls.

In a systematic review of the literature (from 1994 to 2014), Vilgis, Silk, and Vance (2015) identified 33 studies of children and adolescents (age range 6–19 years) with depressive disorders (MDD or dysthymia, according to DSM-IV criteria) in which EFs were tested. All articles met the inclusion criteria of having a nonclinical control group and a sample size of 10 or more participants in the clinical group. The specific EF domains of interest were attention, response inhibition, set-shifting, working memory, planning, and verbal fluency. Results showed that of the nine studies assessing the ability to sustain attention (e.g., Continuous Performance Test) in children and adolescents with depressive disorders, only five reported difficulties in the group of patients with depression. None of the five studies that included measures of selective attention (i.e., target detection in a visual array of similar-looking items) found differences between patients and healthy controls. Only three of the 16 investigations that examined response inhibition (e.g., Stroop test, go/no-go) showed lower scores in the depressed sample compared to controls. It is important to note that only one of the five studies that used the Stroop test as a measure of inhibitory control found worse performance in the clinical group. On the go/no-go task, there was no significant difference between healthy children and patients with MDD and dysthymia, matched for age. Differences in set-shifting (i.e., TMT-B and WCST) between the two groups were observed in three out of ten studies. Two of these studies used the TMT-B, and one used a combined score of the perseverative errors from the WCST and the TMT-B. The TMT-B is a good measure for assessing set-shifting because the patient is required to alternate between numbers and letters (two mental sets) while connecting circles in sequential and alphabetical order. One study that used the WCST alone as a measure of cognitive flexibility did not find differences between the groups. Using the CANTAB set-shifting task, there were no differences in error rate for two of the studies, although differences were detected in reaction time. Five reports were found comparing healthy controls and those diagnosed with depressive disorders in visuospatial working memory tasks (Vilgis et al., 2015). In three of these studies, no differences were observed between groups for adolescents, although one study found more errors for depressed adolescent girls compared to healthy controls. Using the spatial working memory task of the CANTAB, one study reported worse performance from depressed patients.

Moreover, Vilgis et al. (2015) also examined whether depression was associated with reduced verbal working memory. The digit span from the Wechsler Intelligence

Scale for Children (WISC) was used in two of the studies discussed. One of them found a reduced digit span in both adolescents with MDD and those with dysthymia or a depressive disorder not otherwise specified, and the other found no deficits in children with anxiety and depression on digit span compared to the healthy control group. Two of the three studies also reviewed by Vilgis et al. (2015) found difficulties in planning (e.g., Tower of London/Hanoi tasks) in clinical participants with depression. Verbal fluency deficits (e.g., generation of words within phonemic categories) were additionally noted in the depressed groups for two of the four studies.

In terms of attentional bias and affective manipulations of 'cold' EFs, depressed individuals demonstrate attentional biases toward negative stimuli. Neshat-Doost, Moradi, Taghavi, Yule, and Dalgleish (2000) compared the performance of MDD, dysthymia, and controls on the dot-probe task. This is a task of selective attention in which neutral and threatening stimuli are presented simultaneously, and the latency to indicate the location of a dot that is presented after the stimuli is recorded. Performance differences have been observed between clinical and healthy controls, although this was not seen in depressed children utilizing stimuli of emotional words. Depressed groups were biased toward the sad face stimuli, while anxious groups had biases toward both angry and sad faces, with an apparent gender bias for boys but not girls in avoiding happy faces. Four studies found that affective manipulation of stimuli did not show a task performance effect for depressed participants. However, other studies utilizing similar tasks showed shorter reaction times for negative as opposed to positive stimuli only for the acute MDD group, compared to the remitted MDD patients and controls, although this did not correlate with symptom severity.

Vilgis et al. (2015) additionally reviewed studies of 'hot' EFs. They discussed performance on the Iowa gambling task (IGT; a task simulating real-life decision making by sampling four virtual decks of cards that represent reward or punishment) of 31 children diagnosed with MDD compared to 30 controls. There were two studies that showed that boys with dysthymia or MDD selected more disadvantageous cards compared to healthy controls and chose a large reward less often, even when the probability of winning was high. However, one study failed to show differences in IGT comparing self-harming adolescents with MDD and healthy controls. Another study showed no group differences in decision making with betting options across similar groups, although two other studies showed diminished reward seeking and task performance associated with the severity of depressive symptoms. Additionally, Vilgis et al. (2015) cited the study in which incentives were less effective in modulating the performance of adolescents with MDD on a rewarded antisaccade task. Healthy controls showed reductions in the mean 'velocity' or unwanted reflexive saccades/eye movements in reference to punishment or reward compared to patients with MDD, as well as shorter latencies in eye movements for both positive and negative incentive conditions relative to no incentive conditions. No differences were observed in latency by condition for MDD patients.

Wagner, Alloy, and Abramson (2015) observed 486 adolescents in a balanced sample of Caucasians and African Americans with the goal of determining the deficits in EFs associated with rumination and depression among early adolescents (ages 12–13), which is considered a critical developmental period. Rumination is conceptualized under the response styles theory as a way of responding to distress and involves focusing repetitively and passively on present thoughts and events as well as the possible causes and consequences of them. The authors found that the current level of depression was associated with attention, and rumination predicted better-sustained attention in those with low levels of depressive symptoms. Worse-sustained attention was observed in those with high levels of depressive symptoms. The authors found that controlling for depressive symptoms, higher levels of trait rumination (an abstract information processing mode of constantly anticipating present events on future experiences/consequences that remains a stable characteristic throughout changes in depressive symptoms; Kocsel et al., 2017) did not predict poorer attentional set-shifting or better-sustained attention in adolescents. Additionally, rumination was associated with better attentional abilities, only when there was little or no depression present, which contradicted the predicted results. The authors recommended interpreting their findings with caution given the small effect sizes and the small number of significant associations obtained. However, they also offered a possible interpretation of their results, suggesting that trait ruminators, only when not actively depressed/engaging in rumination during task completion, may have a particular cognitive profile that renders them with better performance on certain tasks of EFs possibly due to a narrowed attentional scope, facilitating performance for ignoring distractors and irrelevant information.

Förster et al. (2018) investigated the relationship between EF and social cognitive performance in late adolescence and young adulthood ($M_{\text{age}} = 20.60$ years; $SD_{\text{age}} =$ 3.82 years) with current and remitted depression ($n = 118$) compared to controls ($n = 61$). Social cognitive performance was assessed through three social perception subtests: affect naming, prosody face matching, and prosody pair matching. Four EFs were assessed: set-shifting (or cognitive flexibility; Card Sort Task based on the WCST), planning ability (Tower of London), working memory (updating; n-back task with three different conditions of one-back, two-back, three-back recall), and inhibitory control (Stroop task using the Victoria Stroop Test, a version of the Stroop for French speakers, Bayard, Erkes, & Moroni, 2011; Tremblay et al., 2016). Social cognition and EFs did not significantly differ between healthy and depressed patients. There was no association between EFs and social cognitive function in healthy controls. Depressed adolescents and young adults exhibited lower cognitive flexibility, associated with lower facial-affect recognition and theory of mind. The authors concluded that deficits in cognitive flexibility may lead to a more 'rigid' perception of ambiguous social stimuli.

In summary, many of the studies presented in this section do not demonstrate robust differences in EFs among depressed children and adolescents compared to healthy controls (Vilgis et al., 2015; Wagner, Alloy et al., 2015). Evidence of poorer performance among depressed youths relative to controls has been reported on tests of sustained attention, shifting, planning, verbal memory, and inhibitory control (Wagner, Müller et al., 2015), although other studies have obtained no indication of EF impairments on similar tasks of selective attention as well as mixed findings for visual and verbal working memory measures (e.g., Vilgis et al., 2015). Inconsistencies may be explained partly by methodological limitations, including the use of small and heterogeneous samples, and the fact that many of the samples had differing inclusion criteria for depressed groups, medication use, and other possible comorbid disorders (Vilgis et al., 2015). Further research is needed to establish the role of EFs in depression for children and adolescents to determine whether this influence is dissimilar to the effects of mood states in adults' EFs.

12.2.2 Adult MDD and Executive Dysfunction

Most of the evidence demonstrating that depressive disorders are associated with impairments in EFs has come from studies with adult populations. It is common for adults diagnosed with this mood disorder to present problems in tasks of cognitive inhibition, problem solving, and planning (Fossati, Ergis, & Allilaire, 2002). However, not all EFs are impaired in adults with MDD. Zakzanis et al. (1998) conducted a meta-analysis (726 patients with depression and 795 healthy normal controls) and reported impairments in specific EFs such as verbal fluency (both semantic and phonemic) and inhibition (e.g., Stroop test), but no deficits in shifting (e.g., TMT-B, WCST) or verbal working memory (e.g., backward digit span).

Snyder (2013) conducted another meta-analysis comparing participants with MDD ($M_{age} = 46$) to healthy controls ($M_{age} = 45$) on measures of EFs such as inhibition, shifting, updating, verbal working memory, visuospatial working memory, planning, and verbal fluency. For moderator analyses, they used current depression severity, age, use of psychotropic medication, and the presence of other mental disorders as a comorbidity. They included 113 studies with 7707 participants (3936 patients and 3771 healthy controls, similar in age and gender). MDD was associated with significant impairments on all measures of EFs. Additionally, the use of medication and symptom severity affected EF performance. The use of psychotropic medications predicted greater impairment on the composite score for inhibition, TMT-B, verbal working memory, visuospatial working memory composite scores, and verbal fluency measures, while controlling for symptom severity and age. The severity of depressive symptoms predicted impairment on inhibition composite scores, shifting composite scores, the WCST, verbal working memory manipulation composite scores, backward digit span, and verbal fluency while controlling for age and the use of medication.

Another meta-analysis was conducted by McDermott and Ebmeier (2009), who correlated the severity of depression with cognitive function across 14 studies. Composite scores for timed and untimed tests for each functional domain (episodic memory, EFs, processing speed, semantic memory, and visuospatial memory) were calculated. There were significant correlations between depression severity and episodic memory, EFs, and processing speed, for both timed and untimed measures, in which increased depression severity was associated with reduced cognitive performance. The analyses in this study included patients with major or minor depression according to the DSM-III-R/DSM-IV criteria, leaving uncertainty as to whether these results may apply to MDD, specifically.

Dotson, Resnick, and Zonderman (2008) used a longitudinal design to investigate the relationship between current depressive symptoms and cognitive performance for a sample of older adults. They looked at whether depressive symptoms at baseline predicted cognitive decline and whether chronic or persistent depressive symptoms were associated with cognitive decline in assessments completed at 1- to 2-year intervals for up to 26 years. Their total sample consisted of 1586 participants, but the sample size varied for each cognitive test, ranging from 799 to 1484 participants, and the follow-up interval ranged from 0 to 26 years. Higher average depressive symptoms were related to greater executive dysfunction (measured by letter fluency and TMT-B) and a longitudinal decline in memory (assessed with the California Verbal Learning Test; CVLT), attention (using digits forward), and general cognitive status (using the MMSE). Their results suggested that prolonged/persistent depressive symptoms may have more deleterious effects on cognition than transient ones, with greater association to cognitive decline. Some limitations of this study include lack of information on comorbidities and age of onset of depressive symptoms. Additionally, there was limited diversity in the demographic characteristics of the sample, which mainly consisted of white and highly educated males.

Most studies involving EFs assess the 'cool' or cognitive EFs, but fail to address 'hot' or affective EFs. Studies on executive dysfunction and depression generally have demonstrated deficits specifically in 'cool' EFs. Moreover, deficits in 'cool' EFs have been reported for depressed patients with suicide attempts, in addition to impaired decision making as well as biased attention to negative valence stimuli (Ho et al., 2018). These authors conducted a study comparing MDD with a history of suicide attempts, MDD with no history of suicide attempts, and healthy controls, all of them between 20 to 60 years of age. They computed four indices: general inhibition, general set-shifting, emotion-specific inhibition, and emotion-specific set-shifting. Their results demonstrated that the two MDD groups performed similarly to healthy controls on 'hot' EF tasks and had disrupted 'cool' EFs, which has been consistently shown in previous studies with adolescents in affective decision-making involving reward-seeking behavior (Vilgis et al., 2015). However, there is limited research investigating depressive disorders and 'hot' EFs in adults. Malloy-Diniz, Miranda, and Grassi-Oliveira (2017) reviewed 13 articles describing the relationship between EFs and psychiatric disorders. These authors identified cognitive deficits in bipolar depressed patients, but did not investigate 'hot' EFs.

Despite the numerous studies aimed at understanding the underlying role of EFs in depression, it is still unclear whether executive dysfunction observed in MDD is the result of preexisting trait markers (impairment that remains regardless of severity of symptoms) or if it is state-related deficits that change with depressive symptoms. Additionally, they could be 'scar' impairments that remain during periods of remission and worsen with illness progression (Allott, Fisher, Amminger, Goodall, & Hetrick, 2016). Some studies provide evidence that symptom severity increases EF impairments (Snyder, 2013; McDermott & Ebmeier, 2009), and other studies have observed stable EF impairments even after symptom remission (Paelecke-Habermann, Pohl, & Leplow, 2005). Moreover, there is empirical support for persistent EF impairments in inhibition, switching, and semantic fluency, despite a reduction in depressive symptoms over the course of a 12-month period (Schmid & Hammar, 2013). Finally, other research has observed deficits in sustained attention and EFs (planning, monitoring, cognitive flexibility, and coding) in individuals with MDD even after remission of symptoms, which supports the idea that they are associated with trait markers of depression (Paelecke-Habermann et al., 2005). Therefore, whether aspects of EFs are dependent on symptom severity or whether they are stable traits independent of current depression severity remains unclear (Snyder, 2013).

In summary, there is robust evidence of EF impairment in adults with MDD, particularly at an advanced age. The most frequent deficits are observed in verbal fluency tasks and in tasks that require inhibitory control and shifting. However, it is important to note that there are many methodological limitations in the published studies described above such as a lack of cultural diversity in samples, small sample sizes, absence of uniformity in defining depression and the lack of consideration of comorbid diagnoses, which all need to be accounted for in future studies to confirm these findings.

12.2.2.1 Late-Onset Versus Early-Onset Depression

The age of onset of the depressive disorder seems to be relevant in the characterization of the disorder for older adults and geriatric populations. There are distinctions between early-onset depression (EOD; develops before age 60 with low medical comorbidity, prolonged release of cortisol leading to early hippocampal damage and reduction in neurotrophic factors important for neurogenesis, higher suicidal ideation, and less cognitive impairment) and late-onset depression (LOD; develops after age 60 with high medical comorbidity, increased white matter lesions, faster hippocampal atrophy, fronto-subcortical disruption, lower symptoms of suicidal ideation, and more cognitive impairment). Additionally, it seems that EOD has a better prognosis for treatment (Espinoza & Kaufman, 2014). This is important to distinguish because evidence suggests that the dysexecutive syndrome observed in depressed individuals is more likely to occur among individuals who develop LOD (Herrmann, Goodwin, & Ebmeier 2007).

Moreover, Herrmann et al. (2007) conducted a review comparing individuals with EOD, LOD, and healthy controls. Results suggested that LOD patients suffered mainly from impairments in EFs and processing speed when compared to EOD and controls. Episodic and working memory impairments were similar between LOD and EOD; both groups performed worse on these tasks compared to healthy controls.

Albert, Potter, McQuoid, and Taylor (2017) examined cognitive performance in antidepressant-free depressed adults with early-onset recurrent depression and healthy controls. They analyzed whether the duration of depression was associated with cognitive performance across several cognitive domains (episodic memory, EFs, processing speed, and working memory). Their sample included 91 participants between 20 and 50 years of age that were diagnosed with recurrent MDD according to the DSM-IV and experienced the onset of the first depressive episode before the age of 35. These participants were not currently being treated with psychotherapy and were not using antidepressants within the last month. In addition, their control group was composed of 105 individuals with no history of depression. For measures of EFs, they used the COWAT (verbal fluency), the TMT-B (set-shifting), semantic fluency, and the Stroop Color-Word interference condition (inhibition). No group differences were observed in EF tasks, episodic memory, and working memory, which contrasts with previous findings from studies that mainly analyzed isolated neuropsychological tests and may be explained by deficits in specific cognitive task components. Effects of depression severity on performance were also not significant. There was a significant interaction between depression duration and age with processing speed and EF variables, and no significant interaction between working and episodic memory, which is in line with the cumulative effect of depression on cognition that may interact with age. Older depressed participants with a longer duration of depression exhibited slower processing speed and worse EF performance. Results from this study may be specific to younger adults with EOD. One limitation of this study is that the EF tasks also utilized a timed component, making it difficult to distinguish variance explained by depression on EF tasks separately from processing speed.

12.2.3 Late in Life Depression and Executive Dysfunction

Late-life depression (LLD) is defined as depression occurring after 60 years old with varying age of onset (Espinoza & Kaufman, 2014). The DSM-IV had criteria for LLD, although the DSM-5 no longer makes this distinction by age. Therefore, the clinical criteria for depression remain the same, independent of the individual's age. Some authors have identified the 'depression-executive dysfunction syndrome' (DED) as occurring in late life, characterized by depressive symptoms such as a loss of interest in activities and psychomotor retardation, as well as executive dysfunction (Alexopoulos, Kiosses, Klimstra, Kalayam, & Bruce, 2002). Reduced processing speed appears to be the core of the cognitive difficulties for individuals with LLD (Butters et al., 2004; Koenig, Bhalia, & Butters, 2014). Deficits in tasks such as the TMT-B are found in individuals diagnosed with LLD (Butters et al., 2004) and even in those older than 75 with depression, but without dementia (Jungwirth et al., 2011).

Lockwood et al. (2002) compared 40 adults with MDD and 40 healthy control subjects (half of them were 20–60 years old, and the other half were 61 years or older) in four cognitive domains: selective attention (Connor's Computerized Continuous Performance Test, Visual and Auditory Cancellation Tests, Stroop Color and Word Test, and the CVLT), sustained attention (WAIS-III digit symbol subtest, category fluency test, sustained finger tapping, color-word condition from the Stroop Color and Word Test), inhibitory control (commission errors on the Connor's Computerized Continuous Performance Test, perseverative errors on the WCST, CVLT and category fluency test, and completion time for TMT-B) and focused effort or intensity of directed attention involving working memory, speed of processing, and complex mental operations (e.g., number of items completed for the WAIS-III digit symbol subtest; items completed for the WAIS-III digits backward). It was found that depressed individuals, regardless of age, performed more poorly than non-depressed subjects on selective attention and sustained attention domains. A significant age–depression interaction was found for inhibitory control and focused effort domains. The older depressed adults evidenced significantly greater impairment on tasks requiring set-shifting, problem solving, and initiation of novel responses. The authors concluded that depression-related executive dysfunction is more pronounced during advanced age. Morimoto et al. (2011) observed that deficits in semantic fluency were significantly associated with poorer remission of depressed individuals older than 60 years of age.

Cognitive decline in LLD is associated with structural brain changes. Köhler et al. (2010) conducted a study to observe the level of cortical atrophy and white matter hyperintensities correlating with cognitive deficits for older depressed adults. The differences observed in memory and EFs were associated with white matter hyperintensities (such as lesions in deep white matter and paraventricular regions). Participants with depression who had a higher amount of white matter hyperintensities also had EF and memory scores that were 2–3 standard deviations below the mean compared to healthy controls.

In sum, the studies on LLD emphasize the mediation of age on the negative association between depression and cognitive abilities, particularly with EF skills dependent on the speed of processing. In addition, emotional and cognitive behaviors correlate with structural brain abnormalities.

12.3 Anatomy of Executive Dysfunction in Depression

The behavioral association between depression severity and poor performance on EF tasks suggests a relationship or overlap between the brain circuitries that control both mood disorders and EFs. Rogers et al. (2004) conducted a review of empirical findings related to prefrontal areas and EFs in unipolar depression. Results showed that the regions mainly involved in the various 'cool' EF tasks with depression recruit the prefrontal cortex, particularly, the dorsolateral prefrontal cortex (DLPFC). Hypoactivation of the DLPFC has been reported in cases of depression. Depression also seems to be related to hyperactivation of the anterior cingulate cortex (ACC), an area related to conflict resolution. Ottowitz, Tondo, Dougherty, and Savage (2002) reviewed deficits in attention and EFs in MDD, emphasizing the role of the orbitofrontal cortex (OFC), ACC, and DLPFC in the neurobehavioral domains that are involved in EFs. The meta-analysis of neuroimaging studies by Pizzagalli (2011) described reduced rostral anterior cingulate cortex (rACC) and DLPFC volume for depressed patients compared to healthy controls after 3 years of follow-up; demyelination of these structures, particularly in those with treatment-resistant depression, was also reported. The authors also indicated that reduced gray matter volume in the left DLPFC predicted longer illness duration and increased depression severity. Additionally, reduced right DLPFC volume was associated with worse EFs due to attentional biases toward negative cues. Other studies in this meta-analysis showed blunted activation in neuroimaging of the dorsal anterior cingulate (dACC), rACC, and the left DLPFC, for MDD patients with higher activation in these areas seen during normal performance on EF tasks.

Pizzagalli (2011) aimed to identify regions implicated in frontocingulate dysfunction observed in depression. Heightened activity of the rACC is a promising predictor of treatment outcome for depression. He utilized a three-pronged approach to investigate the reliability of increasing rACC activity for treatment response in depression and the mechanisms that support this relationship. The first prong contained a meta-analysis of the association between resting rACC activity and treatment, arguing that this region plays an important role in treatment due to being the 'hub' of the default mode network or an active network including the posterior cingulate cortex, precuneus, MPFC, and angular gyrus while thinking about the self, others and recalling past events (deactivated during certain tasks). The second prong was the proposal that elevated resting rACC activity led to better treatment outcomes. The third prong provided neuropsychological, electrophysiological, and neuroimaging data for frontocingulate dysfunction in depression in order to confirm the relationship between the rACC and treatment for depression.

Additionally, Pizzagalli (2011) discussed studies with Diffusion Tensor Imaging (DTI) that have also supported the importance of the PFC and ACC in MDD (for adolescents, young adults, and the elderly). DTI measures the flow of water (fractional anisotropy, or FA) in one direction along the myelinated axons allowing for the mapping of connectivity, fiber density, and axonal diameter. Reduced FA within the PFC and ACC white matter tracts for adolescents, young adults, and the elderly has been found. This circuit has also been implicated in EF. Reduced FA in tracts connecting the supragenual ACC and the right amygdala has been additionally demonstrated, which may suggest a possible diminished regulatory input to the amygdala (Cullen et al., 2010). Pizzagalli (2011) described another study in which FA in the left frontal and dACC white matter correlated with total days depressed, indicating an increased disconnection in the frontocingulate pathways due to the duration of depression. Non-remission after a 12-week trial of serotonin reuptake inhibitor (SSRI) medication was associated with reduced FA in the rACC, dACC, and DLPFC, which also supports the importance of these areas and their subcortical connectivity in the presence and maintenance of depressive symptoms. Finally, preserved integrity of myelinated white matter tracts positively correlated with better Stroop performance, suggesting the importance of these tracts for EFs.

In general (for adults and older adults), the most important structures of the prefrontal cortex such as the ACC, DLPFC, OFC and their connection to the amygdala are involved in the mechanisms of depression (Pizzagalli, 2011), overlapping with areas recruited by EFs (the DLPFC, the OFC, and the ACC) related to tasks of working memory, behavioral regulation/monitoring, planning and goal formation (Jurado & Rosselli, 2007). In addition, in late life, depression and deficits on EF tasks are associated with damage to the white matter or the connectivity of the neurons in the prefrontal circuitry, leading to a higher probability of impairment on tasks of EF.

12.4 Executive Functions and Depression in Abnormal Aging

Thomas et al. (2009) discussed executive dysfunction syndrome and risks for the elderly. They indicated that major cognitive deficits in patients with LLD were related to fronto-subcortical circuit dysfunction in disorders of vascular dementia, Alzheimer's disease, Lewy body dementia, fronto-temporal dementia, and mild cognitive impairment (MCI). These disorders may cause damage to the lateral frontal cortices leading to impairment in motor structures such as perseveration/inertia (is defined as disturbance in motor output and compulsive repetition) or the functions related to the 'cool' EFs. Additionally, the orbital/medial areas are linked with limbic/reticular systems leading to disinhibition and changes in affect or function related to the 'hot' EFs. In this study, they examined the dysexecutive dysfunction syndrome (see Sect. 12.2.3 for description), analyzing patients with neurological disorders compared to controls. DED syndrome was associated with a loss of autonomy, risk of fall, and malnutrition. Motivation was additionally altered in depression, and in patients with dementia, depression significantly increased behavioral disorders as well as precipitated the risk of fall and malnutrition.

Thomas and O'Brien (2008) reviewed neurocognitive impairment and depression in MCI. They indicated that neurocognitive impairment persists in older depressed individuals even after recovery from depression, specifically manifesting as slowed information processing speed and executive dysfunction. Additionally, they found that decreased white matter contributes to LLD, and depression also worsens vascular outcomes in this group of patients.

Depression and risk of developing dementia were observed by Byers and Yaffe (2011). In this review, they analyzed evidence linking earlier and late-life depression and dementia, as well as treatment approaches (pharmacological and behavioral interventions). Such interventions for depression may improve cognitive performance (including memory) as well as reduce any pathophysiological alterations that may be associated with dementia and Alzheimer's Disease (AD). Although early-onset depression and/or depressive symptoms have been associated with more than a twofold increase in the risk of dementia, studies remain inconsistent regarding the nature of this association. It is still unclear whether depression is a prodrome (Mosoiu, 2016), a consequence, or a risk factor for dementia (Bennett & Thomas, 2014). The link between depression and dementia may be explained by various underlying biological markers which include vascular diseases, alterations in glucocorticosteroid levels, hippocampal atrophy, increased deposition of beta-amyloid, neurofibrillary tau tangles, inflammatory changes, and deficiency in nerve growth factors. The presence of these biological markers compromises the structural integrity of the prefrontal cortex and its connections with various cortical/subcortical areas, leading to deficits in EFs and depressive symptoms.

Steenland et al. (2012) analyzed 5607 normal subjects ($M_{\text{age}} = 72$) and 2500 with MCI ($M_{\text{age}} = 74$) at 30 Alzheimer Disease Research Center (ADRC) locations in the USA between 2005 and 2011 to observe whether depression played a role in the transition from normal to MCI or MCI to AD. They provided data on depression within the last two years as determined by judgment according to DSM-IV guidelines. Depression diagnoses included MDD, situational depression, bipolar disorder, and other mood disorders. They additionally defined depression based on the pattern across visits as (1) always depressed across all visits, (2) initially depressed and later considered as nondepressed, (3) intermittently depressed across visits, and (4) never depressed across all visits. At baseline, patients with normal cognition that were in one of the depressed categories performed worse on cognitive tests and had an increased risk of progression from normal to MCI, whereas normal subjects with initial depression but later considered nondepressed still had a heightened, yet lower risk of progression. This suggests that improvement in depression may diminish the risk of progression to MCI or AD. The participants who were always depressed also had a modest increased risk of progression from MCI to AD. This indicates that LLD is a strong risk factor for progression to MCI among cognitively normal patients.

Gonzales et al. (2017) investigated the association of cognitive decline and cortical atrophy in individuals with MCI and subsyndromal depression (defined as one depressive symptom such as depression/dysphoria, apathy/indifference, or loss of appetite endorsed by the Neuropsychiatric Inventory—NPI). The subsyndromal depressive (SSD) group had decreased scores in global cognition, memory, information processing, and semantic fluency. Also, the SSD group had accelerated frontal lobe and anterior cingulate atrophy. Paterniti, Verdier-Taillefer, Dufouil, and Alpérovitch (2002) examined depressive symptoms predicting cognitive decline in elderly people with normal cognition utilizing the Mini-Mental State Examination (MMSE). Higher levels of depressive symptoms predicted a higher risk of cognitive decline at the 2- and 4-year follow-up. Therefore, the presence of depressive symptoms has been strongly associated with higher cognitive decline.

12.5 Conclusions

The reviewed literature on executive dysfunction in depressive disorders (MDD) across age, as assessed by EF neuropsychological performance, revealed weak differences between children and adolescents with MDD and controls, failing to support the existence of executive dysfunction in MDD. On the other hand, adults with MDD have lower neuropsychological performance across several EF domains (inhibition, set-shifting, problem solving, planning, verbal fluency, processing speed, sustained attention, and verbal memory). Deficits were negatively correlated with the severity of depression and the duration of the depressive disorder. Age seems to be an additional risk factor for the development of DED in depressed individuals, with elderly patients suffering from more impairments in EFs and processing speed compared to younger depressed individuals. There is an overlap of the brain structures that mediate EFs and those producing functional abnormalities in MDD, including the PFC, the DLPFC, and the ACC. Finally, a heightened level of depression is a risk factor for increased cognitive decline in abnormal aging.

Acknowledgements We would like to express our gratitude to Valeria L. Torres for her comments and editing of this manuscript.

References

Albert, K. M., Potter, G. G., McQuoid, D. R., & Taylor, W. D. (2017). Cognitive performance in antidepressant-free recurrent major depressive disorder. *Depression & Anxiety*, 1–6. https://doi.org/10.1002/da.22747.

Alexopoulos, G. S. (2001). The depression-executive dysfunction syndrome of late life: A specific target for D3 agonists? *The American Journal of Geriatric Psychiatry, 9*(1), 22–29. https://doi.org/10.1097/00019442-200102000-00004.

Alexopoulos, G. S., Kiosses, D. N., Klimstra, S., Kalayam, B., & Bruce, M. L. (2002). Clinical presentation of the "depression–executive dysfunction syndrome" of late life. *The American Journal of Geriatric Psychiatry, 10*(1), 98–106. https://doi.org/10.1176/appi.ajgp.10.1.98.

Allott, K., Fisher, C. A., Amminger, G. P., Goodall, J., & Hetrick, S. (2016). Characterizing neurocognitive impairment in young people with major depression: State, trait, or scar? *Brain and Behavior, 6*(10), e00527. https://doi.org/10.1002/brb3.527.

American Psychiatric Association. (2013). *Diagnostic and statistical manual of mental disorders (DSM-5®)*. Arlington, V.A.: American Psychiatric Publishing.

Ardila, A., & Surloff, C. (2004). *Dysexecutive syndromes*. Medlink Neurology: San Diego, C.A., Arbor Publishing Co.

Ardila, A. (2013). There are two different dysexecutive syndromes. *Journal of Neurological Disorders, 1*(1), 1–4. https://doi.org/10.4172/2329-6895.1000114.

Austin, M. P., Mitchell, P., & Goodwin, G. M. (2001). Cognitive deficits in depression: Possible implications for functional neuropathology. *The British Journal of Psychiatry, 178*(3), 200–206. https://doi.org/10.1192/bjp.178.3.200.

Bayard, S., Erkes, J., & Moroni, C. (2011). Victoria Stroop Test: Normative data in a sample group of older people and the study of their clinical applications in the assessment of inhibition in Alzheimer's disease. *Archives of Clinical Neuropsychology, 26*(7), 653–661. https://doi.org/10.1093/arclin/acr053.

Bennett, S., & Thomas, A. J. (2014). Depression and dementia: Cause, consequence or coincidence? *Maturitas, 79*(2), 184–190.

Butters, M. A., Whyte, E. M., Nebes, R. D., Begley, A. E., Dew, M. A., Mulsant, B. H., … & Reynolds, C. F. (2004). The nature and determinants of neuropsychological functioning in late-life depression. *Archives of General Psychiatry, 61*(6), 587–595. https://doi.org/10.1001/archpsyc.61.6.587.

Byers, A. L., & Yaffe, K. (2011). Depression and risk of developing dementia. *Nature Reviews, Neurology, 7*(6), 323–331. https://doi.org/10.1038/nrneurol.2011.60.

Cullen, K. R., Klimes-Dougan, B., Muetzel, R., Mueller, B. A., Camchong, J., Houri, A., … & Lim, K. O. (2010). Altered white matter microstructure in adolescents with major depression: A preliminary study. *Journal of the American Academy of Child & Adolescent Psychiatry, 49*(2), 173–183. https://doi.org/10.1016/j.jaac.2009.11.005.

Comer, R. J. (2016). *Fundamentals of abnormal psychology* (8th ed.). New York: Worth Publishers.

Dotson, V. M., Resnick, S. M., & Zonderman, A. B. (2008). Differential association of concurrent, baseline, and average depressive symptoms with cognitive decline in older adults. *American Journal of Geriatric Psychiatry, 16*(4), 318–330. https://doi.org/10.1097/JGP.0b013e3181662a9c.

Espinoza, R., & Kaufman, A. H. (2014). Diagnosis and treatment of late-life depression. *Psychiatric Times, 31*(10), 18–23.

Farrar, D. C., Mian, A. Z., Budson, A. E., Moss, M. B., & Killiany, R. J. (2018). Functional brain networks involved in decision-making under certain and uncertain conditions. *Neuroradiology, 60*(1), 61–69. https://doi.org/10.1007/s00234-017-1949-1.

Favre, T., Hughes, C., Emslie, G., Stavinoha, P., Kennard, B., & Carmody, T. (2009). Executive functioning in children and adolescents with major depressive disorder. *Child Neuropsychology, 15*(1), 85–98. https://doi.org/10.1080/09297040802577311.

Fossati, P., Ergis, A. M., & Allilaire, J. F. (2002). Executive functioning in unipolar depression: A review. *L'encéphale, 28*(2), 97–107.

Förster, K., Jörgens, S., Air, T. M., Bürger, C., Enneking, V., Redlich, R., … & Leehr, E. J. (2018). The relationship between social cognition and executive function in Major Depressive Disorder in high-functioning adolescents and young adults. *Psychiatry research, 263*, 139–146. https://doi.org/10.1016/j.psychres.2018.02.046.

Goldman-Rakic, P. S. (1995). Architecture of the prefrontal cortex and the central executive. *Annals of the New York Academy of Sciences, 769,* 71–84. https://doi.org/10.1111/j.1749-6632.1995.tb38132.x.

Gonzales, M. M., Insel, P. S., Nelson, C., Tosun, D., Mattsson, N., Mueller, S. G., … & Alzheimer's Disease Neuroimaging Initiative. (2017). Cortical atrophy is associated with accelerated cognitive decline in mild cognitive impairment with subsyndromal depression. *The American Journal of Geriatric Psychiatry, 25*(9), 980–991. https://doi.org/10.1016/j.jagp.2017.04.011.

Günther, T., Konrad, K., De Brito, S. A., Herpertz-Dahlmann, B., & Vloet, T. D. (2011). Attentional functions in children and adolescents with ADHD, depressive disorders, and the comorbid condition. *Journal of Child Psychology and Psychiatry, 52*(3), 324–331. https://doi.org/10.1111/j.1469-7610.2010.02320.x.

Herrmann, L., Goodwin, G. M., & Ebmeier, K. P. (2007). The cognitive neuropsychology of depression in the elderly. *Psychological Medicine, 37,* 1693–1702. https://doi.org/10.1017/S0033291707001134.

Ho, M. C., Hsu, Y. C., Lu, M. L., Gossop, M., & Chen, V. C. H. (2018). 'Cool' and 'Hot' executive functions in suicide attempters with major depressive disorder. *Journal of Affective Disorders, 235,* 332–340. https://doi.org/10.1016/j.jad.2018.04.057.

Jungwirth, S., Zehetmayer, S., Hinterberger, M., Kudrnovsky-Moser, S., Weissgram, S., Tragl, K. H., et al. (2011). The influence of depression on processing speed and executive function in nondemented subjects aged 75. *Journal of the International Neuropsychological Society, 17*(5), 822–831.

Jurado, M. B., & Rosselli, M. (2007). The elusive nature of executive functions: A review of our current understanding. *Neuropsychology Review, 17*(3), 213–233. https://doi.org/10.1007/s11065-007-9040-z.

Kerr, A., & Zelazo, P. D. (2004). Development of "hot" executive function: The children's gambling task. *Brain and Cognition, 55*(1), 148–157. https://doi.org/10.1016/S0278-2626(03)00275-6.

Kluwe-Schiavon, B., Viola, T. W., Sanvicente-Vieira, B., Malloy-Diniz, L. F., & Grassi-Oliveira, R. (2017). Balancing automatic-controlled behaviors and emotional-salience states: A dynamic executive functioning hypothesis. *Frontiers in Psychology, 7*(2067), 1–12. https://doi.org/10.3389/fpsyg.2016.02067.

Kocsel, N., Szabó, E., Galambos, A., Édes, A., Pap, D., Elliott, R., … & Kökönyei, G. (2017). Trait rumination influences neural correlates of the anticipation but not the consumption phase of reward processing. *Frontiers in Behavioral Neuroscience, 11*(85). 1–10. https://doi.org/10.3389/fnbeh.2017.00085.

Koenig, A. M., Bhalla, R. K., & Butters, M. A. (2014). Cognitive functioning and late-life depression. *Journal of the International Neuropsychological Society, 20*(5), 461–467. https://doi.org/10.1017/S1355617714000198.

Köhler, S., Thomas, A. J., Lloyd, A., Barber, R., Almeida, O. P., & O'brien, J. T. (2010). White matter hyperintensities, cortisol levels, brain atrophy and continuing cognitive deficits in late-life depression. *The British Journal of Psychiatry, 196*(2), 143–149. https://doi.org/10.1192/bjp.bp.109.071399.

Lezak, M. (1983). *Neuropsychological assessment* (2nd ed.). New York: Oxford University Press.

Light, S. N., Heller, A. S., Johnstone, T., Kolden, G. G., Peterson, M. J., Kalin, N. H., et al. (2011). Reduced right ventrolateral prefrontal cortex activity while inhibiting positive affect is associated with improvement in hedonic capacity after 8 weeks of antidepressant treatment in major depressive disorder. *Biological Psychiatry, 70*(10), 962–968. https://doi.org/10.1016/j.biopsych.2011.06.031.

Lockwood, K. A., Alexopoulos, G. S., & van Gorp, W. G. (2002). Executive dysfunction in geriatric depression. *American Journal of Psychiatry, 159*(7), 1119–1126. https://doi.org/10.1176/appi.ajp.159.7.1119.

Malloy-Diniz, L. F., Miranda, D. M., & Grassi-Oliveira, R. (2017). Executive functions in psychiatric disorders. *Frontiers in Psychology, 8,* 1461. https://doi.org/10.3389/fpsyg.2017.01461.

McDermott, L. M., & Ebmeier, K. P. (2009). A meta-analysis of depression severity and cognitive function. *Journal of Affective Disorders, 119*(1–3), 1–8. https://doi.org/10.1016/j.jad.2009.04.022.

Miyake, A., Friedman, N. P., Emerson, M. J., Witzki, A. H., Howerter, A., & Wager, T. D. (2000). The unity and diversity of executive functions and their contributions to complex "frontal lobe" tasks: A latent variable analysis. *Cognitive Psychology, 41*(1), 49–100. https://doi.org/10.1006/cogp.1999.0734.

Morimoto, S. S., Gunning, F. M., Murphy, C. F., Kanellopoulos, D., Kelly, R. E., Jr., & Alexopoulos, G. S. (2011). Executive function and short-term remission of geriatric depression: The role of semantic strategy. *The American Journal of Geriatric Psychiatry, 19*(2), 115–122. https://doi.org/10.1097/JGP.0b013e3181e751c4.

Mosoiu, C. (2016). Depression as a prodrome in Alzheimer's disease. *Acta Medica Transilvanica, 21*(2), 40–42.

Neshat-Doost, H. T., Moradi, A. R., Taghavi, M. R., Yule, W., & Dalgleish, T. (2000). Lack of attentional bias for emotional information in clinically depressed children and adolescents on the dot probe task. *The Journal of Child Psychology and Psychiatry and Allied Disciplines, 41*(3), 363–368. https://doi.org/10.1111/1469-7610.00620.

Ochsner, K. N., & Gross, J. J. (2007). The Neural Architecture of Emotion Regulation. In J. J. Gross (Ed.), *Handbook of emotion regulation* (pp. 87–109). New York, NY, US: The Guilford Press.

Ottowitz, W. E., Tondo, L., Dougherty, D. D., & Savage, C. R. (2002). The neural network basis for abnormalities of attention and executive function in major depressive disorder: Implications for application of the medical disease model to psychiatric disorders. *Harvard Review of Psychiatry, 10*(2), 86–99. https://doi.org/10.1080/10673220216210.

Paelecke-Habermann, Y., Pohl, J., & Leplow, B. (2005). Attention and executive functions in remitted major depression patients. *Journal of Affective Disorders, 89,* 125–135. https://doi.org/10.1016/j.jad.2005.09.006.

Paterniti, S., Verdier-Taillefer, M. H., Dufouil, C., & Alpérovitch, A. (2002). Depressive symptoms and cognitive decline in elderly people: Longitudinal study. *The British Journal of Psychiatry, 181*(5), 406–410. https://doi.org/10.1192/bjp.181.5.406.

Peters, S. L., Fellows, L. K., & Sheldon, S. (2017). The ventromedial frontal lobe contributes to forming effective solutions to real-world problems. *Journal of Cognitive Neuroscience, 29*(6), 991–1001. https://doi.org/10.1162/jocn_a_01088.

Pizzagalli, D. A. (2011). Frontocingulate dysfunction in depression: Toward biomarkers of treatment response. *Neuropsychopharmacology, 36*(1), 183–206. https://doi.org/10.1038/npp.2010.166.

Ravnkilde, B., Videbech, P., Clemmensen, K., Egander, A., Rasmussen, N. A., & Rosenberg, R. (2002). Cognitive deficits in major depression. *Scandinavian Journal of Psychology, 43*(3), 239–251. https://doi.org/10.1111/1467-9450.00292.

Rogers, M. A., Kasai, K., Koji, M., Fukuda, R., Iwanami, A., Nakagome, K., … & Kato, N. (2004). Executive and prefrontal dysfunction in unipolar depression: A review of neuropsychological and imaging evidence. *Neuroscience research, 50*(1), 1–11. https://doi.org/10.1016/j.neures.2004.05.003.

Schmid, M. T., & Hammar, Å. (2013). A follow-up study of first episode major depressive disorder. Impairment in inhibition and semantic fluency—potential predictors for relapse? *Frontiers in psychology*, *4*, 633. https://doi.org/10.3389/fpsyg.2013.00633.

Snyder, H. R. (2013). Major depressive disorder is associated with broad impairments on neuropsychological measures of executive function: A meta-analysis and review. *Psychological Bulletin, 139*(1), 81–132. https://doi.org/10.1037/a0028727.

Steenland, K., Karnes, C., Seals, R., Carnevale, C., Hermida, A., & Levey, A. (2012). Late-life depression as a risk factor for mild cognitive impairment or Alzheimer's disease in 30 US Alzheimer's disease centers. *Journal of Alzheimer's Disease, 31*(2), 265–275. https://doi.org/10.3233/JAD-2012-111922.

Tandon, R. (2015). Bipolar and depressive disorders in diagnostic and statistical manual of mental disorders-5: Clinical implications of revisions from diagnostic and statistical manual of mental disorders-IV. *Indian journal of Psychological Medicine, 37*(1), 1–4. https://doi.org/10.4103/0253-7176.150796.

Thomas, A. J., & O'Brien, J. (2008). Depression and cognition in older adults. *Current Opinion in Psychiatry, 21*(1), 8–13. https://doi.org/10.1097/YCO.0b013e3282f2139b.

Thomas, P., Hazif Thomas, C., Billon, R., Peix, R., Faugeron, P., & Clément, J. P. (2009). Depression and frontal dysfunction: Risks for the elderly? *L'Encephale, 35*(4), 361–369. https://doi.org/10.1016/j.encep.2008.03.012.

Tremblay, M. P., Potvin, O., Belleville, S., Bier, N., Gagnon, L., Blanchet, S., … & Hudon, C. (2016). The victoria stroop test: Normative data in Quebec-French adults and elderly. *Archives of Clinical Neuropsychology, 31*(8), 926–933. https://doi.org/10.1093/arclin/acw029.

Vilgis, V., Silk, T. J., & Vance, A. (2015). Executive function and attention in children and adolescents with depressive disorders: A systematic review. *European Child and Adolescent Psychiatry, 24*(4), 365–384. https://doi.org/10.1007/s00787-015-0675-7.

Wagner, C. A., Alloy, L. B., & Abramson, L. Y. (2015a). Trait rumination, depression, and executive functions in early adolescence. *Journal of Youth and Adolescence, 44*(1), 18–36. https://doi.org/10.1007/s10964-014-0133-8.

Wagner, S., Müller, C., Helmreich, I., Huss, M., & Tadić, A. (2015b). A meta-analysis of cognitive functions in children and adolescents with major depressive disorder. *European Child and Adolescent Psychiatry, 24*(1), 5–19. https://doi.org/10.1007/s00787-014-0559-2.

World Health Organization. (2004). ICD-10: International statistical classification of diseases and related health problems: Tenth revision (2nd ed.). World Health Organization. http://www.who.int/iris/handle/10665/42980.

Zakzanis, K. K., Leach, L., & Kaplan, E. (1998). On the nature and pattern of neurocognitive function in major depressive disorder. *Neuropsychiatry, Neuropsychology, and Behavioral Neurology, 11*(3), 111–119.

Chapter 13
Correlates of Executive Dysfunction in HIV

Roger C. McIntosh and Judy D. Lobo

13.1 Introduction

According to the Center for Disease Control Human Immunodeficiency Virus (HIV) disease may be categorized as (1) asymptomatic, i.e., absence of serious illness and T cell counts above 200, (2) symptomatic, i.e., presenting with non-AIDS-defining illnesses and T-cell counts above 200 or (3) acquired immune deficiency syndrome (AIDS), i.e., having an AIDS-defining opportunistic infection and/or a current or prior T-cell count below 200 (Control & Prevention, 1992). Observations made in the neurological sequel of HIV from the beginning of the epidemic to the late 1990s revealed stark decline in motor functioning, executive skills and information processing speed across the disease spectrum (Reger, Welsh, Razani, Martin, & Boone, 2002). Toward the end of the second decade there was a paradigm shift in the course of the epidemic that was the widespread availability of antiretroviral therapy (ART). Historically, the most commonly reported cognitive domains ART shows an effect are attention, psychomotor speed, verbal learning and memory, as well as global cognitive function. However, early evidence for the effectiveness of ART on executive functions (EF) are inconsistent suggesting disease progression may not be the only contributor to dysexecutive syndromes in persons living with HIV (PLWH) (Cohen et al., 2001; Sacktor et al., 2003; Tozzi et al., 1993, 1999). Nonetheless, the emergence of combination ART (cART) with enhanced features such as central nervous system penetrability has once again changed the course of neurocognitive decline in PLWH, albeit not equally amongst the afore-mentioned cognitive domains (Cysique & Brew, 2009; Heaton et al., 2011). Indeed, rates of neurocognitive impairment before and after widespread cART availability reveal some concerning trends. Notably, rates of mild neurocognitive impairment have risen across the entire disease spectrum; meanwhile, rates of dysfunction in the executive and learning/memory domains are

R. C. McIntosh (✉) · J. D. Lobo
Department of Psychology, University of Miami, Miami, FL, USA
e-mail: r.mcintosh@miami.edu

A. Ardila et al. (eds.), *Dysexecutive Syndromes*,
https://doi.org/10.1007/978-3-030-25077-5_13

being reported at their highest rate (Heaton et al., 2011), particularly in individuals with late-stage HIV disease (Goodkin et al., 2017). Although these trends may be partially attributed to the higher rates of survival into older age (Cohen, Seider, & Navia, 2015; Hardy & Vance, 2009; Valcour, Shikuma, Watters, & Sacktor, 2004; Wendelken & Valcour, 2012), other factors are increasingly being shown to contribute to rates of executive dysfunction in HIV. What follows is a discussion of the various manifestations of executive dysfunction in HIV, their measurement and levels of severity and known associations with central and peripheral biomarkers, psychosocial as well as behavioral risk factors.

13.2 Assessing Executive Dysfunction in HIV

Early efforts to establish the etiology of neurocognitive impairment in HIV focused on polar ends of the spectrum through the identification of primarily asymptomatic individuals with minor cognitive motor disorder (MCMD) and HIV-associated dementia (HAD). Based upon recommendations from a National Institutes of Health (NIH) working group, the nosology for what is now known as HIV-associated neurocognitive disorder (HAND) was revisited and subsequently amended based on performance in at least five domains of neurocognitive functioning typically found to be impacted along the course of HIV infection, i.e., attention/working memory, EFs, episodic memory, speed of information processing, motor skills, language and sensory perception (Antinori et al., 2007). Dependent upon the level of impairment and disease course, HAND may be further subdivided into symptomatic forms of mild neurocognitive disorder (MNCD) and HAD or the asymptomatic form of asymptomatic neurocognitive impairment (ANI). These subtleties pose a unique challenge as patients with ANI often do not experience or report symptoms, yet are at higher risk of developing symptomatic cognitive impairments (Grant et al., 2014). Although the study of HIV-related executive dysfunction has blossomed in recent years, the literature is convoluted with multiple abstractions of EF being reported as outcome measures across studies. While there are several approaches to characterization of EF into core domains such as updating and working memory, set-shifting, and inhibition (Jurado & Rosselli, 2007; Miyake et al., 2000; Stuss & Alexander, 2000), it is widely accepted that there is no unitary EF but rather evidence of varying degrees of frontal lobe involvement with the striatum and limbic system during cognitive task performance (Bechara, Damasio, Tranel, & Anderson, 1998; Lezak, Howieson, Loring, & Fischer, 2004). Those EF domains receiving considerable attention in most recent years include inhibition, updating/working memory, set-shifting and mental flexibility along with decision making (Walker & Brown, 2018).

Inhibition or the ability to withhold or attenuate an action or thought is one of the core functions contributing to performance on attention and complex EF tasks (Hofmann, Schmeichel, & Baddeley, 2012). Because inhibition is tied to many health-related behaviors it has been studied extensively in PLWH. Perhaps the most widely utilized measure of inhibitory control used within this population has been the Stroop task (Hinkin, Castellon, Hardy, Granholm, & Siegle, 1999; Martin et al., 1992). Stroop task indicators of inhibitory control vary widely across studies from vocal reaction time (RT) to time of completion on interference trials (Chang et al., 2002; Cohen et al., 2011; Maki et al., 2015; Martin et al., 2004a). When verbal report is not permissible, such as during an fMRI experiment, the Stroop Match-to-Sample task involving perceptual cueing and repetition has been incorporated to assess PLWH for performance decrements due to cognitive interference (Schulte, Müller-Oehring, Sullivan, & Pfefferbaum, 2011). Also utilized in HIV research is the stop-signal anticipation task as an index of frontostriatal function during inhibitory control (du Plessis et al., 2015).

Updating and working memory are a composite of EFs frequently assessed in PLWH. The most commonly used task design to demonstrate deficits in updating and working memory within PLWH has been the n-back task wherein the two-back condition is most often reported. The sensory domains to which performance outcomes are typically identified include verbal/auditory and visual stimuli (Chang et al., 2008; Hinkin et al., 2002). However, not all post-cART studies have report HIV-related effects within this domain perhaps due to the presence of medical comorbidities such as Hepatitis C Virus (HCV) (Caldwell et al., 2014; Ernst, Chang, Jovicich, Ames, & Arnold, 2002). It is important to note that while the 2-back task provides strong support for HIV-related deficits in working memory modified digit and letter span tasks provide corresponding support in the visual and auditory domain (Farinpour et al., 2000; Hinkin et al., 2002; Martin et al., 2001).

Set-shifting has been described as an individual's ability to reorient attention between different elements of the same task and may be tapped—in part or whole—by complex or resource-dependent EF tasks. Among the tasks most commonly used to assess ability to shift attention is Part B of the Trail Making Test. When controlling for speed of visual processing and fine motor function, this test provides a proxy of mental set-shifting that is integral to EF (Reitan, 1958). Most of the evidence supporting HIV-related effects in set-shifting ability have come from older adult cohorts and substance-abusing PLWH (Bousman et al., 2010a; Chang et al., 2011; Fama, Sullivan, Sassoon, Pfefferbaum, & Zahr, 2016; Kesby et al., 2015, Tang et al., 2015). Nevertheless, some negative findings have been reported in studies comparing performance between PLWH and HIV-negative adults (Manly et al., 2011; Rippeth et al., 2004). The Wisconsin Card Sorting Task (WSCT) is another frequently used complex EF measure that has yielded inconsistent results, potentially confounded by age and SES, regarding deficits in set-shifting ability amongst PLWH (Corrêa et al., 2016; Rippeth et al., 2004). Moreover, composite measures of both WCST and TMT-B suggest HIV-related difficulty in set-shifting (Carter et al., 2003; Reger, Welsh, Razani, Martin, & Boone, 2002). Seldom-used measures of set-shifting further contributing to this heterogeneity in findings amongst PLWH include intra/extra-dimensional shifting tasks and other custom-designed task-switching paradigms (Bousman et al., 2010b; Byrd et al., 2013; Fama et al., 2016; Jiang, Barasky, Olsen, Riesenhuber, & Magnus, 2016; Kesby et al., 2015; Spies, Fennema-Notestine, Cherner, & Seedat, 2017; Tang et al., 2015).

Although not considered by some to be a pure measure of EF decision making ability is heavily dependent upon frontal lobe function and an integral component in behavioral health and disease management in PLWH (Doyle et al., 2016). In the cART era the Iowa gambling task (Bechara, 2007) and the Cambridge gambling task (Sahakian & Owen, 1992) have emerged as the more frequently reported assessments for decision making in PLWH (Iudicello et al., 2013). The vast majority of these studies reveal HIV-related deficits (Hardy, Hinkin, Levine, Castellon, & Lam, 2006; Iudicello et al., 2013; Thames et al., 2012), yet some reports remain inconclusive (Gonzalez et al., 2005; Paydary et al., 2016). IGT performance in PLWH is strongly mitigated by levels of depression implicating affect dysregulation in the etiology of decision-making deficits in this population. Despite this strong tie to affect-related processes such as punishment and reward, IGT performance is shown to be strongly predictive of global EF in PLWH (Thames et al., 2012). Decision making under ambiguity, i.e., when risk and reward contingencies are not explicitly known, appears to be particularly impaired amongst PLWH compared to when risks are explicitly known (Martin et al., 2013). Decision making under explicit risk is less frequently assessed in HIV, but evident in allied tasks such as Game of Dice where peripheral biomarkers such as Nadir CD4+ T-cell count, substance abuse behavior, and psychiatric comorbidities are highly predictive of performance (Gomez, Power, Gill, & Fujiwara, 2017). In another study comparing HIV patients with HIV-negative controls impaired performance on the Game of Dice Task was found suggesting explicit risk decision making impairments in HIV+ individuals are characterized by less advantageous choices and more random choice strategies (Fujiwara, Tomlinson, Purdon, Gill, & Power, 2015). HIV-related deficits in other decision-making assessments such as the balloon analogue task (Paydary et al., 2016) are evident; however, findings from the intertemporal choice Task are null (Meade et al., 2016). Decision-making deficits in PLWH may also be attributable to poor working memory hence more of a syndrome of EF-related deficits; however, results from a study examining IGT performance in HIV-positive and HIV-negative controls with past or current history of substance dependence found delayed non-match to sample task did not relate to decision-making ability (Martin et al., 2004b).

13.3 Peripheral Biomarkers of Executive Dysfunction in HIV

HIV-1 viral RNA and CD4+ counts are among the most commonly used clinical biomarkers of disease progression that are used in conjunction with neurocognitive assessment and diagnosis with HAND. Nonetheless, studies examining the neurocognitive correlates of plasma viral RNA yield inconsistent support for an effect of viral replication on executive dysfunction (Mcguire, Gill, Douglas, & Kolson, 2015; Reger et al., 2005). These and other studies suggest that despite suppression of systemic HIV infection and viral RNA proliferation through cART HIV-related cognitive impairment in the executive domain remains elevated. Despite this, allied measures of viral DNA levels provide some insight into the sequel of executive dysfunction in PLWH in the absence of unhindered viral replication. For example, elevated circulating levels of HIV DNA were linked to poorer performance on a composite measure of EF in older, but not younger, virally suppressed PLWH suggesting an interaction of HIV and age on EF (de Oliveira et al., 2015). Although fraught with inconsistencies, this and other studies inform a paradigm shift in our understanding of peripheral biomarkers predictive of executive dysfunction in PLWH. Of particular interest are peripheral and central biomarkers of inflammation and monocyte activation. One of the main observations made in older adults and individuals with chronic immune suppression is that of inflammation and immune activation, i.e., inflamm-aging (Nasi et al., 2017). In the last several years peripheral monocytes have emerged as a primary reservoir for HIV DNA most closely linked to neurocognitive impairment (Cysique et al., 2015; Kusao et al., 2012; Shiramizu, Williams, Shikuma, & Valcour, 2009; Valcour et al., 2013). Evidence of EF deficits related to peripheral inflammation is common within the literature. For example, along with learning deficits lower performance on a battery of EF tests normed by the HIV Neurobehavioral Research Center (Heaton et al., 2011) yielded an inverse association with higher plasma sCD163 a monocyte/macrophage-specific scavenger receptor shed during the pro-inflammatory response (Burdo et al., 2013).

A host of peripheral biomarkers of inflammation are found to be coincident with inhibitory deficits in PLWH. Reduced performance on the Stroop task has been associated with elevated MIP-1β while evidence of reduced IL-18, MCP-1 and TNF-α concentrations suggesting imbalances in pro- to anti-inflammatory cytokine expression may explain inhibitory deficits in PLWH, particularly those coinfected with other chronic inflammatory immune conditions such as HCV (Cohen et al., 2011). In the Women's Interagency HIV Study (WIHS) higher soluble CD163 and marker of monocyte activation CD14+ was related to EF deficits indexed by the Stroop and Trails Making B task performance. However, circulating IL-6 and another marker of gut microbial translocation were unrelated suggesting a specificity to the effect of inflammatory immune response from different cellular and hence viral reservoirs on EF in PLWH (Imp et al., 2016).

Monocyte activation is also linked to composite measures of working memory performance consisting of the Letter-Number Sequencing Test and Paced Auditory Serial Addition Test (PASAT-50) (Lyons et al., 2011; Woods et al., 2004). Peripheral inflammation, indexed by elevated levels of pro-inflammatory cytokines and reductions in several anti-inflammatory cytokines, is the primary outcome of activated transcription factors such as nuclear factor kappa B in monocyte/macrophage populations. These factors interact in a way that leads to enhanced viral replication in HIV (Thieblemont et al., 1995). Reduced levels of two particular anti-inflammatory cytokine markers, i.e., IL-10 and TRAIL (thought to be involved in activation of cell death/survival signals), were retained among other immunoassayed cytokines as significant predictors of Letter-Number Sequencing performance in a small cohort of HIV-positive and HIV-negative adults (Cohen et al., 2011a). A recent double-blind, placebo-controlled, crossover study examining the time-dependent effects of a single low-dose administration of oral hydrocortisone in 36 HIV-positive women revealed enhanced working memory performance, indexed by the letter-number sequencing task, 30 min after administration (Rubin, Phan, Keating, & Maki, 2018b). Interestingly, these hydrocortisone-related reductions in working memory were mitigated by plasma reductions in tumor necrosis factor (TNF)-α, soluble receptor for TNF type II (TNFRII), MCP-1, MMP9, and sCD14 (Rubin et al., 2018b). Another trial examining the effect of cenicriviroc, a dual C-C chemokine receptor type 2 (CCR2) and type 5 (CCR5) antagonist showed increased working memory performance indexed by the Digit Span Backward, California Verbal Learning Test B, and LNS associated with decreased monocyte activation indexed by sCD163, sCD14, and neopterin (D'Antoni et al., 2018). Among a cohort of low-SES midlife women followed longitudinally, TNF-α and IL-6 predicted poorer global neurocognitive impairment across HIV-positive and HIV-negative individuals while C-reactive protein (CRP) specifically predicted lower attention/working memory indexed by the letter-number sequencing task (Rubin et al., 2018a). Adjacent to these studies Woods and colleagues explored the relationship of peripheral and central biomarkers of inflammation performance on a procedural memory task. Procedural memory is a form of memory for future intentions that involves executive capacities of set-shifting, inhibition, and updating in conjunction with intent and planning (Kliegel et al., 2002; Schnitzspahn, Stahl, Zeintl, Kaller, & Kliegel, 2013). After controlling for HIV disease and treatment-related factors, higher levels of TNFRII, MCP-1 in plasma, and tau in cerebrospinal fluid were associated with greater decrements in prospective memory performance (Woods et al., 2006).

In contrast to this working memory literature, evidence of peripheral biomarkers linked explicitly to set-shifting or mental flexibility domain are more seldomly found. In a cross-sectional study of HIV+/HCV+ adults and HIV-seronegative controls, reduced performance on TMT-B was associated with elevated IL-6 and reduced IL-10 concentrations (Cohen et al., 2011). Genetic sequencing for biomarkers of neurodegeneration derived from peripheral blood yield interesting associations with markers of set-shifting ability. For example, the *APOE* ε4 allele has been associated with poorer Trails B and the Stroop interference task performance within HIV-positive but not HIV-negative individuals (Chang et al., 2011, 2014).

To date, very few studies examining decision-making ability in persons living with HIV compare these indices to peripheral biomarkers. Lower current CD4 cell count has been associated with greater activation of prefrontal brain regions during a decision-making task indirectly suggesting immune suppression is predictive of altered allocation of neural resources during this task (Connolly et al., 2014).

13.4 Central Biomarkers of Executive Dysfunction in HIV

Akin to advancements made in our understanding of the relationship of peripheral immune to executive functioning in HIV, there is now extensive support for the role of immune surveillance in the CNS in the manifestation of neurocognitive impairment among PLWH (Spudich, 2016). CNS metabolites such as glutamate are increasingly linked with HAND and may reflect the indirect damage of neuronal processes via neurotoxic secretions from surveillance cells such as microglia (Dickens et al., 2015; Erdmann et al., 2007; Jiang et al., 2001; Zheng et al., 2001). The damage to neurons in HIV appears to be secondary to the shedding of viral proteins such as TAT and gp120 (Behnisch, Francesconi, & Sanna, 2004; Maragos et al., 2003) or indirectly due to the production of neurotoxic substances from activated astrocytes, monocyte/macrophages, and resident microglia (Benos, Mcpherson, Hahn, Chaikin, & Benveniste, 1994; Brack-Werner, 1999; Chen et al., 2002; Patton, Zhou, Bubien, Benveniste, & Benos, 2000). Indeed, neurons are not directly infected by HIV; rather, greater evidence has been levied in support of the direct infection and activation of these neuroglia and resident immune cells (Epstein and Gendelman, 1993; Trillo-Pazos et al., 2003). This work has traditionally featured pathology of hippocampal regions in the context of HAD; however, exploration into HIV viral proteins and indirect HIV neurotoxicity of midbrain, striatal and cortical dopaminergic neurons yield insight into frontostriatal executive control systems (Bennett et al., 1995; Everall et al., 1999; Itoh, Mehraein, & Weis, 2000; Nath et al., 2000).

There are several magnetic resonance imaging (MRI) modalities used to investigate HIV-related changes in the brain. Magnetic resonance spectroscopy (MRS), for instance, has been used to measure subclinical biochemical abnormalities in the brain that correspond with changes in the metabolic function of underlying cells (Cysique et al., 2013). MRS studies found a Abnormal brain metabolite levels are commonly found in white matter areas underlying executive control (Chang et al., 2002; Ernst et al., 2003). These findings are also consistent with white matter changes detectible by diffusion tensor imaging (DTI) tractography which is an MRI method that measures white matter abnormalities in vivo. In PLWH, average directional movement through white matter, or global functional anisotropy (FA), was also associated with impaired executive function (Tate et al., 2010). The association between EF and HIV extends to the structure and function of gray matter. Structural MRI, which is used to measure the cortical thickness of the brain, consistently reports HIV-related loss in cortical volume (Chang et al., 2011; Pfefferbaum et al., 2012). Functional magnetic resonance imaging (fMRI) is also emerging as a sensitive tool for detecting cerebral pathology related to HIV (Ernst et al., 2002). Blood oxygenated level dependent (BOLD) fMRI measures the brain's hemodynamic response, i.e., delivery of oxygenated blood in response to metabolic activity among neural ensembles. BOLD fMRI studies often investigate changes in functional connectivity (FC), the synchronous activation of spatially distributed brain regions (Biswal, Yetkin, Haughton, & Hyde, 1995). Functional neuroimaging studies of the brain repeatedly show that HIV-associated cognitive function is associated with the FC of the frontostriatal circuits that are involved with attention and working memory (Chang et al., 2001; Ernst et al., 2002). A meta-analysis of fMRI studies concluded that the frontostriatal circuit is generally hyperactive in HIV-positive individuals (Plessis et al., 2014, 2015). Dysfunctional FC between the basal ganglia and frontal regions of the brain was also observed (Ipser et al., 2015; Melrose, Tinaz, Castelo, Courtney, & Stern, 2008; Ortega, Brier, & Ances, 2015; Thomas et al., 2013). In sum, there are generalizable disturbances that can be observed in HIV-positive subjects compared to seronegative in areas involved with EF (Hakkers et al., 2017).

MRS markers of glial functioning (i.e., myo-inositol and creatine) within the frontal white matter have also been found to correlate with reduced inhibitory control, suggesting a possible etiological basis for striatal abnormalities (Chang et al., 2002). As previously mentioned, striatal brain regions in conjunction with frontal lobes are important contributors to EF ability in HIV. In a study comparing treatment-naïve PLWH to HIV-negative controls functional hypoactivation of the right and left putamen was observed while performing the Stop Signal Anticipation Task (SSAT) suggesting poorer inhibitory control (du Plessis et al., 2015). In a follow-up study, reduced functional activity of the left putamen during the modified SSAT was also associated with reduced cortical thickness of the right superior frontal gyrus (du Plessis et al., 2016).

Central biomarkers of neuronal metabolic activity, measured by magnetic resonance spectroscopy (MRS) also relate to working memory deficits in PLWH. For example, working memory deficits were linked to abnormal choline and myo-inositol in frontal white matter and the basal ganglia (Ernst et al., 2003). The neural network most closely implicated in working memory processes in the frontal-parietal attention network. This network has at its core the posterior parietal cortex (PPC) and the prefrontal cortex (PFC). These structures overlap, and the resulting frontoparietal network consistently becomes active during working memory processes (Murray, Jaramillo, & Wang, 2017). Functional abnormalities in frontostriatal and frontoparietal circuitry, which are common in HIV, may also conribute to deficits in working memory (Chang et al., 2001, 2002; Tomasi, Chang, De Castro Caparelli, Telang, & Ernst, 2006). For instance, hyperactivation, particularly in the lateral PFC, was found within and outside the frontoparietal network before and after completing four distinct working memory tasks, suggesting perhaps compensatory challenges for PLWH during working memory task performance (Chang et al., 2001; Ernst et al., 2002). HIV-related deficits in working memory are also found to correlate with BOLD activation in the cerebellum and superior PFC (Tomasi et al., 2006). It should be noted that although most HIV studies report significant differences in cortical activation during working memory tasks, group differences in behavioral performance are not consistently noted suggesting these functional biomarkers are sensitive to compensatory differences in working memory amongst PLWH compared to HIV-negative controls (Caldwell et al., 2014).

Neuroimaging studies in PLWH also suggest that poorer performance in set-shifting ability correlates with structural and functional abnormalities in frontostriatal circuit. HIV-associated changes can be observed in the metabolic activity of global white matter regions of the brain as evidenced by the association of glutamate concentrations with performance on TMT-B (Trillo-pazos et al., 2003). In another study, performance on the TMT-B and the verbal interference task was found to correlate with global FA, (Tate et al., 2010). Lower performance on the WCST is also shown to correspond with lower cortical volume of the bilateral caudate, the left accumbens, right putamen, and globus pallidum of HIV-positive individuals (Correa et al., 2016). Support for set-shifting deficits also extends from the structural literature into the functional domain of neuroimaging studies. In an fMRI study using a task-switching paradigm wherein individuals performed a face-gender or word-semantic task, HIV-related failure to adapt to change was associated with a paucity of activation within the anterior cingulate cortex (ACC), compared to HIV-negative controls (Jiang et al., 2016a). Overall, findings across a host of neuroimaging modalities support abberant brain activity for PLWH during set-shifting tasks.

HIV-related performance decrements on gambling and decision-making tasks are associated with abnormal activation in several brain regions known to support decision-making including the medial PFC, dorsal striatum, ventral striatum, and insula (Connolly et al., 2014; Meade et al., 2016). In an fMRI task there were no behavioral differences found in the rate participants made choices between smaller, more immediate rewards and larger delayed rewards, however, there was an HIV-group effect for activation of the left parietal and bilateral prefrontal cortex during easy trials and soley within the prefrontal cortex during more difficult trials suggesting aberrant allocation of cognitive resources during decision making tasks (Connolly et al., 2014). In addition to the absence of an group effect on behavioral performance the magnitude of HIV-related activation of PFC corresponded with lower CD4 cell nadir count and risk-taking propensity. In another decision-making fMRI task HIV-related differences were noted in behavioral performance, however, greater activation of the basal ganglia, ACC, insula and dorsolateral PFC was found while making risky choices. Additionally, functional neuroimaging has provided evidence of a unique interaction for poly-substance use among primary cocaine abusers in HIV-positive individuals that resulted in aberrant activation in the bilateral PFC and cerebellum during an intertemporal decision-making task (Meade et al., 2017). Lack of behavioral differences to scan tasks. This area of research suggests that there is an adaptive functional response of the frontostriatal loop during decision making processes that may be dysfunctional in HIV despite comparable performance on behavioral indices. Moreover, behavioral factors such as substance abuse can further debilitate these networks to compensate for HIV-related deficits in EF.

13.5 Behavioral Factors Linked to Executive Dysfunction in HIV

Since the beginning of the epidemic, several behavioral factors have aligned with executive difficulties in PLWH, the most intuitive being adherence to ART and the presumed impact of viral suppression on neurocognitive outcomes. Considering the context of this chapter and other text that has covered these relationships in detail (Cysique and Brew, 2009), we turn our focus to other pertinent health behaviors tied to HIV disease management, namely the salient and syndemic effects substance abuse in this population. Despite the widespread availability of cART and lower HIV-related mortality, the number of individuals reporting a history of substance abuse has been on a rise (Control & Prevention, 2005). It is estimated that in the USA over

61.4% of adults under care for HIV report use of substance abuse or mental health services (Burnam et al., 2001). Historically, research in substance-abusing PLWH has focused on intravenous drug users; however, poly-substance-based research on alcohol, psychostimulants, and cannabis use continue to show a rise in usage (Chander, Himelhoch, & Moore, 2006; Hinkin et al., 2004). Recreational and medicinal marijuana use in HIV-positive persons is among the most common forms of substance use (Fogarty et al., 2007). Although still controversial, the largest effects for chronic marijuana use on cognitive functioning in PLWH appears to be within the memory domain (Cristiani, Pukay-Martin, & Bornstein, 2004; Gonzalez, Schuster, Vassileva, & Martin, 2011). Alcohol abuse has substantial impact on most domains of cognitive functioning amongst PLWJ with effects lingering years after sobriety (Gongvatana et al., 2014; Stavro, Pelletier, & Potvin, 2013). While in the presence of alcohol abuse most forms of cognitive functioning show declining trends and are associated with decreased viral resistance, exacerbated metabolic injury, and negative neuropathological, immune, and other treatment outcomes (Azar, Springer, Meyer, & Altice, 2010; Baum et al., 2010; Braithwaite et al., 2007; Conigliaro et al., 2006; Persidsky et al., 2011). Studies examining the effects of stimulant use on neurocognition in HIV have become more expansive with cocaine and methamphetamine use sharing the spotlight in terms of neurobehavioral sequel of psychostimulant abuse among vulnerable populations (Goodkin et al., 1998; Morgan, Iudicello, Weber, & Woods, 2016, Meade, Conn, Skalski, & Safren, 2011; Napier, 2017; Soontornniyomkij et al., 2016).

As our understanding of the neurocognitive sequel of HIV expands, it has also become evident that levels of exercise and physical activity may be important predictors of neurocognitive outcomes in the executive domain (Vancampfort et al., 2018b; Weber, Blackstone, & Woods, 2013). Physical activity and exercise levels in PLWH are among the lowest reported in chronic disease populations due to various factors such as HIV-disease symptomology such as fatigue, medical comorbidities, and socioeconomic barriers for healthy living (Rehm and Konkle-Parker, 2016; Vancampfort et al., 2017, 2018a; Webel et al., 2016). Studies examining the effects of moderate aerobic exercise on health outcomes in PLWH suggest these interventions may be effective in increasing quality of life through enhanced fitness, reduced depression, lower inflammation, and reduced cardiometabolic risk (Chaparro et al., 2018; Cutrono et al., 2016; O'Brien, Tynan, Nixon, & Glazier, 2016; Vancampfort et al., 2016). In healthy populations aerobic, resistance, and multimodal exercise training are all shown to have a positive impact on the preservation of EFs in older age (Barha, Davis, Falck, Nagamatsu, & Liu-Ambrose, 2017). In older adult PLWH higher levels of moderate physical activity were associated with greater EF (Fazeli et al., 2015). In a longitudinal sample of nearly 300 HIV-infected adults, individuals endorsing consistent physical activity, indexed by any activity in which the heart beats rapidly, showed significantly less neurocognitive decline in the broad domain of EF over 30 months than individuals reporting no physical activity (Dufour et al., 2018).

Inhibitory control deficits are found to occur in HIV-positive individuals with co-occurring alcohol (Schulte et al., 2011) or stimulant (Rippeth et al., 2004) use disorders. Notably, Pfefferbaum and collaborators utilized an emotional Stroop task suggesting frontoparietal attention and frontosubcortical emotion systems may be easily taxed in HIV-positive individuals with alcohol abuse (Schulte et al., 2011). It appears that a wide range of drugs have a deleterious effect on cognitive inference in HIV-positive individuals. A recent fMRI study of the Stroop task performance found signal change within a cluster of neurons in the frontoinsular cortex, during cognitive interference, correlated positively with cumulative years of regular marijuana use (Meade et al., 2018). Physical activity proxies are also found to relate to deficits in inhibitory control for PLWH. In a small sample of HIV-positive older adults, higher V02 mL/kg max was associated with greater executive control indexed by the Delis-Kaplan EF System (DKEFS) Color-Word Interference Test (Mapstone et al., 2013). Cross-sectional data from a cohort of over 200 HIV-positive adults from the Multicenter AIDS Cohort Study revealed that compared to individuals reporting low physical activity (Indexed by the International Physical Activity Questionnaire (IPAQ)), those reporting high, but not moderate activity evinced lower likelihood of executive dysfunction indexed by Stroop interference and Trails-B performance (Monroe et al., 2017).

Working memory performance has also been linked with substance abuse and other health behaviors in PLWH. Poly-drug use is found to be associated with poorer delayed non-match-to-sample performance (Martin et al., 2003). Moderate exercise is shown to be among the most highly predictive health behaviors in the modification of neurocognitive function amongst both healthy and chronic disease populations by reducing oxidative stress and other neuro-inflammatory markers while enhancing angiogenesis, neurogenesis, and synaptogenesis (Ahlskog, Geda, Graff-Radford, & Petersen, 2011; Smith et al., 2010). Self-reported exercise was associated with greater working memory (indexed by the PASAT and the WMS-III spatial span test), within a cohort of over 300 community-dwelling HIV-positive adults (Dufour et al., 2013). This coincides with an earlier study showing that in addition to fine-motor control, current exercise was associated with PASAT performance (Honn, Para, Whitacre, & Bornstein, 1999).

Poorer set-shifting ability is also found with co-occur with stimulant use disorders (Bousman et al., 2010b; Rippeth et al., 2004). Meanwhile, activities of daily living, particularly engagement in employment-related activities, predicted poorer Trails B performance. In a study of over 150 adults living with HIV, Trails B performance, along with physical limitations, differentiated employed from unemployed participants (van Gorp, Baerwald, Ferrando, Mcelhiney, & Rabkin, 1999). Although the direction of this effect is not clear greater activities of daily living are supported by preserved EF while job-related activities may support and hence attenuate decline in EF.

Deficits in decision making are present in co-occurring or recent substance dependence including poly-substance dependence in males living with HIV (Martin et al., 2004b). Similarly, history of crack-cocaine and/or heroin use among HIV-infected women is associated with reduced loss aversion (Vassileva et al., 2013). This work begs the question of whether gender differences are present in decision making among persons living with HIV. Indeed, the Game of Dice Task has been used to show decision-making impairments are significantly more impaired amongst women compared to men living with HIV (Martin et al., 2016).

13.6 Psychosocial Factors Linked to Executive Dysfunction in HIV

HIV is a syndemic disease with those infected being disproportionately exposed to life stressors. With an ever-increasing proportion of the HIV population belonging to female or sexual minority group past history of trauma has become a common feature of the HIV syndemic of substance abuse and violence (Israelski et al., 2007; Machtinger, Wilson, Haberer, & Weiss, 2012; McIntosh and Rosselli, 2012; Meyer, Springer, & Altice, 2011; Sullivan, Messer, & Quinlivan, 2015; Whetten et al., 2006). Chronic exposure to stress is increasingly shown to have a negative impact on cognitive performance across the life span (Juster, Mcewen, & Lupien, 2010; McEwen, 2008). Indeed, much of the pathophysiological processes implicated in the effects of childhood adversity on neurocognition, e.g., HPA-axis dysregulation, neuroinflammation and oxidative stress, have been implicated in the multifaceted psychopathology of HAND (Thames et al., 2018). The cascade of neuroendocrine and neurotransmitter activity that occurs in response to repeated and prolonged stress in otherwise healthy individuals may be accelerated in HIV disease. For instance, with regard to the domain of verbal learning and memory, effects for probable PTSD on cognitive impairment in a large group of HIV-positive woman and controls varied depending on whether the PTSD exposure was linked to sexual abuse and/or violence (Rubin et al., 2016a). Moreover, among women living with HIV, the prefrontal lobe of the brain appears to be particularly vulnerable to stress and as a result may provide a pathway to impaired learning and memory processes in this population (Rubin et al., 2016b). Social adversity is a salient psychosocial risk factor. In a mixed sample of HIV-positive and HIV-negative men and women, social adversity predicted reductions in left hippocampus volume which in turn corresponded with deficits in EF including working memory (Thames et al., 2018). Using a composite scale indicating history of trauma, economic hardship (food insecurity and low socioeconomic status), and perceived psychological stress total adversity was correlated with a composite measure of EF (Watson et al., 2019). Perceived stress was also associated with poorer EF indexed by the color-word (interference) condition of the Stroop, Trails B, which measures mental flexibility, and the working memory condition of LNS. Moreover, in predominantly white HIV-infected men who have sex with men, acute stressful life events are associated with an index of worse global EF (Pukay-Martin, Cristiani, Saveanu, & Bornstein, 2003).

Inhibitory deficits, although prevalent, are not readily found associated with psychosocial function in persons living with HIV. However, apathy and irritability ratings were negatively related to inhibitory performance on the Stroop interference task in addition to a dual task (Castellon, Hinkin, & Myers, 2000). Apathy is a neuropsychiatric syndrome that taps frontostriatal circuitry that underpins executive function and is discussed in detail otherwise (McIntosh, Rosselli, Uddin, & Antoni, 2015).

Among a cohort of HIV-positive individuals a combined index of trauma, economic hardship (food insecurity and low socioeconomic status), and stress was related to lower levels of working memory (Watson et al., 2019). Within a cohort of midlife women with and without early life stress (ELS) and HIV infection, greater self-report levels of ELS related to structural atrophy-related attention/working memory were evident between the left frontal lobe volume and Trails Making Test A (Spies, Ahmed-Leitao, Fennema-Notestine, Cherner, & Seedat, 2016). Poorer digit span performance correlated with greater levels of alexithymia, an index of difficulty identifying and describing feelings closely tied to psychological distress, in a small group of asymptomatic HIV+ individuals (Bogdanova, Díaz-Santos, & Cronin-Golomb, 2010). A dual-task paradigm consisting of a visual tracking task interspersed with a digit span task showed performance in 189 HIV-positive adults to covary with an index of apathy and irritability derived from the Neuropsychiatric Inventory (NPI) modified for use with HIV-positive individuals (Cole et al., 2007). Interestingly, apathy, but not depression was found to correlate with working memory performance on a digit span task in HIV-positive individuals across the disease spectrum (Castellon, Hinkin, Wood, & Yarema, 1998). Meanwhile, in another HIV-positive cohort, family-related stress was negatively correlated with performance on the paced auditory serial addition test after controlling for age, education, anxiety, and depression (Pukay-Martin et al., 2003).

As it pertains to set-shifting, a longitudinal cohort of HIV-positive women showed that over the course of 1 year there was an interactive effect of HIV and childhood trauma on their Wisconsin Card Sorting Test performance (Spies et al. 2017). Importantly, greater mood disturbance and medical symptoms are associated with cognitive complaints in HIV-positive individuals but are not neurocognitive performance (Carter et al., 2003). Greater levels of alexithymia were also found to be associated with Trail-B performance, controlling for time of completion on Trails A (McIntosh et al., 2014). A similar finding was made in a small cohort of asymptomatic individuals and HIV-negative controls, albeit only a correlation with the externally oriented thoughts subscale was predicted by longer time of completion on the Trails B (Bogdanova et al., 2010). Studies from international cohorts are also contributing to our understanding of the neurocognitive presentation of HIV in EF. For instance, in a cohort of more clinically advanced HIV-positive women and healthy HIV-negative controls from South Africa history of early life stress was associated with greater decline in WCST performance (Spies et al., 2017). However, among a small sample of HIV + and HIV-negative Iranian men, EF indexed by the WCST and the Tower of London (ToL) task did not relate to PTSD symptoms indexed by the Impact of Event Scale (Moradi, Miraghaei, Parhon, Jabbari, & Jobson, 2013).

13.7 Conclusion

As predictors of HIV-associated executive dysfunction are gradually established in the Western hemisphere it is apparent that efforts must be replicated to elucidate factors contributing to executive dysfunction within the context of the high viral genetic diversity found in other parts of the world. For instance, nearly all of the nine major subtypes of HIV-1 Group M (A–D, F–H, J, and K), in addition to strains of HIV-1 Groups N and O, and HIV-2 are found on the continent of Africa. Roughly 66% of the estimated more than 30 million people living with the virus reside in Africa (Hemelaar, Gouws, Ghys, & Osmanov, 2006). The subtype B HIV-1 strain is most commonly found among US individuals however, those in Cameroon feature groups O and N and unique recombinant forms. A recent study showed executive dysfunction to vary as a function of viral genotype (Kanmogne et al., 2018). Thus, well-validated measures of EF will need to be made available for comparison studies. It is also clear that functional brain abnormalities associated with EF may persist in PLWH despite behavioral differences seldomly being detected. This suggests promise for functional imaging modalities in the detection of changes in neural substrate that predate cognitive impairment in the EF domain. Henceforth, other indices of neurocognitive impairment such as that derived from functional magnetic resonance imaging (fMRI) may emerge as more sensitive screening tools for diagnosis of HAND and its various domains (Hakkers et al., 2017). As fMRI research continues to expand, the field tasked with the challenge of developing sophisticated tools and greater insight to establish the factors related to the neurocognitive sequel of HIV in the executive domain.

References

Ahlskog, J. E., Geda, Y. E., Graff-Radford, N. R., & Petersen, R. C. 2011. Physical exercise as a preventive or disease-modifying treatment of dementia and brain aging. In *Mayo Clinic Proceedings*, (pp. 876–884). Elsevier.

Antinori, A., Arendt, G., Becker, J., Brew, B., Byrd, D., Cherner, M., et al. (2007). Updated research nosology for HIV-associated neurocognitive disorders. *Neurology, 69,* 1789–1799.

Azar, M. M., Springer, S. A., Meyer, J. P., & Altice, F. L. (2010). A systematic review of the impact of alcohol use disorders on HIV treatment outcomes, adherence to antiretroviral therapy and health care utilization. *Drug and Alcohol Dependence, 112,* 178–193.

Barha, C. K., Davis, J. C., Falck, R. S., Nagamatsu, L. S., & Liu-Ambrose, T. (2017). Sex differences in exercise efficacy to improve cognition: A systematic review and meta-analysis of randomized controlled trials in older humans. *Frontiers in Neuroendocrinology, 46,* 71–85.

Baum, M. K., Rafie, C., Lai, S., Sales, S., Page, J. B., & Campa, A. (2010). Alcohol use accelerates HIV disease progression. *AIDS Research and Human Retroviruses, 26,* 511–518.

Bechara, A. (2007). *Iowa gambling task.* Psychological Assessment Resources.

Bechara, A., Damasio, H., Tranel, D., & Anderson, S. W. (1998). Dissociation of working memory from decision making within the human prefrontal cortex. *Journal of Neuroscience, 18,* 428–437.

Behnisch, T., Francesconi, W., & Sanna, P. P. (2004). HIV secreted protein Tat prevents long-term potentiation in the hippocampal CA1 region. *Brain Research, 1012,* 187–189.

Bennett, B. A., Rusyniak, D. E., & Hollingsworth, C. K. (1995). HIV-1 gp120-induced neurotoxicity to midbrain dopamine cultures. *Brain Research, 705,* 168–176.
Benos, D. J., McPherson, S., Hahn, B. H., Chaikin, M. A., & Benveniste, E. N. (1994). Cytokines and HIV envelope glycoprotein gp120 stimulate Na+/H+ exchange in astrocytes. *Journal of Biological Chemistry, 269,* 13811–13816.
Biswal, B., Yetkin, F. Z., Haughton, V. M., & Hyde, J. S. (1995). Functional connectivity in the motor cortex of resting human brain using echo-planar MRI. *Magnetic Resonance in Medicine, 34,* 537–541.
Bogdanova, Y., Díaz-Santos, M., & Cronin-Golomb, A. (2010). Neurocognitive correlates of alexithymia in asymptomatic individuals with HIV. *Neuropsychologia, 48,* 1295–1304.
Bousman, C., Cherner, M., Atkinson, J., Heaton, R., Grant, I., Everall, I., & Group, H. (2010a). COMT Val158Met polymorphism, executive dysfunction, and sexual risk behavior in the context of HIV infection and methamphetamine dependence. *Interdisciplinary Perspectives on Infectious Diseases.*
Bousman, C. A., Cherner, M., Glatt, S. J., Atkinson, J. H., Grant, I., Tsuang, M. T., & Everall, I. P. (2010b). Impact of COMT Val158Met on executive functioning in the context of HIV and methamphetamine. *Neurobehavioral HIV medicine*, 1.
Brack-Werner, R. (1999). Astrocytes: HIV cellular reservoirs and important participants in neuropathogenesis. *Aids, 13,* 1–22.
Braithwaite, R., Conigliaro, J., Roberts, M., Shechter, S., Schaefer, A., McGinnis, K., et al. (2007). Estimating the impact of alcohol consumption on survival for HIV+ individuals. *AIDS care, 19,* 459–466.
Burdo, T. H., Weiffenbach, A., Woods, S. P., Letendre, S., Ellis, R. J., & Williams, K. C. (2013). Elevated sCD163 in plasma but not cerebrospinal fluid is a marker of neurocognitive impairment in HIV infection. *AIDS*, 27.
Burnam, M. A., Bing, E. G., Morton, S. C., Sherbourne, C., Fleishman, J. A., London, A. S., et al. (2001). Use of mental health and substance abuse treatment services among adults with HIV in the United States. *Archives of General Psychiatry, 58,* 729–736.
Byrd, D. A., Robinson-Papp, J., Mindt, M. R., Mintz, L., Elliott, K., Lighty, Q. & Morgello, S. J. J. O. T. I. N. S. (2013). Isolating cognitive and neurologic HIV effects in substance-dependent, confounded cohorts: A pilot study. *19,* 463–473.
Caldwell, J., Gongvatana, A., Navia, B., Sweet, L., Tashima, K., Ding, M., et al. (2014). Neural dysregulation during a working memory task in human immunodeficiency virus-seropositive and hepatitis C coinfected individuals. *Journal of Neurovirology, 20,* 398–411.
Carter, S. L., Rourke, S. B., Murji, S., Shore, D., & Rourke, B. P. (2003). Cognitive complaints, depression, medical symptoms, and their association with neuropsychological functioning in HIV infection: A structural equation model analysis. *Neuropsychology, 17,* 410.
Castellon, S. A., Hinkin, C. H., & Myers, H. F. (2000). Neuropsychiatric disturbance is associated with executive dysfunction in HIV-1 infection. *Journal of the International Neuropsychological Society, 6,* 336–347.
Castellon, S. A., Hinkin, C. H., Wood, S., & Yarema, K. T. (1998). Apathy, depression, and cognitive performance in HIV-1 infection. *The Journal of Neuropsychiatry and Clinical Neurosciences, 10,* 320–329.
Chander, G., Himelhoch, S., & Moore, R. D. (2006). Substance abuse and psychiatric disorders in HIV-positive patients. *Drugs, 66,* 769–789.
Chang, L., Andres, M., Sadino, J., Jiang, C., Nakama, H., Miller, E., et al. (2011). Impact of apolipoprotein E ε4 and HIV on cognition and brain atrophy: antagonistic pleiotropy and premature brain aging. *Neuroimage, 58,* 1017–1027.
Chang, L., Ernst, T., Witt, M. D., Ames, N., Gaiefsky, M. & Miller, E. (2002). Relationships among brain metabolites, cognitive function, and viral loads in antiretroviral-naıve HIV patients. *Neuroimage*, 17, 1638–1648.
Chang, L., Jiang, C., Cunningham, E., Buchthal, S., Douet, V., Andres, M., et al. (2014). Effects of APOE ε4, age, and HIV on glial metabolites and cognitive deficits. *Neurology, 82,* 2213–2222.

Chang, L., Speck, O., Miller, E. N., Braun, J., Jovicich, J., Koch, C., et al. (2001). Neural correlates of attention and working memory deficits in HIV patients. *Neurology, 57,* 1001–1007.

Chang, L., Wong, V., Nakama, H., Watters, M., Ramones, D., Miller, E. N., et al. (2008). Greater than age-related changes in brain diffusion of HIV patients after 1 year. *Journal of Neuroimmune Pharmacology, 3,* 265–274.

Chaparro, C. G. A. P., Zech, P., Schuch, F., Wolfarth, B., Rapp, M., & Heiβel, A. (2018). Effects of aerobic and resistance exercise alone or combined on strength and hormone outcomes for people living with HIV. A meta-analysis. *PloS one, 13,* e0203384.

Chen, W., Sulcove, J., Frank, I., Jaffer, S., Ozdener, H., & Kolson, D. L. (2002). Development of a human neuronal cell model for human immunodeficiency virus (HIV)-infected macrophage-induced neurotoxicity: apoptosis induced by HIV type 1 primary isolates and evidence for involvement of the Bcl-2/Bcl-xL-sensitive intrinsic apoptosis pathway. *Journal of Virology, 76,* 9407–9419.

Cohen, R. A., Boland, R., Paul, R., Tashima, K. T., Schoenbaum, E. E., Celentano, D. D., et al. (2001). Neurocognitive performance enhanced by highly active antiretroviral therapy in HIV-infected women. *Aids, 15,* 341–345.

Cohen, R. A., De La Monte, S., Gongvatana, A., Ombao, H., Gonzalez, B., Devlin, … Tashima, K. T. (2011). Plasma cytokine concentrations associated with HIV/hepatitis C coinfection are related to attention, executive and psychomotor functioning. *Journal of neuroimmunology*, 233, 204–210.

Cohen, R. A., Seider, T. R., & Navia, B. (2015). HIV effects on age-associated neurocognitive dysfunction: Premature cognitive aging or neurodegenerative disease? *Alzheimer's Research and Therapy, 7,* 37.

Cole, M. A., Castellon, S. A., Perkins, A. C., Ureno, O. S., Robinet, M. B., Reinhard, M. J., et al. (2007). Relationship between psychiatric status and frontal–subcortical systems in HIV-infected individuals. *Journal of the International Neuropsychological Society, 13,* 549–554.

Conigliaro, J., Justice, A. C., Gordon, A. J., Bryant, K., Alcohol, V., & Group, B. C. R. (2006). Role of alcohol in determining human immunodeficiency virus (HIV)-relevant outcomes: a conceptual model to guide the implementation of evidence-based interventions into practice. *Medical Care*, S1–S6.

Connolly, C. G., Bischoff-Grethe, A., Jordan, S. J., Woods, S. P., Ellis, R. J., Paulus, M. P., … Group, T. M. A. R. C. (2014). Altered functional response to risky choice in HIV infection. *PloS one, 9*, e111583.

Control, C. F. D., & Prevention. (1992). 1993 revised classification system for HIV infection and expanded surveillance case definition for AIDS among adolescents and adults. *MMWR Recommendations and Reports, 41*, 1–19.

Control, C. F. D., & Prevention, (2005). Cases of HIV infection and AIDS in the United States, 2002. *HIV/AIDS Surveillance Report*, 16, 14.

Corrêa, D. G., Zimmermann, N., Netto, T. M., Tukamoto, G., Ventura, N., De Castro Bellini Leite, S., … Gasparetto, E. L. (2016). Regional cerebral gray matter volume in HIV-positive patients with executive function deficits. *Journal of Neuroimaging, 26*, 450–457.

Cristiani, S. A., Pukay-Martin, N. D., & Bornstein, R. A. (2004). Marijuana use and cognitive function in HIV-infected people. *The Journal of Neuropsychiatry and Clinical Neurosciences, 16,* 330–335.

Cutrono, S. E., Lewis, J. E., Perry, A., Signorile, J., Tiozzo, E., & Jacobs, K. A. (2016). The effect of a community-based exercise program on inflammation, metabolic risk, and fitness levels among persons living with HIV/AIDS. *AIDS and Behavior, 20,* 1123–1131.

Cysique, L. A., & Brew, B. J. (2009). Neuropsychological functioning and antiretroviral treatment in HIV/AIDS: A review. *Neuropsychology Review, 19,* 169–185.

Cysique, L. A., Hey-Cunningham, W. J., Dermody, N., Chan, P., Brew, B. J., & Koelsch, K. K. (2015). Peripheral blood mononuclear cells HIV DNA levels impact intermittently on neurocognition. *PLoS ONE, 10,* e0120488.

Cysique, L. A., Moffat, K., Moore, D. M., Lane, T. A., Davies, N. W., Carr, A., et al. (2013). HIV, vascular and aging injuries in the brain of clinically stable HIV-infected adults: A (1)H MRS study. *PLoS ONE, 8,* e61738.
D'Antoni, M. L., Paul, R. H., Mitchell, B. I., Kohorn, L., Fischer, L., Lefebvre, E., et al. (2018). Improved cognitive performance and reduced monocyte activation in virally suppressed chronic HIV after dual CCR51 and CCR51 antagonism. *JAIDS Journal of Acquired Immune Deficiency Syndromes, 79,* 108–116.
de Oliveira, M. F., Murrell, B., Pérez-Santiago, J., Vargas, M., Ellis, R. J., Letendre, S., et al. (2015). Circulating HIV DNA correlates with neurocognitive impairment in older HIV-infected adults on suppressive ART. *Scientific Reports, 5,* 17094.
Dickens, A. M., Anthony, D. C., Deutsch, R., Mielke, M. M., Claridge, T. D., Grant, I., et al. (2015). Cerebrospinal fluid metabolomics implicate bioenergetic adaptation as a neural mechanism regulating shifts in cognitive states of HIV-infected patients. *AIDS (London, England), 29,* 559.
Doyle, K. L., Woods, S. P., Morgan, E. E., Iudicello, J. E., Cameron, M. V., Gilbert, P. E., … Group, H. N. R. P. (2016). Health-related decision-making in HIV disease. *Journal of Clinical Psychology in Medical Settings, 23,* 135–146.
du Plessis, S., Vink, M., Joska, J. A., Koutsilieri, E., Bagadia, A., Stein, D. J., et al. (2015). HIV infection is associated with impaired striatal function during inhibition with normal cortical functioning on functional MRI. *Journal of the International Neuropsychological Society, 21,* 722–731.
du Plessis, S., Vink, M., Joska, J. A., Koutsilieri, E., Bagadia, A., Stein, D. J., et al. (2016). Prefrontal cortical thinning in HIV infection is associated with impaired striatal functioning. *Journal of Neural Transmission (Vienna), 123,* 643–651.
Dufour, C. A., Marquine, M. J., Fazeli, P. L., Henry, B. L., Ellis, R. J., Grant, I., … Group, H. (2013). Physical exercise is associated with less neurocognitive impairment among HIV-infected adults. *Journal of neurovirology, 19,* 410–417.
Dufour, C. A., Marquine, M. J., Fazeli, P. L., Umlauf, A., Henry, B. L., Zlatar, Z., et al. (2018). A longitudinal analysis of the impact of physical activity on neurocognitive functioning among hiv-infected adults. *AIDS and Behavior, 22,* 1562–1572.
Epstein, L. G., & Gendelman, H. E. (1993). Human immunodeficiency virus type 1 infection of the nervous system: Pathogenetic mechanisms. *Annals of Neurology: Official Journal of the American Neurological Association and the Child Neurology Society, 33,* 429–436.
Erdmann, N., Zhao, J., Lopez, A. L., Herek, S., Curthoys, N., Hexum, T. D., et al. (2007). Glutamate production by HIV-1 infected human macrophage is blocked by the inhibition of glutaminase. *Journal of Neurochemistry, 102,* 539–549.
Ernst, T., Chang, L., & Arnold, S. (2003). Increased glial metabolites predict increased working memory network activation in HIV brain injury. *Neuroimage, 19,* 1686–1693.
Ernst, T., Chang, L., Jovicich, J., Ames, N., & Arnold, S. (2002). Abnormal brain activation on functional MRI in cognitively asymptomatic HIV patients. *Neurology, 59,* 1343–1349.
Everall, I., Heaton, R., Marcotte, T., Ellis, R., Mccutchan, J., Atkinson, J., … Group, H. (1999). Cortical synaptic density is reduced in mild to moderate human immunodeficiency virus neurocognitive disorder. *Brain Pathology, 9,* 209–217.
Fama, R., Sullivan, E. V., Sassoon, S. A., Pfefferbaum, A., & Zahr, N. M. (2016). Impairments in component processes of executive function and episodic memory in alcoholism, HIV infection, and HIV infection with alcoholism comorbidity. *Alcoholism: Clinical and Experimental Research, 40,* 2656–2666.
Farinpour, R., Martin, E. M., Seidenberg, M., Pitrak, D. L., Pursell, K. J., Mullane, K. M., et al. (2000). Verbal working memory in HIV-seropositive drug users. *Journal of the International Neuropsychological Society, 6,* 548–555.
Fazeli, P. L., Marquine, M. J., Dufour, C., Henry, B. L., Montoya, J., Gouaux, B., et al. (2015). Physical activity is associated with better neurocognitive and everyday functioning among older adults with HIV disease. *AIDS and Behavior, 19,* 1470–1477.

Fogarty, A., Rawstorne, P., Prestage, G., Crawford, J., Grierson, J., & Kippax, S. (2007). Marijuana as therapy for people living with HIV/AIDS: Social and health aspects. *AIDS Care, 19,* 295–301.

Fujiwara, E., Tomlinson, S. E., Purdon, S. E., Gill, M. J., & Power, C. (2015). Decision making under explicit risk is impaired in individuals with human immunodeficiency virus (HIV). *Journal of Clinical and Experimental Neuropsychology, 37,* 733–750.

Gomez, D., Power, C., Gill, M. J., & Fujiwara, E. (2017). Determinants of risk-taking in HIV-associated neurocognitive disorders. *Neuropsychology, 31,* 798.

Gongvatana, A., Morgan, E. E., Iudicello, J. E., Letendre, S. L., Grant, I., Woods, S. P. & Group, H. N. R. P. (2014). A history of alcohol dependence augments HIV-associated neurocognitive deficits in persons aged 60 and older. *Journal of Neurovirology, 20,* 505–513.

Gonzalez, R., Schuster, R. M., Vassileva, J., & Martin, E. M. (2011). Impact of HIV and a history of marijuana dependence on procedural learning among individuals with a history of substance dependence. *Journal of Clinical and Experimental Neuropsychology, 33,* 735–752.

Gonzalez, R., Vassileva, J., Bechara, A., Grbesic, S., Sworowski, L., Novak, R. M., et al. (2005). The influence of executive functions, sensation seeking, and HIV serostatus on the risky sexual practices of substance-dependent individuals. *Journal of the International Neuropsychological Society, 11,* 121–131.

Goodkin, K., Miller, E. N., Cox, C., Reynolds, S., Becker, J. T., Martin, E., ... Study, M. A. C. (2017). Effect of ageing on neurocognitive function by stage of HIV infection: Evidence from the Multicenter AIDS Cohort Study. *The Lancet HIV, 4,* e411–e422.

Goodkin, K., Shapshak, P., Metsch, L. R., McCoy, C. B., Crandall, K. A., Kumar, M., et al. (1998). Cocaine abuse and HIV-1 infection: Epidemiology and neuropathogenesis. *Journal of Neuroimmunology, 83,* 88–101.

Grant, I., Franklin, D. R., Jr, Deutsch, R., Woods, S. P., Vaida, F., Ellis, R. J., ... CHARTER Group (2014). Asymptomatic HIV-associated neurocognitive impairment increases risk for symptomatic decline. *Neurology*, *82*(23), 2055–2062. https://doi.org/10.1212/WNL.0000000000000492.

Hakkers, C. S., Arends, J. E., Barth, R. E., Du Plessis, S., Hoepelman, A. I., & Vink, M. (2017). Review of functional MRI in HIV: effects of aging and medication. *Journal of neurovirology*, *23*(1), 20–32. https://doi.org/10.1007/s13365-016-0483-y.

Hardy, D. J., Hinkin, C. H., Levine, A. J., Castellon, S. A., & Lam, M. N. (2006). Risky decision making assessed with the gambling task in adults with HIV. *Neuropsychology, 20,* 355.

Hardy, D. J., & Vance, D. E. (2009). The neuropsychology of HIV/AIDS in older adults. *Neuropsychology Review, 19,* 263.

Heaton, R. K., Franklin, D. R., Ellis, R. J., McCutchan, J. A., Letendre, S. L., Leblanc, S., et al. (2011). HIV-associated neurocognitive disorders before and during the era of combination antiretroviral therapy: differences in rates, nature, and predictors. *Journal of Neurovirology, 17,* 3–16.

Hemelaar, J., Gouws, E., Ghys, P. D., & Osmanov, S. (2006). Global and regional distribution of HIV-1 genetic subtypes and recombinants in 2004. *Aids, 20,* W13–W23.

Hinkin, C. H., Castellon, S. A., Hardy, D. J., Granholm, E., & Siegle, G. (1999). Computerized and traditional stroop task dysfunction in HIV-l infection. *Neuropsychology, 13,* 306–316.

Hinkin, C. H., Hardy, D. J., Mason, K. I., Castellon, S. A., Durvasula, R. S., Lam, M. N., et al. (2004). Medication adherence in HIV-infected adults: Effect of patient age, cognitive status, and substance abuse. *AIDS (London, England), 18,* S19.

Hinkin, C. H., Hardy, D. J., Mason, K. I., Castellon, S. A., Lam, M. N., Stefaniak, M., et al. (2002). Verbal and spatial working memory performance among HIV-infected adults. *Journal of the International Neuropsychological Society, 8,* 532–538.

Hofmann, W., Schmeichel, B. J., & Baddeley, A. D. (2012). Executive functions and self-regulation. *Trends in Cognitive Sciences, 16,* 174–180.

Honn, V. J., Para, M. F., Whitacre, C. C., & Bornstein, R. A. (1999). Effect of exercise on neuropsychological performance in asymptomatic HIV infection. *AIDS and Behavior, 3,* 67–74.

Imp, B. M., Rubin, L. H., Tien, P. C., Plankey, M. W., Golub, E. T., French, A. L., & Valcour, V. G. (2016). Monocyte activation is associated with worse cognitive performance in virologically suppressed HIV-infected women. *The Journal of Infectious Diseases*, jiw506.

Ipser, J. C., Brown, G. G., Bischoff-Grethe, A., Connolly, C. G., Ellis, R. J., Heaton, R. K., et al. (2015). HIV infection is associated with attenuated frontostriatal intrinsic connectivity: A preliminary study. *Journal of the International Neuropsychological Society, 21,* 203–213.

Israelski, D., Prentiss, D., Lubega, S., Balmas, G., Garcia, P., Muhammad, M., et al. (2007). Psychiatric co-morbidity in vulnerable populations receiving primary care for HIV/AIDS. *Aids Care, 19,* 220–225.

Itoh, K., Mehraein, P., & Weis, S. (2000). Neuronal damage of the substantia nigra in HIV-1 infected brains. *Acta Neuropathologica, 99,* 376–384.

Iudicello, J. E., Woods, S. P., Cattie, J. E., Doyle, K., Grant, I., & Group, H. N. R. P. (2013). Risky decision-making in HIV-associated neurocognitive disorders (HAND). *The Clinical Neuropsychologist, 27,* 256–275.

Jiang, X., Barasky, R., Olsen, H., Riesenhuber, M., & Magnus, M. (2016). Behavioral and neuroimaging evidence for impaired executive function in "cognitively normal" older HIV-infected adults. *AIDS Care, 28,* 436–440.

Jiang, Z.-G., Piggee, C., Heyes, M., Murphy, C., Quearry, B., Bauer, M., et al. (2001). Glutamate is a mediator of neurotoxicity in secretions of activated HIV-1-infected macrophages. *Journal of Neuroimmunology, 117,* 97–107.

Jurado, M. B., & Rosselli, M. (2007). The elusive nature of executive functions: A review of our current understanding. *Neuropsychology Review, 17,* 213–233.

Juster, R.-P., McEwen, B. S., & Lupien, S. J. (2010). Allostatic load biomarkers of chronic stress and impact on health and cognition. *Neuroscience and Biobehavioral Reviews, 35,* 2–16.

Kanmogne, G. D., Fonsah, J. Y., Tang, B., Doh, R. F., Kengne, A. M., Umlauf, A., ... Franklin, D. (2018). Effects of HIV on executive function and verbal fluency in Cameroon. *Scientific Reports, 8.*

Kesby, J. P., Heaton, R. K., Young, J. W., Umlauf, A., Woods, S. P., Letendre, S. L., ... Semenova, S. (2015). Methamphetamine exposure combined with HIV-1 disease or gp120 expression: Comparison of learning and executive functions in humans and mice. *Neuropsychopharmacology, 40,* 1899.

Kliegel, M., Martin, M., McDaniel, M. A., & Einstein, G. O. (2002). Complex prospective memory and executive control of working memory: A process model. *Psychological Test and Assessment Modeling, 44,* 303.

Kusao, I., Shiramizu, B., Liang, C.-Y., Grove, J., Agsalda, M., Troelstrup, D., et al. (2012). Cognitive performance related to HIV-1-infected monocytes. *The Journal of Neuropsychiatry and Clinical Neurosciences, 24,* 71–80.

Lezak, M. D., Howieson, D. B., Loring, D. W., & Fischer, J. S. (2004). *Neuropsychological assessment.* USA: Oxford University Press.

Lyons, J. L., Uno, H., Ancuta, P., Kamat, A., Moore, D. J., Singer, E. J., ... Gabuzda, D. (2011). Plasma sCD14 is a biomarker associated with impaired neurocognitive test performance in attention and learning domains in HIV infection. *Journal of Acquired Immune Deficiency Syndromes, 57,* 371.

Machtinger, E., Wilson, T., Haberer, J. E., & Weiss, D. (2012). Psychological trauma and PTSD in HIV-positive women: A meta-analysis. *AIDS and Behavior, 16,* 2091–2100.

Maki, P. M., Rubin, L. H., Valcour, V., Martin, E., Crystal, H., Young, M., ... Alden, C. J. N. (2015). Cognitive function in women with HIV Findings from the Women's Interagency HIV Study. *84,* 231–240.

Manly, J. J., Smith, C., Crystal, H. A., Richardson, J., Golub, E. T., Greenblatt, R., et al. (2011). Relationship of ethnicity, age, education, and reading level to speed and executive function among HIV+ and HIV−women: The Women's Interagency HIV Study (WIHS) Neurocognitive Substudy. *Journal of Clinical and Experimental Neuropsychology, 33,* 853–863.

Mapstone, M., Hilton, T. N., Yang, H., Guido, J. J., Luque, A. E., Hall, W. J., et al. (2013). Poor aerobic fitness may contribute to cognitive decline in HIV-infected older adults. *Aging and disease, 4,* 311.

Maragos, W., Tillman, P., Jones, M., Bruce-Keller, A., Roth, S., Bell, J., et al. (2003). Neuronal injury in hippocampus with human immunodeficiency virus transactivating protein, Tat. *Neuroscience, 117,* 43–53.

Martin, E., Gonzalez, R., Vassileva, J., Maki, P. M., Bechara, A., & Brand, M. (2016). Sex and HIV serostatus differences in decision making under risk among substance-dependent individuals. *Journal of Clinical and Experimental Neuropsychology, 38,* 404–415.

Martin, E. M., Dehaan, S., Vassileva, J., Gonzalez, R., Weller, J., & Bechara, A. (2013). Decision making among HIV+ drug using men who have sex with men: A preliminary report from the Chicago Multicenter AIDS Cohort Study. *Journal of Clinical and Experimental Neuropsychology, 35,* 573–583.

Martin, E. M., Novak, R. M., Fendrich, M., Vassileva, J., Gonzalez, R., Grbesic, S., … Sworowski, L. J. J. O. T. I. N. S. (2004a). Stroop performance in drug users classified by HIV and hepatitis C virus serostatus. *10,* 298–300.

Martin, E. M., Pitrak, D. L., Rains, N., Grbesic, S., Pursell, K., Nunnally, G., et al. (2003). Delayed nonmatch-to-sample performance in HIV-seropositive and HIV-seronegative polydrug abusers. *Neuropsychology, 17,* 283.

Martin, E. M., Pitrak, D. L., Weddington, W., Rains, N. A., Nunnally, G., Nixon, H., … Bechara, A. (2004b). Cognitive impulsivity and HIV serostatus in substance dependent males. *Journal of the International Neuropsychological Society, 10,* 931–938.

Martin, E. M., Robertson, L. C., Edelstein, H. E., Jagust, W. J., Sorensen, D. J., Giovanni, D. S., et al. (1992). Performance of patients with early HIV-1 infection on the Stroop task. *Journal of Clinical and Experimental Neuropsychology, 14,* 857–868.

Martin, E. M., Sullivan, T. S., Reed, R. A., Fletcher, T. A., Pitrak, D. L., Weddington, W., et al. (2001). Auditory working memory in HIV-1 infection. *Journal of the International Neuropsychological Society, 7,* 20–26.

McEwen, B. S. (2008). Central effects of stress hormones in health and disease: Understanding the protective and damaging effects of stress and stress mediators. *European Journal of Pharmacology, 583,* 174–185.

McGuire, J. L., Gill, A. J., Douglas, S. D., & Kolson, D. L. (2015). Central and peripheral markers of neurodegeneration and monocyte activation in HIV-associated neurocognitive disorders. *Journal of neurovirology, 21,* 439–448.

McIntosh, R. C., Ironson, G., Antoni, M., Kumar, M., Fletcher, M. A., & Schneiderman, N. (2014). Alexithymia is linked to neurocognitive, psychological, neuroendocrine, and immune dysfunction in persons living with HIV. *Brain, Behavior, and Immunity, 36,* 165–175.

McIntosh, R. C., & Rosselli, M. (2012). Stress and coping in women living with HIV: A meta-analytic review. *AIDS and Behavior, 16,* 2144–2159.

McIntosh, R. C., Rosselli, M., Uddin, L. Q., & Antoni, M. (2015). Neuropathological sequelae of human immunodeficiency virus and apathy: A review of neuropsychological and neuroimaging studies. *Neuroscience and Biobehavioral Reviews, 55,* 147–164.

Meade, C. S., Bell, R. P., Towe, S. L., Chen, N. K., Hobkirk, A. L., & Huettel, S. A. (2018). Synergistic effects of marijuana abuse and HIV infection on neural activation during a cognitive interference task. *Addiction Biology*.

Meade, C. S., Conn, N. A., Skalski, L. M., & Safren, S. A. (2011). Neurocognitive impairment and medication adherence in HIV patients with and without cocaine dependence. *Journal of Behavioral Medicine, 34,* 128–138.

Meade, C. S., Cordero, D. M., Hobkirk, A. L., Metra, B. M., Chen, N. K., & Huettel, S. A. (2016). Compensatory activation in fronto-parietal cortices among HIV-infected persons during a monetary decision-making task. *Human Brain Mapping, 37,* 2455–2467.

Meade, C. S., Hobkirk, A. L., Towe, S. L., Chen, N.-K., Bell, R. P., & Huettel, S. A. (2017). Cocaine dependence modulates the effect of HIV infection on brain activation during intertemporal decision making. *Drug and Alcohol Dependence, 178,* 443–451.

Melrose, R. J., Tinaz, S., Castelo, J. M., Courtney, M. G., & Stern, C. E. (2008). Compromised fronto-striatal functioning in HIV: An fMRI investigation of semantic event sequencing. *Behavioural Brain Research, 188,* 337–347.

Meyer, J. P., Springer, S. A., & Altice, F. L. (2011). Substance abuse, violence, and HIV in women: A literature review of the syndemic. *Journal of Women's Health, 20,* 991–1006.

Miyake, A., Friedman, N. P., Emerson, M. J., Witzki, A. H., Howerter, A., & Wager, T. D. (2000). The unity and diversity of executive functions and their contributions to complex "frontal lobe" tasks: A latent variable analysis. *Cognitive Psychology, 41,* 49–100.

Monroe, A., Zhang, L., Jacobson, L. P., Plankey, M., Brown, T. T., Miller, E., et al. (2017). The association between physical activity and cognition in men with and without HIV infection. *HIV Medicine, 18,* 555–563.

Moradi, A. R., Miraghaei, M. A., Parhon, H., Jabbari, H., & Jobson, L. (2013). Posttraumatic stress disorder, depression, executive functioning, and autobiographical remembering in individuals with HIV and in carers of those with HIV in Iran. *AIDS Care, 25,* 281–288.

Morgan, E. E., Iudicello, J. E., Weber, E., & Woods, S. P. (2016). Neuropsychological aspects of methamphetamine use disorders and human immunodeficiency virus disease. In *Neuropathology of drug addictions and substance misuse.* Elsevier.

Murray, J. D., Jaramillo, J., & Wang, X. J. (2017). Working memory and decision-making in a frontoparietal circuit model. *Journal of Neuroscience, 37,* 12167–12186.

Napier, T. C. (2017). Impact on cortical function of cocaine abuse co-occurring with HIV. *Neuropsychopharmacology, 42,* 365.

Nasi, M., de Biasi, S., Gibellini, L., Bianchini, E., Pecorini, S., Bacca, V., et al. (2017). Ageing and inflammation in patients with HIV infection. *Clinical and Experimental Immunology, 187,* 44–52.

Nath, A., Anderson, C., Jones, M., Maragos, W., Booze, R., Mactutus, C., et al. (2000). Neurotoxicity and dysfunction of dopaminergic systems associated with AIDS dementia. *Journal of Psychopharmacology, 14,* 222–227.

O'Brien, K. K., Tynan, A.-M., Nixon, S. A., & Glazier, R. H. (2016). Effectiveness of aerobic exercise for adults living with HIV: Systematic review and meta-analysis using the Cochrane Collaboration protocol. *BMC Infectious Diseases, 16,* 182.

Ortega, M., Brier, M. R., & Ances, B. M. (2015). Effects of HIV and combination antiretroviral therapy on cortico-striatal functional connectivity. *Aids, 29,* 703–712.

Patton, H. K., Zhou, Z.-H., Bubien, J. K., Benveniste, E. N., & Benos, D. J. (2000). gp120-induced alterations of human astrocyte function: Na+/H+ exchange, K+ conductance, and glutamate flux. *American Journal of Physiology-Cell Physiology, 279,* C700–C708.

Paydary, K., Mahin Torabi, S., Seyedalinaghi, S., Noori, M., Noroozi, A., Ameri, S., & Ekhtiari, H. (2016). Impulsivity, sensation seeking, and risk-taking behaviors among HIV-positive and HIV-negative heroin dependent persons. *AIDS Research and Treatment.*

Persidsky, Y., Ho, W., Ramirez, S. H., Potula, R., Abood, M. E., Unterwald, E., et al. (2011). HIV-1 infection and alcohol abuse: Neurocognitive impairment, mechanisms of neurodegeneration and therapeutic interventions. *Brain, Behavior, and Immunity, 25,* S61–S70.

Pfefferbaum, A., Rosenbloom, M. J., Sassoon, S. A., Kemper, C. A., Deresinski, S., Rohlfing, T., et al. (2012). Regional brain structural dysmorphology in human immunodeficiency virus infection: Effects of acquired immune deficiency syndrome, alcoholism, and age. *Biological Psychiatry, 72,* 361–370.

Plessis, S., Vink, M., Joska, J. A., Koutsilieri, E., Bagadia, A., Stein, D. J., et al. (2015). HIV infection results in ventral-striatal reward system hypo-activation during cue processing. *AIDS, 29,* 1335–1343.

Plessis, S. D., Vink, M., Joska, J. A., Koutsilieri, E., Stein, D. J., & Emsley, R. (2014). HIV infection and the fronto-striatal system: A systematic review and meta-analysis of fMRI studies. *AIDS, 28,* 803–811.

Pukay-Martin, N. D., Cristiani, S. A., Saveanu, R., & Bornstein, R. A. (2003). The relationship between stressful life events and cognitive function in HIV-infected men. *The Journal of Neuropsychiatry and Clinical Neurosciences, 15,* 436–441.

Reger, M., Welsh, R., Razani, J., Martin, D. J., & Boone, K. B. (2002). A meta-analysis of the neuropsychological sequelae of HIV infection. *Journal of the International Neuropsychological Society, 8,* 410–424.

Reger, M. A., Martin, D. J., Cole, S. L., & Strauss, G. (2005). The relationship between plasma viral load and neuropsychological functioning in HIV-1 infection. *Archives of Clinical Neuropsychology, 20,* 137–143.

Rehm, K. E., & Konkle-Parker, D. (2016). Physical activity levels and perceived benefits and barriers to physical activity in HIV-infected women living in the deep south of the United States. *AIDS Care, 28,* 1205–1210.

Reitan, R. M. (1958). Validity of the trail making test as an indicator of organic brain damage. *Perceptual and Motor Skills, 8,* 271–276.

Rippeth, J. D., Heaton, R. K., Carey, C. L., Marcotte, T. D., Moore, D. J., Gonzalez, R., … Group, H. (2004). Methamphetamine dependence increases risk of neuropsychological impairment in HIV infected persons. *Journal of the International Neuropsychological Society, 10,* 1–14.

Rubin, L. H., Benning, L., Keating, S. M., Norris, P. J., Burke-Miller, J., Savarese, A., et al. (2018a). Variability in C-reactive protein is associated with cognitive impairment in women living with and without HIV: A longitudinal study. *Journal of Neurovirology, 24,* 41–51.

Rubin, L. H., Phan, K. L., Keating, S. M., & Maki, P. M. (2018b). A single low dose of hydrocortisone enhances cognitive functioning in HIV-infected women. *AIDS, 32,* 1983–1993.

Rubin, L. H., Pyra, M., Cook, J. A., Weber, K. M., Cohen, M. H., Martin, E., et al. (2016a). Post-traumatic stress is associated with verbal learning, memory, and psychomotor speed in HIV-infected and HIV-uninfected women. *Journal of Neurovirology, 22,* 159–169.

Rubin, L. H., Wu, M., Sundermann, E. E., Meyer, V. J., Smith, R., Weber, K. M., et al. (2016b). Elevated stress is associated with prefrontal cortex dysfunction during a verbal memory task in women with HIV. *Journal of Neurovirology, 22,* 840–851.

Sacktor, N., Skolasky, R., Tarwater, P., Mcarthur, J., Selnes, O., Becker, J., … Study, M. A. C. (2003). Response to systemic HIV viral load suppression correlates with psychomotor speed performance. *Neurology, 61,* 567–569.

Sahakian, B. J., & Owen, A. (1992). Computerized assessment in neuropsychiatry using CANTAB: Discussion paper. *Journal of the Royal Society of Medicine, 85,* 399.

Schnitzspahn, K. M., Stahl, C., Zeintl, M., Kaller, C. P., & Kliegel, M. (2013). The role of shifting, updating, and inhibition in prospective memory performance in young and older adults. *Developmental Psychology, 49,* 1544.

Schulte, T., Müller-Oehring, E. M., Sullivan, E. V., & Pfefferbaum, A. (2011). Disruption of emotion and conflict processing in HIV infection with and without alcoholism comorbidity. *Journal of the International Neuropsychological Society, 17,* 537–550.

Shiramizu, B., Williams, A. E., Shikuma, C., & Valcour, V. (2009). Amount of HIV DNA in peripheral blood mononuclear cells is proportional to the severity of HIV-1-associated neurocognitive disorders. *The Journal of Neuropsychiatry and Clinical Neurosciences, 21,* 68–74.

Smith, P. J., Blumenthal, J. A., Hoffman, B. M., Cooper, H., Strauman, T. A., Welsh-Bohmer, K., et al. (2010). Aerobic exercise and neurocognitive performance: A meta-analytic review of randomized controlled trials. *Psychosomatic Medicine, 72,* 239.

Soontornniyomkij, V., Kesby, J. P., Morgan, E. E., Bischoff-Grethe, A., Minassian, A., Brown, G. G., … Group, T. M. A. R. C. (2016). Effects of HIV and methamphetamine on brain and behavior: Evidence from human studies and animal models. *Journal of Neuroimmune Pharmacology, 11,* 495–510.

Spies, G., Ahmed-Leitao, F., Fennema-Notestine, C., Cherner, M., & Seedat, S. (2016). Effects of HIV and childhood trauma on brain morphometry and neurocognitive function. *Journal of Neurovirology, 22,* 149–158.

Spies, G., Fennema-Notestine, C., Cherner, M., & Seedat, S. (2017). Changes in cognitive function in women with HIV infection and early life stress. *AIDS Care, 29,* 14–23.

Spudich, S. (2016). Immune activation in the central nervous system throughout the course of HIV infection. *Current Opinion in HIV and AIDS, 11,* 226.

Stavro, K., Pelletier, J., & Potvin, S. (2013). Widespread and sustained cognitive deficits in alcoholism: A meta-analysis. *Addiction Biology, 18,* 203–213.

Stuss, D. T., & Alexander, M. P. (2000). Executive functions and the frontal lobes: A conceptual view. *Psychological Research, 63,* 289–298.

Sullivan, K. A., Messer, L. C., & Quinlivan, E. B. (2015). Substance abuse, violence, and HIV/AIDS (SAVA) syndemic effects on viral suppression among HIV positive women of color. *AIDS Patient Care and STDs, 29,* S42–S48.

Tang, V. M., Lang, D. J., Giesbrecht, C. J., Panenka, W. J., Willi, T., Procyshyn, R. M., et al. (2015). White matter deficits assessed by diffusion tensor imaging and cognitive dysfunction in psychostimulant users with comorbid human immunodeficiency virus infection. *BMC Research Notes, 8,* 515.

Tate, D. F., Conley, J., Paul, R. H., Coop, K., Zhang, S., Zhou, W., et al. (2010). Quantitative diffusion tensor imaging tractography metrics are associated with cognitive performance among HIV-infected patients. *Brain Imaging and Behavior, 4,* 68–79.

Thames, A., Kuhn, T., Mahmood, Z., Bilder, R., Williamson, T., Singer, E., et al. (2018). Effects of social adversity and HIV on subcortical shape and neurocognitive function. *Brain imaging and behavior, 12,* 96–108.

Thames, A. D., Streiff, V., Patel, S. M., Panos, S. E., Castellon, S. A., & Hinkin, C. H. (2012). The role of HIV infection, cognition, and depression in risky decision-making. *The Journal of Neuropsychiatry and Clinical Neurosciences, 24,* 340–348.

Thieblemont, N., Haeffner-Cavaillon, N., Haeffner, A., Cholley, B., Weiss, L., & Kazatchkine, M. D. (1995). Triggering of complement receptors CR173 (CD35) and CR173 (CD11b/CD18) induces nuclear translocation of NF-kappa B (p50/p65) in human monocytes and enhances viral replication in HIV-infected monocytic cells. *The Journal of Immunology, 155,* 4861–4867.

Thomas, J. B., Brier, M. R., Snyder, A. Z., Vaida, F. F., & Ances, B. M. (2013). Pathways to neurodegeneration: Effects of HIV and aging on resting-state functional connectivity. *Neurology, 80,* 1186–1193.

Tomasi, D., Chang, L., De Castro Caparelli, E., Telang, F., & Ernst, T. (2006). The human immunodeficiency virus reduces network capacity: acoustic noise effect. *Annals ofNeurology, 59,* 419–423.

Tozzi, V., Balestra, P., Galgani, S., Narciso, P., Ferri, F., Sebastiani, G., et al. (1999). Positive and sustained effects of highly active antiretroviral therapy on HIV-1-associated neurocognitive impairment. *Aids, 13,* 1889–1897.

Tozzi, V., Narciso, P., Galgani, S., Sette, P., Balestra, P., Gerace, C., … CAMPORIONDO, M. P. (1993). Effects of zidovudine in 30 patients with mild to end-stage AIDS dementia complex. *Aids.*

Trillo-Pazos, G., Diamanturos, A., Rislove, L., Menza, T., Chao, W., Belem, P., et al. (2003). Detection of HIV-1 DNA in microglia/macrophages, astrocytes and neurons isolated from brain tissue with Hiv-1 encephalitis by laser capture microdissection. *Brain Pathology, 13,* 144–154.

Valcour, V. G., Ananworanich, J., Agsalda, M., Sailasuta, N., Chalermchai, T., Schuetz, A., et al. (2013). HIV DNA reservoir increases risk for cognitive disorders in cART-naive patients. *PLoS ONE, 8,* e70164.

Valcour, V. G., Shikuma, C. M., Watters, M. R., & Sacktor, N. C. (2004). Cognitive impairment in older HIV-1-seropositive individuals: Prevalence and potential mechanisms. *AIDS (London, England), 18,* S79.

van Gorp, W. G., Baerwald, J. P., Ferrando, S. J., McElhiney, M. C., & Rabkin, J. G. (1999). The relationship between employment and neuropsychological impairment in HIV infection. *Journal of the International Neuropsychological Society, 5,* 534–539.
Vancampfort, D., Mugisha, J., de Hert, M., Probst, M., Firth, J., Gorczynski, P., et al. (2018a). Global physical activity levels among people living with HIV: A systematic review and meta-analysis. *Disability and Rehabilitation, 40,* 388–397.
Vancampfort, D., Mugisha, J., Richards, J., de Hert, M., Lazzarotto, A., Schuch, F., et al. (2017). Dropout from physical activity interventions in people living with HIV: a systematic review and meta-analysis. *AIDS Care, 29,* 636–643.
Vancampfort, D., Mugisha, J., Richards, J., de Hert, M., Probst, M., & Stubbs, B. (2018b). Physical activity correlates in people living with HIV/AIDS: A systematic review of 45 studies. *Disability and Rehabilitation, 40,* 1618–1629.
Vancampfort, D., Mugisha, J., Rosenbaum, S., Firth, J., de Hert, M., Probst, M., et al. (2016). Cardiorespiratory fitness levels and moderators in people with HIV: A systematic review and meta-analysis. *Preventive Medicine, 93,* 106–114.
Vassileva, J., Ahn, W.-Y., Weber, K. M., Busemeyer, J. R., Stout, J. C., Gonzalez, R., et al. (2013). Computational modeling reveals distinct effects of HIV and history of drug use on decision-making processes in women. *PLoS ONE, 8,* e68962.
Walker, K. A., & Brown, G. G. (2018). HIV-associated executive dysfunction in the era of modern antiretroviral therapy: A systematic review and meta-analysis. *Journal of Clinical and Experimental Neuropsychology, 40,* 357–376.
Watson, C. W.-M., Sundermann, E. E., Hussain, M. A., Umlauf, A., Thames, A. D., Moore, R. C., et al. (2019). Effects of trauma, economic hardship, and stress on neurocognition and everyday function in HIV. *Health Psychology, 38,* 33.
Webel, A. R., Perazzo, J., Decker, M., Horvat-Davey, C., Sattar, A., & Voss, J. (2016). Physical activity is associated with reduced fatigue in adults living with HIV/AIDS. *Journal of Advanced Nursing, 72,* 3104–3112.
Weber, E., Blackstone, K., & Woods, S. P. (2013). Cognitive neurorehabilitation of HIV-associated neurocognitive disorders: a qualitative review and call to action. *Neuropsychology Review, 23,* 81–98.
Wendelken, L. A., & Valcour, V. (2012). Impact of HIV and aging on neuropsychological function. *Journal of Neurovirology, 18,* 256–263.
Whetten, K., Leserman, J., Lowe, K., Stangl, D., Thielman, N., Swartz, M., et al. (2006). Prevalence of childhood sexual abuse and physical trauma in an HIV-positive sample from the deep south. *American Journal of Public Health, 96,* 1028–1030.
Woods, S. P., Morgan, E. E., Marquie-Beck, J., Carey, C. L., Grant, I., & Letendre, S. L. (2006). Markers of macrophage activation and axonal injury are associated with prospective memory in HIV-1 disease. *Cognitive and Behavioral Neurology: Official Journal of the Society for Behavioral and Cognitive Neurology, 19,* 217.
Woods, S. P., Rippeth, J. D., Frol, A. B., Levy, J. K., Ryan, E., Soukup, V. M., et al. (2004). Interrater reliability of clinical ratings and neurocognitive diagnoses in HIV. *Journal of Clinical and Experimental Neuropsychology, 26,* 759–778.
Zheng, J., Thylin, M. R., Persidsky, Y., Williams, C. E., Cotter, R. L., Zink, W., et al. (2001). HIV-1 infected immune competent mononuclear phagocytes influence the pathways to neuronal demise. *Neurotoxicity Research, 3,* 461–484.

Part VI
Assessment of Executive Dysfunction

Chapter 14
Neuropsychological Assessment of Executive Functions

Feggy Ostrosky Shejet and Asucena Lozano Gutiérrez

14.1 Introduction

The frontal lobes are the brain structures of more recent development and evolution in the human brain. From the neuropsychological point of view, these structures represent a system of planning, regulation and control of psychological processes (Luria, 1986): They allow the coordination and selection of multiple processes and of the different options of behavior and strategies available; they organize behaviors based on motivations and interests toward achieving goals that can only be reached through non-fixed procedures or rules (Miller & Cohen, 2001). They also participate decisively in the formation of intentions and programs, as well as in the regulation and verification of the most complex forms of human behavior (Luria, 1989). Due to this ability to regulate, to plan and to monitor the most complex psychological processes of the human being, it is considered that the frontal lobes represent the "executive center of the brain" (Goldberg, 2001; Goldstein, Naglieri, Princiotta, & Otero, 2014; Logue & Gould, 2014).

It has been proposed that the prefrontal region of frontal lobes regulates executive functions (EF). Although there are a number of theories regarding the nature of EF, this term has been defined as a construct that comprises several functions that allow the control, regulation and planning of behavior and cognitive processes in order to develop independent, proactive and productive activities (Lezak, Howieson, Bigler, & Tranel, 2012). These functions are within the most complex human functions (Goldberg, 2001) that are responsible for regulating and controlling more basic cognitive skills; these skills or cognitive routines are processes learned through practice or repetition and include motor and cognitive skills such as reading, memory or language. In addition, Zelazo and Müller (2002) proposed that executive functions

F. Ostrosky Shejet (✉) · A. Lozano Gutiérrez
Laboratorio de Psicofisiología y Neuropsicología, Facultad de Psicología, Universidad Nacional Autonoma de Mexico, Av. Universidad 3004 Copilco-Universidad 04510, Edificio D Cubículo 211, Mexico City, Mexico
e-mail: feggy@unam.mx

A. Ardila et al. (eds.), *Dysexecutive Syndromes*,
https://doi.org/10.1007/978-3-030-25077-5_14

may also be seen in motivational and affective situations, in contrast to the decontextualized, abstract and non-affective EF. Thus, the term of EF has undergone a broader conceptualization that has not only theoretical implications but also clinical assessment issues.

EF include inhibitory control, working memory, flexibility, planning and metacognition. Inhibitory control refers to the ability to regulate and control the tendencies to generate impulsive or automatized responses originated in other cerebral regions, which in turn is important to control the behavior and attention. Mental flexibility refers to the change of a set of strategies or responses which are not appropriate for a specific task and/or context, and it is necessary then to avoid persistence in a strategy/activity and disengage from it so as to explore other forms of cognitive procedures. Planning has been defined as the sequential order in which a series of cognitive procedures or strategies must be implemented; in this way, the execution of the action plans allows the goal-oriented behavior in a shorter time with less effort and cognitive dispersion. Working memory refers to keeping information online while it is processed (analyzed, selected and integrated semantically), so it is essential for a number of basic skills such as language comprehension or learning (Barkley, 2012).

Recently, metacognition has been studied within the field of neuropsychology because of its close relationship with the prefrontal cortex (PFC) and EF (Fernández-Duque, Baird, & Posner, 2000). This function controls and regulates EF in the same way that these functions regulate others of lower cognitive hierarchy. Metacognition is defined as the ability to monitor and control one's cognitive processes and is considered as a higher level process (Shimamura, 2000).

These EF have been related to different regions of the PFC; the region anterior to the motor and premotor cortex is called the prefrontal cortex (PFC). Its most anterior portion (Brodmann's area [BA] 10) presents a developmental and functional organization, exclusive of the human species (Stuss & Levine 2002). These regions are considered supramodal or, since they do not process direct sensory stimuli (Fuster, 2002, 2017). A higher ratio of white matter to gray matter has been found in the PFC in humans than in other non-human primates, an important finding for the functional connections between the different zones of the PFC, as well as their connections with posterior cortex and subcortical structures (Schoenemann, Seehan, & Glotzer, 2005).

The dorsolateral region of the PFC is functionally divided into two parts: dorsolateral and anterior, which in turn have three regions: upper, lower and frontal pole. This region is closely related to the processes of planning, working memory, fluency (design and verbal), complex problem solving, mental flexibility, generation of hypotheses, strategies, seriation and sequencing (Stuss & Alexander, 2000). The anterior (polar) portions of the dorsolateral prefrontal cortex are related to processes of greater cognitive hierarchy, such as metacognition, that is, self-assessment (monitoring) and adjustment (control) of activity based on continuous performance, and to the most recent evolutionary psychological aspects of humans, such as social cognition and autonoetic consciousness (integration between self-awareness and autobiographical knowledge). In this way, DLPFC allows a complete integration of the emotional and cognitive experiences of individuals (Fernández-Duque et al., 2000).

The orbitofrontal cortex (OFC) is part of the arquicortical mantle that comes from the olfactory caudal orbital cortex (Stuss & Levine, 2002) and is closely related to the limbic system. Its main function is the processing and regulation of emotions and affective states, as well as the regulation and control of behavior (Damasio, 1998). It is involved in the detection of changes in negative and positive environmental conditions (risky or beneficial situations to the subject), which allows adjustments to behavioral patterns in relation to quick or sudden environmental changes (Hunt, Turner, Polatajko, Bottari, & Dawson, 2013).

This cortex is related to decision making based on the risk–benefit estimation (Bechara, Damasio, & Damasio, 2000), or in uncertain, unspecific or unpredictable situations. Its role is to point to the emotional relevance of a particular scheme of action among many other options that are available for the given situation. In particular, its ventromedial region (BA 13) has been related to the detection of risky situations, while the lateral region (BA 47–12) has been related to the processing of negative–positive emotions (Verdejo-García & Bechara, 2010).

The frontomedial cortex (FMC) participates actively in the processes of inhibition, in the detection and resolution of conflicts, as well as in regulating attentional control. It also intervenes in the regulation of aggression and motivational states. It is considered that anterior cingulate cortex (BA 24) works in an integrated manner with this region (McKlveen, Myers, & Herman, 2015). Its inferior portion (infero-medial: BA 32) is closely related to autonomic control, visceral responses, motor reactions and changes in skin conductance to affective stimuli (Ongur, Ferry, & Price, 2003), while the upper (upper-medial) portion is more related to cognitive processes. The most anterior portions of the FMC are involved in the processes of mentalization (theory of mind) (Shallice, 2001).

Additionally, there are important differences between left and the right PFC functioning. The left PFC is more related to the processes of sequential planning, mental flexibility, verbal fluency, working memory (verbal information), memory strategies (verbal material), semantic memory coding and inverse sequence, as well as the establishment and consolidation of frequently used routines or action schemes. In contrast, right PFC is related to visuoconstruction, design of objects and figures, visual working memory, the appreciation of humor, episodic memory, behavior and social cognition, and detection and processing of new information and situations (Vallesi, 2012).

14.2 Neuropsychological Assessment of EF

Neuropsychological assessment is a complex procedure that requires a multidimensional approach, which seeks to estimate the cognitive and behavioral consequences of brain dysfunction, therefore taking into account issues such as patient history, medical findings, informal observations and application of neuropsychological tests. This evaluation process must be flexible and adapted to the characteristics of each patient that is, to their handicaps, abilities and needs derived from the magnitude and nature of his impairment. The interpretation of the results obtained from the neuropsychological assessment should be framed within the knowledge about mental functioning and the neurobiological bases of cognition and the behavior, thus allowing an accurate picture of the problem (Ardila & Ostrosky, 2012).

The neuropsychological assessment of the cognitive processes supported by the frontal lobes, among them the EF, continues to be a challenge both in clinical settings and in neuropsychological research. The diversity and complexity of these functions impose an important challenge to researchers and clinical professionals of the area, since they face the questions: what EF to evaluate? and, how to do it? In addition, there is a lack of adapted and standardized tests for non-English-speaking population and within the clinical scope, not until recently, has it been acknowledged the relevance to assess EF in different stages of development (Godefroy et al. 2018).

It has also been pointed out that despite the importance of various regions of the prefrontal cortex (PFC) for human behavior and cognition, even in adults they are not satisfactorily evaluated by the usual methods of neuropsychological assessment (Stuss & Levine, 2002).

EF are characterized by presenting an important diversity of deficits, since the damage in different brain regions or pathologies of neurodevelopment can affect different EF (Zelazo & Müller, 2002). In adults, damage to the frontal lobes conveys heterogeneous and important consequences that affect behavior and cognition, ranging from deficits of emotion regulation and social behavior, to deficits in abstract thinking and metacognition (Stuss & Levine, 2002). This damage is common in different pathologies, for example, head trauma (Hunt et al., 2013), attention deficit disorder (Kamradt, Ullsperger, & Nikolas, 2014), cerebrovascular accidents (Keil & Kaszniak, 2002) or in normal aging (Overdorp, Kessels, Claassen, & Oosterman, 2016).

The complexity–precision relationship in neuropsychology represents a type of negative correlation: the more complex the test, the less function accuracy. That is, the more complex the test, more areas of the PFC and the brain are needed to perform it, and vice versa. The relatively lower cognitive complexity of frontal tests allows maximizing area accuracy, which is one of the most important objectives in frontal lobe neuropsychology. It is important to clarify that the concept "main area" does not mean exclusive area. Several areas of the PFC and the brain in general are required for performing a test, and the more complex it is, the greater number of areas is needed; however, it is suggested that the main components of a test are particularly sensitive to damage in a specific brain region (Goldstein et al., 2014; Stuss & Alexander, 2000).

The lack of agreement among the different theoretical perspectives in relation to the different processes that can be considered as EF has impacted on the consensus about how many and which of these processes should be evaluated. For example, it is increasingly common to find references to a possible dichotomy in the components of EF with an association to neuronal structures; hence, "cold" or cognitive components based on mechanical and logical operations have been conceptualized (Zelazo & Müller, 2002) and the "hot" components that are related to those functions that involve emotional and motivational aspects (Peterson & Welsh, 2014).

The connections between the dorsolateral prefrontal cortex and subcortical structures mediate the functioning of cold EF such as planning, conceptual reasoning, flexibility or working memory, while the ventromedial and orbitofrontal prefrontal cortex and the basal ganglia and thalamus are related to the hot FE (self-control and regulation of the processing and emotional response) (Peterson & Welsh, 2014).

Other studies about the conceptualization and development of the FE have revealed two perspectives about its nature. On the one hand, it has been postulated that EF can be considered as a single cognitive process of a higher order, which has been referred to as "the central executive" (Baddeley, 1996), "attentional control" (Engle, 2002) or "supervisory attention system" (Norman & Shallice, 1986). From this perspective, a single latent factor would explain the performance in tasks that demand this type of processing.

Another point of view considers the FE as a conceptual umbrella that includes different interrelated processes that are put into play when the task demands a guide, direction and control of both thought and emotion and behavior to reach a goal in new or changing tasks (Gioia, Isquith, Guy, & Kenworthy, 2000) where automatic behavior is not effective (Diamond, 2006).

This diversity of concepts and theoretical approaches to EF reflects the little consensus about the processes involved in the regulation of behavior and emotions which in turn implies a difficulty in their measurement.

Currently, there are a wide variety of tasks created to evaluate the development of EF in subjects of different ages (Welsh & Peterson, 2014). These tasks measure multiple skills simultaneously, which has been called "impurity of the task" (Miyake et al., 2000); however, it has been considered that this reflects the nature of the construct that is intended to be measured; in this case, EF imply the coordination of multiple processes necessary for the execution of a specific task. As mentioned above, EF tasks generally involve more than one function; however, they can be organized according to the main component they evaluate.

14.3 EF Assessment in Spanish-Speaking Population

Cognitive assessment, of both healthy and pathological populations, requires the use of objective and reliable neuropsychological instruments designed and adapted to appropriately evaluate the populations we are interested in. Moreover, appropriate normative data must be developed in order to establish an accurate clinical picture about the nature of the impairments. Therefore, it is important to have neuropsychological tests that are developed and standardized for Spanish-speaking populations. It is not only important to have data collected in Spanish-speaking populations, but also, given the influence that educational factors have on cognitive performance, norms for neuropsychological tests should represent persons with different educational levels

As Ardila, Ostrosky, Rosselli and Gómez (2000) pointed out, the educational effect in not linear, but rather is a negatively accelerated curve, tending to a plateau. Differences between 0 and 3 years of education are highly significant, differences between 3 and 6 years of education are lower, between 6 and 9 are even lower and virtually no differences are expected to be found between 12 and 15 years of education.

In this context, the Neuropsychological Battery of Executive Functions and Frontal Lobes (Batería de Funciones Ejecutivas y Lóbulos Frontales BANFE; Flores, Ostrosky, & Lozano, 2014) was developed in order to assess these functions in Spanish-speaking population. The tests included in the battery were selected and organized based on the anatomo-functional criterion and in relation to the relative lower–higher complexity of the evaluated processes: those that evaluate functions that depend on the orbitofrontal cortex (OFC), medial prefrontal cortex (MPFC), dorsolateral prefrontal cortex (DLPFC) and the anterior prefrontal cortex (APFC). Thus, the tests are characterized by having little cognitive complexity in favor of specificity of area.

The application and interpretation of each test is based on a quantitative and qualitative analysis of accuracy and errors. The qualitative analysis of the execution considers the concept of functional system postulated by Luria (1986), according to which higher psychic functions can only exist thanks to the interaction of highly differentiated structures, each of which makes a specific contribution to the whole dynamic function so the damage in some link of the functional system causes a very specific type of disorder in these complex behavioral processes. Standardization and norms were obtained from 300 normal subjects between 6 and 85 years of age. According to age, the sample was divided into nine groups: 6–7, 8–9, 10–11, 12–13, 14–15, 16–30, 31–55, 56–64 and 65–85; and adults were divided according to two levels of education: 4–9 years and 10–24 years of education.

The battery comprises 14 tests that assess several frontal and executive functions related to the three main prefrontal areas:

Tests that depend mainly on the OFC and the MPFC:

1. Stroop effect. Evaluates inhibitory control.
2. Gambling task. Estimates the ability to detect and avoid risk selections, as well as to detect and maintain beneficial selections.
3. Labyrinths. Ability to respect limits and follow rules.

Tests that depend mainly on the DLPFC:

4. Self-directed signaling. Evaluates the ability to use the visuospatial working memory to indicate a series of figures in a self-directed way.
5. Visuospatial working memory. Estimates the ability to actively retain and reproduce the sequential visuospatial order of a series of figures.
6. Alphabetic word ordering. Ability to manipulate and mentally ordering of verbal information contained in working memory.
7. Card sorting. Evaluates the ability to generate a classification hypothesis, and to change (mental flexibility) the classification criterion.
8. Labyrinths. Ability to plan and anticipate visuospatial behavior.
9. Tower of Hanoi. Ability to anticipate actions in both progressive and regressive order (sequential planning).

10. Serial addition and subtraction. Ability to develop sequences in reverse order (inverse sequencing).
11. Verbal fluency. Ability to produce the most verbs in a fluid way and within a reduced margin of time.

Tests that depend mainly on the APFC:

12. Semantic classifications. Evaluates the productivity of semantic groups, and the capacity of abstract attitude: the number of abstract categories spontaneously produced.
13. Sayings. Ability to understand, compare and select answers with figurative meaning.
14. Metamemory. Evaluates the ability to develop a memory strategy (metacognitive monitoring), as well as to make performance judgments (metacognitive judgments) and to make adjustments between performance judgments and actual performance.

These tests were also selected in relation to the relative lower–higher complexity of the evaluated processes, that is, metacognition (metamemory, figurative meaning, abstract attitude), executive functions (verbal fluency, productivity, mental flexibility, visuospatial) and basic functions (inhibitory control, rule-guided goals and decision making).

14.4 EF Assessment in Spanish-Speaking Children

In recent years, there has been a growing interest in the study of EF during childhood (Garon, Bryson, & Smith, 2008) largely due to a series of studies that show the rapid development of these functions during the first year of life (Diamond, 2006). These data are not only relevant for the identification of EF characteristics during this stage of development, but also emphasize the importance of having appropriate assessment instruments adapted to the level of development of children.

During childhood, there are structural and functional changes of the PFC, which do not guarantee by themselves the appearance and adequate development of the cognitive functions associated with this brain region. The development of EF depends both on maturation through biological processes and on the quantity and quality of the learning experiences provided by the environment, so it has been postulated that factors such as sociocultural factors can influence their development (Hackman, Farah, & Meaney, 2010).

The neuropsychological assessment of FE in preschool children has been characterized by the creation of appropriate and sensitive tasks to this stage of development and by the adaptation of tasks used with adults. These tasks have tried to minimize the role of language in output responses and emphasize motor-type responses. The growing interest in FE during this period has marked the need to have instruments that allow identifying their characteristics as well as the deficits that may be associated with a disorder (Baron & Anderson, 2012).

The Neuropsychological Battery for Preschoolers (BANPE) (Ostrosky, Lozano, & González, 2016) aims to evaluate the normal and pathological course of the neuropsychological development of various cognitive processes in the preschool stage such as attention, memory, language, motor skills and executive functions, all considering various aspects such as variability in the attentional amplitude, linguistic competences and degree of knowledge, minimizing the complexity of the instructions, as well as the demand for verbal response, and this battery uses material and knowledge familiar to the children's daily experience, such as crayons, candies, colors and animals. The assessment of these functions includes techniques that reflect the specific characteristics of the process and incorporates recent findings of neuroanatomical research and developmental neuropsychology.

Regarding EF, this battery includes the following tasks:

- Inhibition. It includes subtests of motor and cognitive inhibition and delayed gratification.
- Work memory. It includes subtests of auditory-verbal modality and visuospatial modality.
- Flexibility. It includes a card sorting task.
- Planning. It includes labyrinths and a sequential planning task.
- Abstraction. It includes an error detection in nonsense pictures
- Theory of mind. It includes false belief tasks.
- Decision making. It includes a gambling task.

In order to obtain norms, a convenience sampling was conducted and 485 healthy children between 3 and 5 years 11 months of age were selected. This battery allows to obtain an index of performance of: orientation, attention and concentration, memory, language (articulation, comprehension and expression), motor coordination, academic skills, inhibition, working memory, flexibility, planning, abstraction, theory of mind and decision making.

14.5 Conclusion

Neuropsychological assessment of EF, both in adults and in children, remains a challenge in clinical settings. New findings in research regarding the nature of EF have contributed to the development of tests which are sensible enough to detect deficits associated with frontal lobe damage.

In Latin America and in Spanish-speaking countries, there is a need for brief, reliable and norm-based neuropsychological instruments to assess cognitive abilities of geriatric, neurological and general medical populations. Standardized neuropsychological instruments in Spanish are still few.

The Battery of Executive Functions and the Preschool Neuropsychological Battery provide the possibility to obtain an index of performance of different frontal areas that are related to different EF, thus allowing for a better clinical description and analysis of a patient's cognitive status.

Funding This work was partially supported by PAPIIT UNAM (IN302016)

References

Ardila, A., & Ostrosky, F. (2012). *Guía para el diagnóstico Neuropsicológico*. http://ineuro.cucba.udg.mx/libros/bv_guia_para_el_diagnostico_neuropsicologico.pdf.

Ardila, A., Ostrosky, F., Rosselli, M., & Gómez, C. (2000). Age related cognitive decline during normal aging: The complex effect of education. *Archives of Clinical Neuropsychology, 15,* 495–514.

Baddeley, A. D. (1996). Exploring the central executive. *The Quarterly Journal of Experimental Psychology, 49,* 5–28.

Barkley, R. A. (2012). *Executive functions: What they are, how they work, and why they evolved*. London: The Guilford Press.

Baron, I. S., & Anderson, P. J. (2012). Neuropsychological assessment of preschoolers. *Neuropsychological Review, 22,* 311–312. https://doi.org/10.1007/s11065-012-9221-2.

Bechara, A., Damasio, H., & Damasio, A. R. (2000). Emotion, decision making and the orbitofrontal cortex. *Cerebral Cortex, 10,* 295–307.

Damasio, A. R. (1998). The somatic marker hypothesis and the possible functions of the prefrontal cortex. In A. C. Roberts, T. W. Robbins, & L. Weiskrantz (Eds.), *The prefrontalcortex, executive and cognitive functions* (pp. 36–50). Nueva York: Oxford University Press.

Diamond, A. (2006). The early development of executive functions. In E. Bialystok & F. Craik (Eds.), *Lifespan cognition: Mechanisms of change* (pp. 70–95). New York: Oxford University Press.

Engle, R. W. (2002). Working memory capacity as executive attention. *Current Directions in Psychological Science, 11,* 19–23.

Fernández-Duque, D., Baird, J. A., & Posner, M. (2000). Executive attention and metacognitive regulation. *Consciousnes and Cognition, 9,* 288–307.

Flores, J. C., Ostrosky, F., & Lozano, A. (2014). *Batería de Funciones Ejecutivas y Lóbulos Frontales BANFE*. México: Manual Moderno.

Fuster, J. (2017). Prefrontal executive functions predict and preadapt. In E. Goldberg (Ed.). *Executive functions in health and disease*. Academic Press. https://doi.org/10.1016/b978-0-12-803676-1.00001.

Fuster, J. M. (2002). Frontal lobe and cognitive development. *Journal ofNeurocitology, 31,* 373–385.

Garon, N., Bryson, S. E., & Smith, I. M. (2008). Executive function in preschoolers: A review using an integrative framework. *Psychological Bulletin, 134,* 31–60.

Gioia, G. A., Isquith, P. K., Guy, S. C., & Kenworthy, L. (2000). Behavior rating inventory of executive function. *Child Neuropsychology: A Journal on Normal and Abnormal Development in Childhood and Adolescence, 6*(3), 235–238.

Godefroy, O., Martinaud, O., Narme, P., Joseph, P. A., Mosca, C., Lhommée, E., et al. (2018). Dysexecutive disorders and their diagnosis: A position paper. *Cortex, 109,* 322–335.

Goldberg, E. (2001). *The executive brain, frontal lobes and the civilized mind*. Nueva York: Oxford University Press.

Goldstein, S., Naglieri, J., Princiotta, D., & Otero, T. (2014). Introduction: A history of executive functioning as a theoretical and clinical construct. In S. Goldstein & J. Naglieri (Eds.), *Handbook of executive functioning* (pp. 3–12). New York, NY: Springer.

Hackman, D. A., Farah, M. J., & Meaney, M. J. (2010). Socioeconomic status and the brain: mechanistic insights from human and animal research. *Nature Reviews Neuroscience, 11*(9), 651–659.

Hunt, A. W., Turner, G. R., Polatajko, H., Bottari, C., & Dawson, D. R. (2013). Executive function, self-regulation and attribution in acquired brain injury: A scoping review. *Neuropsychological Rehabilitation, 23*(6), 914–932.

Kamradt, J. M., Ullsperger, J. M., & Nikolas, M. A. (2014). Executive function assessment and adult attention-deficit/hyperactivity disorder: Tasks versus ratings on the Barkley deficits in executive functioning scale. *Psychological Assessment, 26*(4), 1095–1105.

Keil, K., & Kaszniak, A. W. (2002). Examining executive function in individuals with brain injury: A review. *Aphasiology, 16*(3), 305–335. https://doi.org/10.1080/02687030143000654.

Lezak, M. D., Howieson, D. B., Bigler, E. D., & Tranel, D. (2012). *Neuropsychological assessment* (5th ed.). USA: Oxford University Press.

Logue, S. F., & Gould, T. J. (2014). The neural and genetic basis of executive function: Attention, cognitive flexibility, and response inhibition. *Pharmacology, Biochemistry and Behavior, 123,* 45–54.

Luria, A. R. (1986). *Las funciones corticales superiores del hombre*. México: Fontamara.

Luria, A. R. (1989). *El cerebro en acción*. Barcelona: Fontanella.

McKlveen, J. M., Myers, B., & Herman, J. P. (2015). The medial prefrontal cortex: coordinator of autonomic, neuroendocrine and behavioural responses to stress. *Journal of Neuroendocrinology, 27,* 446–456.

Miller, E. K., & Cohen, J. D. (2001). An integrative theory of prefrontal cortex function. *Annual Review of Neuroscience, 24,* 67–202.

Miyake, A., Friedman, N. P., Emerson, M. J., Witzki, A. H., Howerter, A., & Wager, T. D. (2000). The unity and diversity of executive functions and their contributions to complex frontal lobe tasks: A latent variable analysis. *Cognitive Psychology, 41,* 49–100.

Norman, D. A., & Shallice, T. (1986). Attention to action: Willed and automatic control of behavior. In R. J. Davidson, G. E. Schwartz, & D. Shapiro (Eds.), *Consciousness and Self-Regulation* (Vol. 4, pp. 1–18)., Advances in Research and Theory New York: Plenum Press.

Ongur, D., Ferry, A. T., & Price, J. L. (2003). Architectonic subdivision of the human orbital and medial prefrontal cortex. *Journal of Comparative Neurology, 460,* 425–449.

Ostrosky, F., Lozano, A., & González, M. G. (2016). *Batería neuropsicológica para preescolares*. México: Manual Moderno.

Overdorp, E. J., Kessels, R. P., Claassen, J. A., & Oosterman, J. M. (2016). The combined effect of neuropsychological and neuropathological deficits on instrumental activities of daily living in older adults: A systematic review. *Neuropsychology Review, 26*(1), 92–106.

Peterson, E., & Welsh, M. (2014). The development of hot and cool executive functions: Are we getting warmer? In S. Goldstein & J. A. Naglieri (Eds.), *Handbook of executive functions*. New York, NY: Springer.

Schoenemann, P. T., Seehan, M. J., & Glotzer, L. D. (2005). Prefrontalwhite matter volume is disproportionately larger in humans than in other primates. *Nature Neuroscience, 8,* 242–252.

Shallice, T. (2001). "Theory of mind" and the prefrontal cortex. *Brain, 124,* 247–248.

Shimamura, A. P. (2000). Toward a cognitive neurosicence of metacognition. *Consciousness and Cognition, 9,* 313–323.

Stuss, D. T., & Alexander, M. P. (2000). Executive functions and the frontal lobes: A conceptual view. *Psychology Research, 63,* 289–298.

Stuss, D. T., & Levine, B. (2002). Adult Clinical Neuropsychology: lessons from studies of the frontal lobes. *Annual Review of Psychology, 53,* 401–433.

Vallesi, A. (2012). Organisation of executive functions: Hemispheric asymmetries. *Journal of Cognitive Psychology, 24*(4), 367–386.

Verdejo-García, A., & Bechara, A. (2010). Neuropsychology of executive functions. *Psicothema, 22*(2), 227–235.

Welsh, M., & Peterson, E. (2014). Issues in the conceptualization and assessment of hot executive functions in childhood. *Journal of the International Neuropsychological Society, 20*(2), 152–156.
Zelazo, P. D., & Muller, U. (2002). Executive function in typical and atypical development. In U. Goswami (Ed.), *Handbook of child cognitive development* (pp. 445–469). Oxford: Blackwell.

Chapter 15
The Assessment of Executive Dysfunction in Bilinguals

Mónica Rosselli, Idaly Vélez-Uribe and Valeria L. Torres

15.1 Introduction

Dictionaries define bilingualism as the habitual use of two languages by one person or one region (*Diccionario de la Real Academia Española*, 2001) and the ability to speak (understand and produce) two languages (Merriam-Webster Dictionary, https://www.merriam-webster.com). From these definitions, it seems simple to categorize individuals into bilingual or monolingual. However, bilingualism is not dichotomous (yes or no), but rather, it is a continuous variable. Bilinguals encompass a heterogeneous group of individuals with diverse degrees of language proficiency. In addition, proficiency can be domain-specific as individuals might present different levels of competence across different domains, for instance, school versus personal (Gollan, Weissberger, Runnqvist, Montoya, & Cera, 2012). These language dissimilarities among bilinguals depend, among other variables, on the age of acquisition of each language, the frequency of use, and the context in which both languages are used (which can, in turn, affect the levels of proficiency across domains).

Age of acquisition (AoA) refers to the age at which each language is learned, regardless of its context. Usually, L1 refers to the language that is learned first, L2 to the second, and so on. Additionally, the context in which the languages are acquired is relevant; a language learned at home, for example, will include a different vocabulary from a language learned at school (naturalistic vs. instructional context; Pavlenko, 2007). The methods of acquisition of the language, either naturalistic or instructional, will be reflected on an individual's vocabulary. Furthermore, it is important to assess

M. Rosselli (✉) · I. Vélez-Uribe · V. L. Torres
Department of Psychology, Florida Atlantic University, Davie, FL, USA
e-mail: mrossell@fau.edu

I. Vélez-Uribe
e-mail: ivelezuribe@gmail.com

V. L. Torres
e-mail: vtorres2015@fau.edu

A. Ardila et al. (eds.), *Dysexecutive Syndromes*,
https://doi.org/10.1007/978-3-030-25077-5_15

how well each language has been acquired through a measure of language proficiency. The level of proficiency needs to be quantified in each language in at least two main aspects: expression/production and understanding/comprehension; differences in the level of proficiency may exist between and within the bilinguals' languages. For example, a bilingual speaker may develop the phonology of a native speaker and a limited level of comprehension in one language, whereas in the other language, the levels of comprehension and expression might be equivalent. The characterization of bilingualism also relates to the frequency of use of each language; how often the individual is exposed to a bilingual environment using both languages (e.g., on a daily or weekly bases) influences the bilingual's language fluency.

Understanding the pattern of language use over the life span could be important, as well. It is common to encounter individuals who were active bilinguals during childhood but became monolinguals (in terms of language use) in adulthood. Due to the levels of proficiency and the frequency of use, one language may become dominant. These varying proficiency and frequency of use characteristics may result in the non-native language (L2) becoming the dominant language (Ardila, Lopez-Recio, Sakowitz, Sanchez, & Sarmiento, 2018; Ardila, Rosselli, Ortega, Lang, & Torres, 2019). Therefore, it is not always the case that a bilingual's first or native language is the preferred/dominant language.

Another relevant variable in bilingualism is the person's level of identification with the culture associated with a language. This cultural/social attitude could influence the motivation to learn the language and the frequency with which the speakers will use it (Fienberg & Meyer, 1992). Additionally, the social context will determine the pattern of use of each language. As stated above, bilinguals who use their native language in a family environment and the second language at school and/or work will develop different vocabularies and distinctive levels of proficiency in each language.

A final pertinent variable in the characterization of bilingualism refers to the linguistic distance between two languages. We can consider a case of strong bilingualism in which the two languages are linguistically distant from each other (e.g., in Chinese/Spanish bilinguals), whereas weak bilingualism may exist when the two languages are closer in their linguistic systems (e.g., in Italian/Spanish bilinguals) (Ardila, 2007). It has been documented that the linguistic distance between the learned languages influences the bilingual learning process (Hoff & Core, 2018). When children are acquiring a L2, they use the structural properties of their L1 to do so. For example, children whose L1 has no articles make article omissions when acquiring English (Zdorenko & Paradis, 2012). Therefore, bilingual development differs depending on the particular languages being acquired (Hoff & Core, 2018).

Bilingualism has been identified as a potential generator of cognitive advantages and disadvantages, as well as a modulator of brain plasticity (Bialystok, 2017; Bialystok, Craik, & Luk, 2012; Rosselli & Ardila, 2018). Speaking two languages has been shown to influence the individual's cognitive skills beyond linguistic capabilities. Executive functions (EFs) seem to be the most affected (Bialystok, 2001). Fluent bilinguals rely extensively on cognitive control during language switching; they have to monitor the situation to select the appropriate language, activate the target language, all while inhibiting the nontarget language. This continuous practice may serve to enhance cognitive control in ways that appear to extend beyond language control (Rosselli & Ardila, 2018). These abilities are manifested in advantages on EF tests, particularly the nonverbal types. Bilingualism can also generate a disadvantage, specifically regarding verbal learning. There is evidence of lower (Bialystok, 2001) or differential (Kohnert, 2010) performance on verbal tasks in bilingual children (Bialystok, 2001) and adults (Gollan, Montoya, & Werner, 2002) compared to monolinguals. This disadvantage seems to be related to the cross-language interference that occurs when the two languages are activated (Rosselli et al., 2000). Code-switching (switching between languages) is a process that requires executive processes mostly related to inhibition of the nontarget language. Active bilinguals cannot simply "shut off" one language and function as monolinguals. Overall, it is unknown whether the benefits of bilingualism outweigh its disadvantages and whether any effects are reflected on neuropsychological tasks.

The cognitive differences between bilinguals and monolinguals described above are related to differences in brain organization (Abutalebi & Green, 2016; Abutalebi et al., 2012, 2013). Evidence shows that a dual language experience is a brain modifier across the life span (for a review, see Bialystok, 2017; Rosselli & Ardila, 2018). In other words, bilingualism seems to act as a plasticity variable, generating changes in brain structures (Borsa et al., 2018; Del Maschio et al., 2018) and in the patterns of brain activation during task performance (Berroir et al., 2017).

Due to the reported cognitive, structural, and functional effects of a dual language experience, the neuropsychological assessment of bilingual individuals may differ from that of monolinguals and requires special psychometric and clinical considerations. Moreover, bilinguals with neurological disorders might present a cognitive profile, course of recovery, and compensatory mechanisms, that are dissimilar to those of monolinguals with the same neurological conditions. Clinical adjustments may be recommended for the most valid and accurate assessment of this population.

The aim of this chapter is to examine the relevant issues around the neuropsychological assessment of bilingual individuals, particularly in association with EFs. First, we will consider the subtypes of bilingualism, followed by the instruments used in the evaluation of language proficiency, as well as the empirical evidence that relates bilingualism to measures of EF. The chapter ends with a description of the research findings connecting the assessment of EFs in bilinguals with neurological disorders and with conclusions and directions for further research.

15.2 Subtypes of Bilingualism

There is diversity in the characterization of bilingualism. The cognitive and brain effects of bilingualism might vary according to the type of bilingualism (Ardila, 2007; Kousaie, Chai, Sander, & Klein, 2017; Luk, De Sa, & Bialystok, 2011; Tao, Marzecová, Taft, Asanowicz, & Wodniecka, 2011). Three kinds of bilingualism (depending on AoA and proficiency) have been described: coordinated, compound, and subordinated (Weinreich, 1953). In coordinated bilingualism, the individual learns two languages independently of each other, with each language having its autonomous semantic and production units. These bilinguals have difficulties translating from one language to other, which could be due to their independent development. In most cases, coordinated bilinguals learn both languages early in life (before age 3) simultaneously and in parallel. In compound bilingualism, there is a combined semantic unit (there is a common semantic system) and two production units (words), which usually characterizes early bilinguals but not simultaneous bilinguals. In subordinated bilingualism, learning L2 is mediated by the previously well-learned native language; in these cases, there is one semantic system in the native language, with two production systems, one for each language. Subordinated bilingualism is characteristic of late bilinguals. Subordinated bilingualism may become compound bilingualism as L2 proficiency improves. This change is frequently seen in bilinguals who learn L2 during adolescence or early adulthood.

Bilinguals have also been distinguished according to the AoA of L2, separating them into early and late bilinguals. Early bilingualism occurs when the person learned both languages early in life, for example, before age seven (Pelham & Abrams, 2014) or ten (Luk et al., 2011). A person can be considered a late bilingual if L2 was acquired after 13 years of age (Pelham & Abrams, 2014). In these cases, the first language learned is L1 and the second language is L2. This classification is related to another dichotomy used in bilingualism: simultaneous versus successive bilingualism. Researchers have used simultaneous bilingualism to refer to bilinguals who learned both languages at the same time, and successive bilingualism when the learning of the two languages occurred one after the other. Instances of simultaneous bilingualism are always considered early bilingualism, and they occur when the two languages are learned during the child's first three years.

Depending on the degree of use of a bilingual's languages, researchers have used terms such as active bilinguals to describe individuals who use both languages on a daily or weekly basis, as opposed to passive bilinguals who may have learned a language that is not currently in practice.

A final way of categorizing dual language speakers is between balanced and unbalanced bilinguals. Balanced bilinguals are described as those individuals who are equally proficient in both languages, whereas unbalanced bilinguals include those with a differential degree of proficiency between the two languages. It is important to clarify that balanced bilingualism is not equivalent to proficient bilingualism. For example, Rosselli, Ardila, Jurado, and Salvatierra (2014) evaluated a sample of balanced bilinguals who had low proficiency and compared them to balanced and highly proficient bilinguals. The former group had equivalently low naming scores in both languages (using the Spanish and English Boston Naming Test) while the latter had equivalently high scores in both languages. These findings highlight the variability and the importance of clarifying the aspects of bilingualism being explored.

In summary, the bilingual population is heterogeneous, with diverse language experiences that result in specific types of bilingualism. The accurate characterization of bilingualism will help evaluators to more accurately interpret the results of bilinguals' performance on neuropsychological evaluations.

15.3 The Assessment of Bilingualism

The neuropsychological assessment of bilinguals differs from that of monolinguals. Initially, decisions related to the language used for assessment and whether this is conducted in a monolingual or a bilingual mode must be made. A monolingual mode of assessment implies the exclusive use of one of the bilingual's languages and presumes that similar results would be expected regardless of the language of administration. Assessment in a bilingual mode takes place when the evaluator speaks the two languages of the person who is being evaluated and the use of either language is permitted throughout the evaluation process, including the test responses, without penalization. This is particularly important during the evaluation of children with suspected language impairment. Due the challenging nature of these types of evaluations, it has been suggested that using parental questionnaires with unbiased language measures (e.g., the Nonword Repetition task and the Multilingual Assessment Instrument for Narratives) is also adequate (Boerma & Blom, 2017).

A crucial question in the assessment of dual language learners recently tested by Ardila et al. (2019) is whether the language used the evalutaion affects cognitive test scores. The authors used a within-subject design to compare the performance of Spanish/English bilinguals on seven verbal subtests from the WAIS-III, with assessments completed in both languages. Results showed a significantly superior performance on the vocabulary subtest in English (dominant language) compared to Spanish (primary language). These results were found despite participants reporting that Spanish was L1. The authors emphasized the importance of properly selecting the testing language in clinical practice to obtain reliable results regarding the capabilities of bilinguals.

Typically, the dominant language is preferred by participants during cognitive testing (Cummins & Swain, 2014; Gathercole & Thomas, 2009). However, only using the dominant language during language tests may not reflect the bilingual's entire linguistic ability (Ardila et al., 2018). Bilinguals may learn different words in each language, and therefore, a more comprehensive (and fair) assessment is performed with a bilingual evaluation. A bilingual is not two monolinguals in one person (Grosjean, 1989) and therefore, it is unreliable and unfair to treat bilinguals' assessment as if they were monolinguals of the dominant language. Moreover, assessment of both languages is recognized as the best practice (Bilingual Service Delivery, 2017). In addition, the question of language dominance can yield inaccurate responses. Language dominance (like proficiency) can be domain-specific, meaning that bilinguals might have different levels of proficiency and dominance in different domains. Alternative scoring, which counts items produced in either language as valid, has shown the potential for improving scores in bilingual individuals (Gollan, Fennema-Notestine, Montoya, & Jernigan, 2007), including those diagnosed with Alzheimer's disease (AD; Gollan, Salmon, Montoya, & da Pena, 2010).

In order to properly assess an individual's bilingual abilities, various methods have been used in clinical practice or in research designs. For example, Li, Sepanski, and Zhao (2006) developed a Web-based L2 language history questionnaire by including the most relevant dimensions of bilingualism from 41 published questionnaires. The following are the nine most frequent questionnaire items across studies (presented in order of frequency after excluding demographic variables): years of residence in the country where L2 is spoken, age at which L2 learning started, self-assessment in reading ability in L1 and L2, self-assessment in speaking ability in L1 and L2, years of L2 instruction received, self-assessment in writing ability in L1 and L2, language spoken at home, self-assessment in comprehension ability in L1 and L2, and a question identifying the native language. This questionnaire has three parts. Part A includes general questions related to the participant's language history and the participant's proficiency in each language in terms of reading, writing, speaking, and understanding abilities. Part B includes language-specific questions related to linguistic environment and language use, and Part C allows for the researcher to customize the questionnaire by adding bilingual questions that suit their study needs. Subjects can enter the information online, and results are automatically generated as an RTF output file.

Another reliable, valid, and commonly used assessment tool is the Language Experience and Proficiency Questionnaire (LEAP-Q; Marian, Blumenfeld, & Kaushanskaya, 2007), developed to assess the linguistic profile of healthy adults while considering language competence (proficiency, dominance, and preference) and current language use (prior language exposure and current language use) in different environments (family and work). The LEAP-Q is a self-rated measure of linguistic abilities that includes proficiency scores in four areas speaking, understanding spoken language, reading, and writing. These are rated on a 0–10 Likert-type scale (0 = none, 1 = very low, 2 = low, 3 = fair, 4 = slightly less than adequate, 5 = adequate, 6 = slightly more than adequate, 7 = good, 8 = very good, 9 = excellent, 10 = perfect).

Using objective methods to assess bilingualism rather than self-report measures (or in combination with) may more accurately capture proficiency levels across languages as well as the degree of bilingualism. Researchers may use interviews (conducted by native speakers of the language) to determine the bilinguals' ability to maintain conversations in each language (Pelham & Abrams, 2014). Using confrontation naming tests, such as the Multilingual Naming Test (MINT; Gollan et al., 2012) and the Boston Naming Test (BNT; Kaplan, Goodglass, & Weintraub, 1983), allows researchers to more objectively examine language abilities in bilinguals and to compare their proficiency in each language (Gollan, Salmon, Montoya, & Galasko, 2011; Salvatierra & Rosselli, 2011). Additionally, the Bilingual Verbal Ability Test (BVAT; Muñoz-Sandoval, Cummins, Alvarado, & Ruef, 1998) is often used to evaluate Spanish/English bilinguals' vocabulary, comprehension, and communication skills in their languages and can be used to determine how balanced/unbalanced a bilingual is (Rosselli, Ardila, Lalwani, & Vélez-Uribe, 2016).

Gollan et al. (2011) calculated an index of bilingualism by dividing the non-dominant language scores on the BNT by the dominant language scores, yielding an index that ranged from 0 (monolingual) to 1 (bilingual). Rosselli et al. (2019) used a similar measure to determine the degree of bilingualism by dividing participants' lower average LEAP-Q score (speaking, understanding, and reading in one language, English or Spanish) by the higher average LEAP-Q score (speaking, understanding, and reading of the other language, Spanish or English). Similar indices have been calculated using questionnaires that consider the competence and use of both languages across the life span. Martínez-Horta et al. (2019) used the modified version of the bilingualism questionnaire created by Anderson, Mak, Chahi, and Bialystok (2018) to compute an index relative to use (BIuse) and competence (BIcomp) with the formula [$BI = 1 - (\%L1 - \%L2)$] (% corresponded to the number of answers given for the numbered items). BIuse was considered a measure of how a person used both languages throughout life, with a value of 1 indicating the equal use of both languages (i.e., speaking each language half of the time). BIcomp evaluated the level of language proficiency, with a value of 1 indicating that the participant was equally proficient in both languages.

15.4 The Assessment of Executive Functions in Bilinguals

When assessing EF in bilinguals, it is relevant for the evaluator to understand the potential performance difference between bilinguals and monolinguals. In proficient bilinguals, both languages are constantly active, requiring the inhibition of one language at all times. This could cause delays in the processing of verbal information (Green, 1998). Green has proposed the existence of a supervisory attentional system (SAS) that will be used when there is parallel activation of lexical items associated with a particular concept between languages, and this system inhibits the nontarget language (Hilchey & Klein, 2011). When simultaneous semantic information is activated for speech or word retrieval, SAS allows for the retrieval of a word in the target language after resolving the conflict via inhibition of the word in the nontarget language.

Conforming to this model, bilinguals will develop extensive experience in inhibiting and switching, which has been suggested to depend on general executive control (EC) abilities (Abutalebi & Green, 2007). This constant practice could lead to an EF advantage over monolinguals and has been reported in some tasks in bilingual children and adults (Pelham & Abrams, 2014; Thomas-Sunesson, Hakuta, & Bialystok, 2018). These advantages have been described in different aspects of nonverbal EF, such as conflict resolution (Costa, Hernández, & Sebastián-Gallés, 2008; Thomas-Sunesson et al., 2018), suppression of irrelevant information (Bialystok, Craik, Klein, & Viswanathan, 2004; Bialystok, Craik, & Luk, 2008; Ransdell, Barbier, & Niit, 2006), shifting between mental sets (Garbin et al., 2010; Prior & MacWhinney, 2010), and working memory (Thomas-Sunesson et al., 2018). However, recent research suggests that these effects might be true only for some types of bilinguals under specific circumstances, and only in certain EF tasks (Bak, 2016; Paap, Johnson, & Sawi, 2016). Rosselli et al. (2016) suggested that linguistic proficiency might influence this advantage independent of bilingual status, a conclusion that has been supported by neuroimaging studies (Abutalebi, Cappa, & Perani, 2001). In Rosselli et al.'s (2016) study, highly proficient monolingual adults performed at the level of highly proficient balanced bilinguals on the Block Design task and on verbal (Stroop,

Digit span) and nonverbal EF (Simon task, Corsi Blocks) tasks, while the low proficiency groups (bilinguals and monolinguals) had different performances. Similarly, Thomas-Sunesson et al. (2018) reported a significant association between higher EF performance (conflict resolution was evaluated with the Flanker task and nonverbal working memory was evaluated with the Frog Recall task) and level of bilingualism in Spanish/English bilingual children, with more balanced bilingualism being associated with better performance.

The language-control mechanisms required for the efficient use of languages in bilinguals may not necessarily generalize to domain-general EF mechanisms (Gollan & Goldrick, 2016). Consequently, some research has failed to support differences between bilinguals and monolinguals. Within elderly passive Telugu/English bilinguals (active users of Telugu), Mishra, Padmanabhuni, Bhandari, Viswambharan, and Prasad (2018) failed to find an association between language proficiency and increased performance on a range of EF neuropsychological tasks (numerical Stroop task, Attention Network task, Dimensional Change Card Sorting task, and stop-signal task). Furthermore, null findings by meta-analytic reviews (e.g., Lehtonen et al., 2018) suggest that the positive effects and advantages in several EF tasks may be influenced, at least in part, by publication bias or other nonlinguistic variables (e.g., nonverbal intelligence; Rosselli et al., 2016).

Although the manipulation of two languages can be advantageous for the performance on some nonverbal EF tasks, it can also present a disadvantage on EF tasks that rely on verbal abilities (Gollan et al., 2002; Rosselli et al., 2000). Research shows that adult bilinguals produce a smaller number of words than monolinguals on semantic verbal fluency tasks; the simple act of retrieving a common word with limited time seems to be more effortful for bilinguals. Also, when bilinguals function in a bilingual mode (both languages are simultaneously activated), the increased interference during word recall results in lower scores (Rosselli et al., 2000).

The assessment outcomes described above are unique to bilinguals. Activating both languages might result in dual language users presenting cross-linguistic effects, meaning that one language can affect the other. Support for this idea has been documented with the use of cognates in bilinguals. Cognates are cross-language word pairs that are alike in both meaning and form. For example, "elephant" in English and "elefante" in Spanish are a cognate pair, as they refer to the same object and have a high degree of similarity in their phonological (and orthographic) composition (Potapova & Pruitt-Lord, 2019). The "cognate facilitation effect" refers to the advantage in the recognition and production of cognate words over non-cognates during the performance of oral and written language tasks. Rosselli et al. (2014) demonstrated that although the cognate effect in balanced bilinguals is similar in both languages, the unbalanced group showed a more prominent cognate effect in the non-preferred language.

Finally, another important issue in the assessment of bilinguals relates to the lack of appropriate norms. As documented above, bilingualism may act as a cognitive modifier of EF measures, therefore, it is inaccurate to compare the performance of a bilingual to monolingual standards. Neuropsychological tests and normative data developed for monolingual speakers are inappropriate for bilinguals and might need to be adapted accordingly.

15.5 Executive Dysfunction in Bilinguals with Neurological Conditions

Additional challenges are faced when evaluating bilinguals with neurological conditions, since the consequences of these disorders may affect executive mechanisms of language control, thereby influencing both languages. For example, Ratiu and Azuma (2017) evaluated English–Spanish bilinguals with mild traumatic brain injury (mTBI) and healthy Spanish–English bilinguals with tasks intended to measure inhibition (Flanker task), task switching (color-shape switching task), simple memory (digit span forward, digit span backward, and Corsi blocks task), working memory (Operation Span, Symmetry Span tasks), and language control abilities. Their results showed that bilinguals with mTBI performed worse in some conditions of the Flanker task; they had slower response times than the healthy bilingual group on the Go/no-go condition (response inhibition), but not in the conflict condition (interference inhibition). No group differences were observed on other EF measures, however, the mTBI group made more language control errors (cross-language intrusions and pronouncing words in the nontarget language) in the reading aloud task, especially when switching between languages was required. While the results of this study suggest that inhibitory difficulties are characteristic of bilinguals, the lack of monolingual control groups is problematic.

15.5.1 Neurodegenerative Disorders

One of the most important developments in the field of bilingualism and neurological disorders is findings suggesting that bilingualism may have a protective effect over abnormal aging. It has been proposed that actively using two languages increases cognitive reserve (CR) among bilinguals and may delay the emergence of dementia (Fischer & Schweizer, 2014; Perani & Abutalebi, 2015; Perani et al., 2017). Cognitive reserve (Stern, 2009) is defined as a discrepancy between the observed behavioral and/or cognitive functioning and the anticipated (reduced) levels shown with typical aging (Barulli & Stern, 2013).

Bialystok, Craik, and Freedman (2007) found that among Canadian bilinguals, the onset of dementia occurred on average 4.1 years later than dementia onset among English-speaking monolinguals. However, this was not a longitudinal study but a retrospective review of patient charts. Similarly, Alladi et al. (2013) studied an Indian bilingual sample and reported a 4.5-year delay in the onset of AD, frontotemporal, and vascular dementia. In addition, they found a trend toward a delay in the onset of

Lewy body and mixed dementias. In support of these findings, Woumans et al. (2015) obtained similar results after controlling for possible confounding variables such as sex, education, occupation, and initial Mini-Mental State Examination (MMSE; Folstein, Folstein, & McHugh, 1975) scores. Others have demonstrated that a greater number of languages spoken by participants was associated with increased delays in cognitive decline (Chertkow et al., 2010; Kavé, Eyal, Shorek, & Cohen-Mansfield, 2008).

Bialystok, Craik, Binns, Ossher, and Freedman (2014) evaluated monolinguals and bilinguals in EF tasks over the course of one year and found that bilinguals were older than monolinguals when they initially reported symptoms of cognitive impairment. These symptoms were assessed via a questionnaire establishing when the patients or their families noted changes in memory or other cognitive domains, as well as changes in the ability to concentrate and communicate. During the baseline evaluation, both groups performed similarly, and despite bilinguals being older than monolinguals, their performance on EF tasks was comparable.

In a cross-sectional study, Rosselli et al. (2019) compared verbal and nonverbal memory performance between bilinguals and monolinguals with amnestic Mild Cognitive Impairment (aMCI). Results demonstrated a superior performance of aMCI bilinguals over aMCI monolinguals on the cued recall of words in a measure that is sensitive to recovery from proactive semantic interference (observed when old verbal learning interferes with new learning of semantically related information). The memory advantage in bilinguals on these measures was associated with higher inhibitory control as measured by the Stroop Color-Word test. In a longitudinal study among a large sample of Spanish–English-speaking elderly individuals tested over 23 years, memory and executive function were better in bilinguals compared to monolinguals at baseline, while rates of progression to dementia were comparable (Zahodne, Schofield, Farrell, Stern, & Manly 2014). These authors suggested that bilingualism in community-dwelling adults is associated with higher cognitive function in individuals who are cognitively normal and in the early stages of abnormal aging.

The CR theory of bilingualism and dementia has numerous critics, as other factors related to bilingualism also appear to influence dementia onset (e.g., immigrant status and education). Yeung, St John, Menec, and Tyas (2014) did not find bilingualism effects on the risk of developing dementia in a sample of older adults that was followed for 5 years. Other researchers (Calvo, García, Manoiloff, & Ibáñez, 2015) described additional challenges to this research due to small sample sizes with vastly differing linguistic profiles. In addition to these criticisms, Paap, Johnson, and Sawi (2016) highlighted flaws in the design of studies showing this delay, including the lack of a monolingual control group (Kavé et al., 2008), or poor matching of study groups (Alladi et al., 2013). Recent reviews have failed to support this theory (Yeung, St John, Menec, & Tyas, 2014) and stress the idea that retrospective studies are more likely to find delays in dementia due to multiple confounding factors and the reliance on self-reported memory complaints (Mukadam, Sommerlad, & Livingston, 2017). To reconcile these discrepant results, several authors suggested that the effects of bilingualism on normal and abnormal aging may be restricted to specific tasks of executive control in a limited group of bilinguals (Paap & Greenberg, 2013; von Bastian, Souza, & Gade, 2016). Moreover, Zahodne et al. (2014) proposed that bilingualism is related to higher cognitive function in individuals who are cognitively normal or in the early stages of abnormal aging.

Besides AD, bilingual language control has been studied in Parkinson's disease (PD), a neurodegenerative disease that involves the degeneration of the nigrostriatal (from the substantia nigra to the striatum in the basal ganglia) system. Cattaneo et al. (2015) evaluated highly proficient Catalan–Spanish bilinguals diagnosed with PD compared to a healthy bilingual group to examine the language control processes that manage cross-language interference, allowing for the successful communication in one language. Participants underwent neuropsychological assessments of cognitive status, memory, EFs, language production, and naming, in each language. The authors argued that structures involved in PD may also modulate language control in bilinguals; however, the relationship between domain-general executive control and bilingual language control was not apparent. This study did not include monolingual control groups, and therefore, the question of the relationship between basal ganglia dysfunction in PD and domain-general executive control was not fully explored.

The effect of bilingualism has also been explored in individuals with Huntington's disease, an inherited neurodegenerative disease, which primarily affects the caudate nucleus and putamen of the basal ganglia and leads to degeneration of the frontal and temporal lobes. Martínez-Horta et al. (2019) evaluated a sample of Catalan–Spanish bilinguals who were diagnosed with Huntington's disease and were either in the early or mild stages of the disease. A bilingualism index was calculated considering the use and competence of the two languages. Patients underwent cognitive evaluation of EFs which included verbal fluency (semantic and phonemic), the symbol digit modality test, the Stroop test, and Trail-Making Test (TMT) A and B. Results suggested that greater lifelong use of bilingualism has positive effects on the functional and structural integrity in the brains of Huntington's disease patients, with higher degrees of bilingualism associated with increased performance on the TMT-B and the Stroop test. However, this study did not include a sample of monolingual Huntington's disease participants, therefore restricting the validity of these results.

15.5.2 Vascular Disorders

The literature about focal brain damage in bilinguals is restricted to aphasia and aspects of recovery of linguistic abilities in both languages, and how the trajectories differ (or not) between languages. In addition, it explores whether word-retrieval deficits in bilingual aphasia can be attributed to broader issues of cognitive control. Balancing two languages in the bilingual brain and effectively using one at the time requires complex activation and inhibition processes (Adrover-Roig et al., 2011) which can be considered executive in nature. In the context of bilingual EF, some aspects of language control can be impaired in cases of subcortical aphasia (resulting from damage to the thalamus or the basal ganglia). The symptoms may include a selective impairment of one language resulting from the inability to appropriately inhibit the nontarget language, or the inability to activate the target language. Lalor and Kirsner (2001) indicated that this impairment may be due to damage to the connections between the basal ganglia and the frontal lobe. The deficits would be most evident in code-switching (switching between languages) failures, or uncontrolled code-switching, which were reported in a case study after damage to the left basal ganglia (Ansaldo, Marcotte, Scherer, & Raboyeau, 2008) and have received support from studies of patients with PD (Cattaneo et al., 2015). Accordingly, fMRI evidence supports a relationship between networks that include the basal ganglia, the anterior cingulate cortex, and the prefrontal cortex, with code-switching (Abutalebi & Green, 2007). Others have demonstrated the involvement of the dorsolateral prefrontal cortex instead, which would strongly support the idea of an executive component in language switching (Rubinstein, Meyer, & Evans, 2001). In addition, pathological code-switching has been detected as the sole aspect of language impaired after damage to the frontal lobe which slightly extended to the anterior cingulate gyrus (Fabbro, 2001). In a case study of a patient with damage to the left basal ganglia, Adrover-Roig et al. (2011) reported a greater impairment in L1 (Basque) than in L2 (Spanish), with decreased verbal fluency and impaired cognitive flexibility. The authors suggested that this may indicate a deficit in inhibitory control.

Van Der Linden et al. (2018) compared patients with parallel (when both languages follow similar trajectories of recovery) and differential aphasia (when one language recovers better/faster than the other), as defined by Paradis (2004). The authors postulated that the mechanism underlying differential aphasia could be more related to cognitive control than to the loss of access to word representations in the most impaired language, as previously proposed. The comparison between the two groups in a Flanker task indicated that the group with differential aphasia had much greater impairments of non-linguistic cognitive control than the group with parallel aphasia.

Furthermore, in bilinguals, word retrieval in the target language requires the successful inhibition of lexical competitors from the nontarget language. Faroqi-Shah, Sampson, Pranger, and Baughman (2018) studied the relationship between word retrieval and cognitive control in aphasics and found impairments reflected by the inability to recover from interference on the Stroop test. However, these findings were not affected by bilingual status, indicating that cognitive control is equally affected in bilinguals and monolinguals and does not seem to relate to how word-finding difficulties vary in differential aphasia. Even though all the patients with aphasia in this study had a left middle cerebral artery stroke, it is unclear whether these lesions encompassed subcortical structures that have been implicated in language control impairments.

It is essential for clinicians to be aware of the variation in the degree of impairment and recovery within bilinguals. Lesion studies have reported cases in which after brain insult, one language is affected while the other is spared (Paradis, 2004). Furthermore, neuroimaging evidence indicates that the bilingual language system does not appear as two distinct systems (one for each language) but is more complex and highly influenced by individual variability, depending particularly on proficiency

(Abutalebi, Cappa, & Perani, 2001). Nevertheless, the differences in cortical representation indicate that dual language exposure modifies the brain of bilinguals, which seems to support the hypothesis that these cortical changes could be reflected in cognitive functioning. However, the question of how it is reflected in cognitive abilities, particularly in EFs, remains controversial.

15.6 Conclusions

The characterization of the bilingual ability is incredibly complex and includes multiple dimensions. Accordingly, numerous questionnaires, scales, and indices have been created, each with its own strengths and disadvantages. It is important for researchers and clinicians to understand how this ability can impact neuropsychological assessment, including the language in which evaluations are conducted and the use of language-appropriate normative data. While evaluating bilingual individuals in a bilingual mode is not always feasible, doing so may be the fairest way to assess this population. Additionally, considering other factors that are often present in bilinguals (e.g., immigrant status and different levels of quality of education as well as different learning trajectories across languages) will ensure a fair evaluation. The assessment of bilinguals with neurological disorders presents greater challenges, including the differential impact of the lesion across languages and their recovery. Furthermore, disorders that affect structures related to language control may lead to difficulties with code-switching.

Bilinguals may show some advantages and disadvantages on specific EF tasks despite the discrepancy regarding the bilingual cognitive advantage. The idea that the active use of two languages is a proxy for CR is still controversial; several studies report a delayed onset of dementia in bilinguals (e.g., Bialystok et al., 2007), while others argue that this benefit is due to the retrospective design of studies and confounding variables (Mukadam et al., 2017). Much like the purported EF advantage, these conflicting results may be due to the influence of other variables. It is imperative for the field to devise methods that allow for the direct examination of linguistic influences while effectively controlling for other variables.

References

Abutalebi, J., Cappa, S. F., & Perani, D. (2001). The bilingual brain as revealed by functional neuroimaging. *Bilingualism: Language and Cognition, 4*(2), 179–190.

Abutalebi, J., Della Rosa, P. A., Ding, G., Weekes, B., Costa, A., & Green, D. W. (2013). Language proficiency modulates the engagement of cognitive control areas in multilinguals. *Cortex; A Journal Devoted to the Study of the Nervous System and Behavior, 49*(3), 905–911. https://doi.org/10.1016/j.cortex.2012.08.018.

Abutalebi, J., Della Rosa, P. A., Green, D. W., Hernandez, M., Scifo, P., Keim, R., & Costa, A. (2012). Bilingualism tunes the anterior cingulate cortex for conflict monitoring. *Cerebral Cortex (New York, N.Y.: 1991), 22*(9), 2076–2086. https://doi.org/10.1093/cercor/bhr287.

Abutalebi, J., & Green, D. (2007). Bilingual language production: The neurocognition of language representation and control. *Journal of Neurolinguistics, 20,* 242–275.

Abutalebi, J., & Green, D. W. (2016). Neuroimaging of language control in bilinguals: Neural adaptation and reserve. *Bilingualism: Language and Cognition, 19*(4), 689–698. https://doi.org/10.1017/S1366728916000225.

Adrover-Roig, D., Galparsoro-Izagirre, N., Marcotte, K., Ferré, P., Wilson, M. A., & Inés Ansaldo, A. (2011). Impaired L1 and executive control after left basal ganglia damage in a bilingual Basque-Spanish person with aphasia. *Clinical Linguistics & Phonetics, 25*(6–7), 480–498.

Alladi, S., Bak, T. H., Duggirala, V., Surampudi, B., Shailaja, M., Shukla, A. K., et al. (2013). Bilingualism delays age at onset of dementia, independent of education and immigration status. *Neurology, 81*(22), 1938–1944. https://doi.org/10.1212/01.wnl.0000436620.33155.a4.

Anderson, J. A., Mak, L., Chahi, A. K., & Bialystok, E. (2018). The language and social background questionnaire: Assessing degree of bilingualism in a diverse population. *Behavior Research Methods, 50*(1), 250–263.

Ansaldo, A. I., Marcotte, K., Scherer, L., & Raboyeau, G. (2008). Language therapy and bilingual aphasia: Clinical implications of psycholinguistic and neuroimaging research. *Journal of Neurolinguistics, 21*(6), 539–557.

Ardila, A. (2007). Bilingualism in the contemporary world. In A. Ardila & E. Ramos (Eds.), *Speech and language disorders in bilinguals* (pp. 1–20). New York: Nova Science Publishers.

Ardila, A., Lopez-Recio, A., Sakowitz, A., Sanchez, E., & Sarmiento, S. (2018). Verbal intelligence in bilinguals when measured in L1 and L2. *Applied Neuropsychology: Adult,* 1–6.

Ardila, A., Rosselli, M., Ortega, A., Lang, M., & Torres, V. L. (2019). Oral and written language abilities in young Spanish/English bilinguals. *International Journal of Bilingualism, 23*(1), 296–312.

Bak, T. (2016). Cooking pasta in La Paz: Bilingualism, bias and the replication crisis. *Linguistic Approaches to Bilingualism, 6*(5), 699–717. https://doi.org/10.1075/lab.16002.bak.

Barulli, D., & Stern, Y. (2013). Efficiency, capacity, compensation, maintenance, plasticity: Emerging concepts in cognitive reserve. *Trends in Cognitive Sciences, 17*(10), 502–509. https://doi.org/10.1016/j.tics.2013.08.012.

Berroir, P., Ghazi-Saidi, L., Dash, T., Adrover-Roig, D., Benali, H., & Ansaldo, A. I. (2017). Interference control at the response level: Functional networks reveal higher efficiency in the bilingual brain. *Journal of Neurolinguistics, 43,* 4–16.

Bialystok, E. (2001). *Bilingualism in development: Language, literacy, and cognition.* Cambridge University Press.

Bialystok, E. (2017). The bilingual adaptation: How minds accommodate experience. *Psychological Bulletin, 143*(3), 233.

Bialystok, E., Craik, F. I., Binns, M. A., Ossher, L., & Freedman, M. (2014). Effects of bilingualism on the age of onset and progression of MCI and AD: Evidence from executive function tests. *Neuropsychology, 28*(2), 290–304. https://doi.org/10.1037/neu0000023.

Bialystok, E., Craik, F. I., & Freedman, M. (2007). Bilingualism as a protection against the onset of symptoms of dementia. *Neuropsychologia, 45*(2), 459–464. https://doi.org/10.1016/j.neuropsychologia.2006.10.009.

Bialystok, E., Craik, F. I., Klein, R., & Viswanathan, M. (2004). Bilingualism, aging, and cognitive control: Evidence from the Simon task. *Psychology and Aging, 19*(2), 290–303. https://doi.org/10.1037/0882-7974.19.2.290.

Bialystok, E., Craik, F., & Luk, G. (2008). Cognitive control and lexical access in younger and older bilinguals. *Journal of Experimental Psychology. Learning, Memory, and Cognition, 34*(4), 859–873. https://doi.org/10.1037/0278-7393.34.4.859.

Bialystok, E., Craik, F. I., & Luk, G. (2012). Bilingualism: Consequences for mind and brain. *Trends in Cognitive Sciences, 16*(4), 240–250.

Bilingual Service Delivery. (2017). *Asha.org*. Retrieved from http://www.asha.org/Practice-Portal/Professional-Issues/Bilingual-Service-Delivery.

Boerma, T., & Blom, E. (2017). Assessment of bilingual children: What if testing both languages is not possible? *Journal of Communication Disorders, 66,* 65–76. https://doi.org/10.1016/j.jcomdis.2017.04.001.

Borsa, V. M., Perani, D., Della Rosa, P. A., Videsott, G., Guidi, L., Weekes, B. S., et al. (2018). Bilingualism and healthy aging: Aging effects and neural maintenance. *Neuropsychologia, 111,* 51–61.

Calvo, N., García, A. M., Manoiloff, L., & Ibáñez, A. (2015). Bilingualism and cognitive reserve: A critical overview and a plea for methodological innovations. *Frontiers in Aging Neuroscience, 7,* 249. https://doi.org/10.3389/fnagi.2015.00249.

Cattaneo, G., Calabria, M., Marne, P., Gironell, A., Abutalebi, J., & Costa, A. (2015). The role of executive control in bilingual language production: A study with Parkinson's disease individuals. *Neuropsychologia, 66,* 99–110.

Chertkow, H., Whitehead, V., Phillips, N., Wolfson, C., Atherton, J., & Bergman, H. (2010). Multilingualism (but not always bilingualism) delays the onset of Alzheimer disease: Evidence from a bilingual community. *Alzheimer Disease and Associated Disorders, 24*(2), 118–125. https://doi.org/10.1097/WAD.0b013e3181ca1221.

Costa, A., Hernández, M., & Sebastián-Gallés, N. (2008). Bilingualism aids conflict resolution: Evidence from the ANT task. *Cognition, 106*(1), 59–86. https://doi.org/10.1016/j.cognition.2006.12.013.

Cummins, J., & Swain, M. (2014). *Bilingualism in education: Aspects of theory, research and practice*. Routledge.

Del Maschio, N., Sulpizio, S., Gallo, F., Fedeli, D., Weekes, B. S., & Abutalebi, J. (2018). Neuroplasticity across the lifespan and aging effects in bilinguals and monolinguals. *Brain and Cognition, 125,* 118–126.

Fabbro, F. (2001). The bilingual brain: Bilingual aphasia. *Brain and Language, 79,* 201–210.

Faroqi-Shah, Y., Sampson, M., Pranger, M., & Baughman, S. (2018). Cognitive control, word retrieval and bilingual aphasia: Is there a relationship? *Journal of Neurolinguistics, 45,* 95–109.

Fienberg, S. E., & Meyer, M. M. (1992). *The case of bilingual education strategies*. National Academy Press.

Fischer, C. E., & Schweizer, T. A. (2014). How does speaking another language reduce the risk of dementia? *Expert Review of Neurotherapeutics, 14*(5), 469–471. https://doi.org/10.1586/14737175.2014.892831.

Folstein, M. F., Folstein, S. E., & McHugh, P. R. (1975). "Mini-mental state": A practical method for grading the cognitive state of patients for the clinician. *Journal of psychiatric research, 12*(3), 189–198.

Garbin, G., Sanjuan, A., Forn, C., Bustamante, J. C., Rodriguez-Pujadas, A., Belloch, V., et al. (2010). Bridging language and attention: Brain basis of the impact of bilingualism on cognitive control. *NeuroImage, 53*(4), 1272–1278. https://doi.org/10.1016/j.neuroimage.2010.05.078.

Gathercole, V. C. M., & Thomas, E. M. (2009). Bilingual first-language development: Dominant language takeover, threatened minority language take-up. *Bilingualism: Language and Cognition, 12*(2), 213–237. https://doi.org/10.1017/S1366728909004015.

Gollan, T. H., Fennema-Notestine, C., Montoya, R. I., & Jernigan, T. L. (2007). The bilingual effect on Boston Naming Test performance. *Journal of the International Neuropsychological Society: JINS, 13*(2), 197–208. https://doi.org/10.1017/S1355617707070038.

Gollan, T. H., & Goldrick, M. (2016). Grammatical constraints on language switching: Language control is not just executive control. *Journal of Memory and Language, 90,* 177–199. https://doi.org/10.1016/j.jml.2016.04.002.

Gollan, T. H., Montoya, R. I., & Werner, G. A. (2002). Semantic and letter fluency in Spanish–English bilinguals. *Neuropsychology, 16*(4), 562–576.

Gollan, T. H., Salmon, D. P., Montoya, R. I., & Galasko, D. R. (2011). Degree of bilingualism predicts age of diagnosis of Alzheimer's disease in low-education but not in highly educated

Hispanics. *Neuropsychologia, 49*(14), 3826–3830. https://doi.org/10.1016/j.neuropsychologia.2011.09.041.

Gollan, T. H., Salmon, D. P., Montoya, R. I., & da Pena, E. (2010). Accessibility of the nondominant language in picture naming: A counterintuitive effect of dementia on bilingual language production. *Neuropsychologia, 48*(5), 1356–1366. https://doi.org/10.1016/j.neuropsychologia.2009.12.038.

Gollan, T. H., Weissberger, G. H., Runnqvist, E., Montoya, R. I., & Cera, C. M. (2012). Self-ratings of spoken language dominance: A Multi-lingual Naming Test (MINT) and preliminary norms for young and aging Spanish–English bilinguals. *Bilingualism (Cambridge, England), 15*(3), 594–615. https://doi.org/10.1017/S1366728911000332.

Green, D. W. (1998). Mental control of the bilingual lexico-semantic system. *Bilingualism: Language and Cognition, 1*(2), 67–81. https://doi.org/10.1017/S1366728998000133.

Grosjean, F. (1989). Neurolinguists, beware! The bilingual is not two monolinguals in one person. *Brain and Language, 36*(1), 3–15. https://doi.org/10.1016/0093-934x(89)90048-5.

Hilchey, M. D., & Klein, R. M. (2011). Are there bilingual advantages on nonlinguistic interference tasks? Implications for the plasticity of executive control processes. *Psychonomic Bulletin & Review, 18*(4), 625–658. https://doi.org/10.3758/s13423-011-0116-7.

Hoff, E., Core, C. (2018). Advances in the assessment of young bilinguals: Comments on floccia. *Monographs of the Society for Research in Child Development, 83*(1), 109–123.

Kaplan, E. F., Goodglass, H., & Weintraub, S. (1983). *The Boston Naming Test* (2nd ed.). Philadelphia: Lea & Febiger.

Kavé, G., Eyal, N., Shorek, A., & Cohen-Mansfield, J. (2008). Multilingualism and cognitive state in the oldest old. *Psychology and Aging, 23*(1), 70–78. https://doi.org/10.1037/0882-7974.23.1.70.

Kohnert, K. (2010). Bilingual children with primary language impairment: Issues, evidence and implications for clinical actions. *Journal of Communication Disorders, 43*(6), 456–473.

Kousaie, S., Chai, X. J., Sander, K. M., & Klein, D. (2017). Simultaneous learning of two languages from birth positively impacts intrinsic functional connectivity and cognitive control. *Brain and Cognition, 117,* 49–56.

Lalor, E., & Kirsner, K. (2001). The representation of false cognates in the bilingual lexicon. *Psychonomic Bulletin & Review, 8,* 552–559.

Lehtonen, M., Soveri, A., Laine, A., Järvenpää, J., de Bruin, A., & Antfolk, J. (2018). Is bilingualism associated with enhanced executive functioning in adults? A meta-analytic review. *Psychological Bulletin, 144*(4), 394–425. https://doi.org/10.1037/bul0000142.

Li, P., Sepanski, S., & Zhao, X. (2006). Language history questionnaire: A web-based interface for bilingual research. *Behavior Research Methods, 38*(2), 202–210. https://doi.org/10.3758/BF03192770.

Luk, G., De Sa, E., & Bialystok, E. (2011). Is there a relation between onset age of bilingualism and enhancement of cognitive control? *Bilingualism: Language and Cognition, 14*(4), 588–595.

Marian, V., Blumenfeld, H. K., & Kaushanskaya, M. (2007). The Language Experience and Proficiency Questionnaire (LEAP-Q): Assessing language profiles in bilinguals and multilinguals. *Journal of Speech, Language, and Hearing Research: JSLHR, 50*(4), 940–967. https://doi.org/10.1044/1092-4388(2007/067).

Martínez-Horta, S., Moreu, A., Perez-Perez, J., Sampedro, F., Horta-Barba, A., Pagonabarraga, J., et al. (2019). The impact of bilingualism on brain structure and function in Huntington's disease. *Parkinsonism & Related Disorders, 60,* 92–97. https://doi.org/10.1016/j.parkreldis.2018.09.017.

Mishra, R. K., Padmanabhuni, M., Bhandari, P., Viswambharan, S., & Prasad, S. G. (2018). Language proficiency does not modulate executive control in older bilinguals. *Neuropsychology, Development, and Cognition. Section B, Aging, Neuropsychology and Cognition,* 1–32. https://doi.org/10.1080/13825585.2018.1562029.

Mukadam, N., Sommerlad, A., & Livingston, G. (2017). The relationship of bilingualism compared to monolingualism to the risk of cognitive decline or dementia: A systematic review and meta-analysis. *Journal of Alzheimer's Disease: JAD, 58*(1), 45–54. https://doi.org/10.3233/JAD-170131.

Muñoz-Sandoval, A. F., Cummins, J., Alvarado, C. G., & Ruef, M. L. (1998). *Bilingual verbal ability tests: Comprehensive manual*. Itasca, IL: Riverside Publishing.

Paap, K. R., & Greenberg, Z. I. (2013). There is no coherent evidence for a bilingual advantage in executive processing. *Cognitive Psychology, 66*(2), 232–258. https://doi.org/10.1016/j.cogpsych.2012.12.002.

Paap, K. R., Johnson, H. A., & Sawi, O. (2016). Should the search for bilingual advantages in executive functioning continue? *Cortex; A Journal Devoted to the Study of the Nervous System and Behavior, 74,* 305–314. https://doi.org/10.1016/j.cortex.2015.09.010.

Paradis, M. (2004). *A neurolinguistic theory of bilingualism* (Vol. 18). John Benjamins Publishing.

Pavlenko, A. (2007). *Emotions and multilingualism*. Cambridge University Press.

Pelham, S. D., & Abrams, L. (2014). Cognitive advantages and disadvantages in early and late bilinguals. *Journal of Experimental Psychology. Learning, Memory, and Cognition, 40*(2), 313–325. https://doi.org/10.1037/a0035224.

Perani, D., & Abutalebi, J. (2015). Bilingualism, dementia, cognitive and neural reserve. *Current Opinion in Neurology, 28*(6), 618–625. https://doi.org/10.1097/WCO.0000000000000267.

Perani, D., Farsad, M., Ballarini, T., Lubian, F., Malpetti, M., Fraccheti, A., et al. (2017). The impact of bilingualism on brain reserve and metabolic connectivity in Alzheimer's dementia. *Proceedings of National Academy of Sciences of the United States of America, 114*(7), 1690–1695. https://doi.org/10.1073/pnas.1610909114.

Potapova, I., & Pruitt-Lord, S. L. (2019). Towards understanding the bilingual profile in typical and atypical language development: A tutorial. *International Journal of Speech-Language Pathology,* 1–11.

Prior, A., & Macwhinney, B. (2010). A bilingual advantage in task switching. *Bilingualism: Language and Cognition, 13*(2), 253–262. https://doi.org/10.1017/S1366728909990526.

Ransdell, S., Barbier, M.-L., & Niit, T. (2006). Metacognitions about language skill and working memory among monolingual and bilingual college students: When does multilingualism matter? *International Journal of Bilingual Education and Bilingualism, 9*(6), 728–741. https://doi.org/10.2167/beb390.0.

Ratiu, I., & Azuma, T. (2017). Language control in bilingual adults with and without history of mild traumatic brain injury. *Brain and Language, 166,* 29–39.

Real Academia Española. (2001). *Diccionario de la lengua española [Dictionary of the Spanish language]* (22nd ed.). Madrid, Spain.

Rosselli, M., & Ardila, A. (2018). Neuropsychology of bilingualism. In J. P. Lantolf, M. E. Poehner, & M. Swain (Eds.), *The Routledge handbook of sociocultural theory and second language development*. Routledge.

Rosselli, M., Ardila, A., Araujo, K., Weekes, V. A., Caracciolo, V., Padilla, M., et al. (2000). Verbal fluency and repetition skills in healthy older Spanish–English bilinguals. *Applied Neuropsychology, 7*(1), 17–24. https://doi.org/10.1207/S15324826AN0701_3.

Rosselli, M., Ardila, A., Jurado, M. B., & Salvatierra, J. L. (2014). Cognate facilitation effect in balanced and non-balanced Spanish–English bilinguals using the Boston Naming Test. *International Journal of Bilingualism, 18*(6), 649–662.

Rosselli, M., Ardila, A., Lalwani, L. N., & Vélez-Uribe, I. (2016). The effect of language proficiency on executive functions in balanced and unbalanced Spanish–English bilinguals. *Bilingualism: Language and Cognition, 19*(3), 489–503. https://doi.org/10.1017/S1366728915000309.

Rosselli, M., Loewenstein, D. A., Curiel, R. E., Penate, A., Torres, V. L., Lang, M., et al. (2019). Effects of bilingualism on verbal and nonverbal memory measures in mild cognitive impairment. *Journal of the International Neuropsychological Society, 25*(1), 15–28.

Rubinstein, J. S., Meyer, D. E., & Evans, J. E. (2001). Executive control of cognitive processes in task switching. *Journal of Experimental Psychology: Human Perception and Performance, 4,* 763–797.

Salvatierra, J., & Rosselli, M. (2011). The effect of bilingualism and age on inhibitory control. *International Journal of Bilingualism, 15*(1), 26–37.

Stern, Y. (2009). Cognitive reserve. *Neuropsychologia, 47*(10), 2015–2028. https://doi.org/10.1016/j.neuropsychologia.2009.03.004.

Tao, L., Marzecová, A., Taft, M., Asanowicz, D., & Wodniecka, Z. (2011). The efficiency of attentional networks in early and late bilinguals: The role of age of acquisition. *Frontiers in Psychology, 2,* 123.

Thomas-Sunesson, D., Hakuta, K., & Bialystok, E. (2018). Degree of bilingualism modifies executive control in Hispanic children in the USA. *International Journal of Bilingual Education and Bilingualism, 21*(2), 197–206. https://doi.org/10.1080/13670050.2016.1148114.

Van der Linden, L., Laurence, D., De Letter, M., Wouter, D., de Partz, M. P., Adrian, I., et al. (2018). A case study about the interplay between language control and cognitive abilities in bilingual differential aphasia: Behavioral and brain correlates. *Journal of Neurolinguistics, 46,* 37–68.

von Bastian, C. C., Souza, A. S., & Gade, M. (2016). No evidence for bilingual cognitive advantages: A test of four hypotheses. *Journal of Experimental Psychology: General, 145*(2), 246–258. https://doi.org/10.1037/xge0000120.

Weinreich, Uriel. (1953). *Languages in contact: Findings and problems*. The Hague: Mouton.

Woumans, E., Santens, P., Sieben, A., Versijpt, J., Stevens, M., & Duyck, W. (2015). Bilingualism delays clinical manifestation of Alzheimer's disease. *Bilingualism: Language and Cognition, 18*(3), 568–574. https://doi.org/10.1017/S136672891400087X.

Yeung, C. M., St John, P. D., Menec, V., & Tyas, S. L. (2014). Is bilingualism associated with a lower risk of dementia in community-living older adults? Cross-sectional and prospective analyses. *Alzheimer Disease and Associated Disorders, 28*(4), 326–332. https://doi.org/10.1097/WAD.0000000000000019.

Zahodne, L. B., Schofield, P. W., Farrell, M. T., Stern, Y., & Manly, J. J. (2014). Bilingualism does not alter cognitive decline or dementia risk among Spanish-speaking immigrants. *Neuropsychology, 28*(2), 238–246. https://doi.org/10.1037/neu0000014.

Zdorenko, T., & Paradis, J. (2012). Articles in child L2 English: When L1 and L2 acquisition meet at the interface. *First Language, 32*(1–2), 38–62.

Chapter 16
The Assessment of Executive Functions in Cross-Cultural Context

Shameem Fatima and Humera Sharif

16.1 Introduction

Executive functioning is an umbrella term referring to a wide range of cognitive processes and behavioral competencies. These functions include verbal reasoning, working memory, attentional control, problem solving, inhibition, cognitive flexibility, multitasking, and the ability to sustain attention, resist interference, utilize feedback, and deal with novelty. These processes allow successful adaptation by facilitating us in breaking out maladaptive habits, planning for future goals, prioritizing and sequential processing of actions, decision making, risk evaluation, and flexible adaptation.

As executive functions are defined to encompass a series of abilities which are necessary for self-regulated and goal-directed behavior, assessment of these cognitive functions requires multiple measures. Although the field of cognitive neuroscience has attained an accelerated growth during the last few decades, the neuropsychological assessment of executive functions and related dysexecutive syndromes faces inherent difficulties. Among these, the accurate, valid, cultural free, and cultural fair assessment has now become the most important one. Even though several books and papers have been published for the last 2–3 decades on the brain organization of human cognition, the knowledge in the field is not only partial but also biased because majority of the existing literature is based on Westernized, industrialized, educated, rich and particularly middle class urban samples (Ardila, 2007).

Assessment of human behavior is meaningful only when viewed in its context. As the neuropsychologists deal with assessment and rehabilitation of human cognition and behavior, consideration of the cultural context becomes very important

S. Fatima (✉)
COMSATS University Islamabad, Lahore, Pakistan
e-mail: shameemfatima@cuilahore.edu.pk

H. Sharif
University of Lahore, Lahore, Pakistan

A. Ardila et al. (eds.), *Dysexecutive Syndromes*,
https://doi.org/10.1007/978-3-030-25077-5_16

for them. The concept of cultural diversity had been commonly overlooked in neuropsychological assessment in the past, but fortunately, the situation is now changing to recognize and consider cultural influences on neuropsychological assessment and rehabilitation. Significant interest in cross-cultural neuropsychology has started since the last decade of the twentieth century (Ardila, 2007). Due to increasing interest of cognitive psychologists in cultural effects, they have started sorting out why and how does culture influence cognitive processes. For clearer understating of cultural effects on neurocognitive development and neuropsychological assessment, it would be important to first describe the concept of culture.

16.2 Culture

Culture is defined as a set of learned values, traditions, and living styles which are common to the members of a particular society. This set of learned values comprises the modes of thinking, feeling, and acting (Harris, 1983). More simply, the culture can be defined as a particular way of living of a human group sharing a particular region. It represents a specific way of adaptation and survival in a specific context. Particularly, the culture provides a worldly and a contextual insight into apparently universal human processes. Anthropologists describe a several thousands of different cultures in the world, and humans in the contemporary world speak around 7000 different languages (Lewis, 2009).

Ardila (2018) describes three dimensions of culture including the internal dimension, behavioral dimension, and the cultural elements. The internal dimension is the subjective or psychological representation of culture in terms of thinking, feeling, knowledge, values, attitudes, and beliefs. The behavioral dimension is described as ways of social interaction, meetings, behaving in different contexts, celebrations, and festivals. The third dimension refers to cultural elements including physical and symbolic elements of a particular human group such as clothes, ornaments, buildings, instruments, and weapons.

16.2.1 Characteristics of Culture

Ardila (2018) has described several characteristics of cultures. These and certain other characteristics of the culture have been explained in this section. First, cultural differences are clearly associated with environmental conditions. For example, differences in urban and rural cultures can be significantly attributed to environmental, physical, and geographical differences. Internal and behavioral aspects as well as cultural elements in two cultures are clearly associated with environmental conditions in two locations. Second, cultures are not static but dynamic. Cultures are continuously evolving, and cultural changes are observed throughout history. Many factors are responsible for cultural evolution including continuously changing environmental conditions, global development, contact between different cultures, and internal cultural revolution. Third, cultures can be separated into subcultures using some specific criteria. Norms and values of the subcultures within a wider culture are different from the main cultures based on some criteria. For example, in the major Pakistani culture, there are many subcultures including Punjabi, Saraiki, Kashmiri cultures in the East region; Makrani culture in the South region; Balochi and Pashtun cultures in the West region; and Dards, Baltis, and Shinki cultures in the north region. These Pakistani subcultures have been significantly influenced by their neighbor cultures such as by the Indian, Chinese, Turkish, and Irani cultures.

Fourth, comparison between two cultures can be made using some *relative distance*. For example, the relative distance of Mediterranean cultures from Anglo-Saxon cultures is lesser than its distance from the Amerindian cultures, indicating that Mediterranean people have more cultural elements in common with Anglo-Saxons than with Amerindians. In the Asian context, the relative distance of Pakistani culture from Indian culture is lesser than its distance from Chinese culture. Fifth, cultures are generally in contact, which may lead to cultural diffusion. Certain cultural elements have been particularly successful and have a strong tendency to diffuse across different cultures. For example, science and technology as a highly successful cultural element has an extremely strong tendency to diffuse to almost all cultures in the world. So far as the science and technology is concerned, the modern man has become more homogenous as compared to earlier times when science and technology was not so common. Also, due to increasing trend of science and technology all over the world, communication has become faster, which may further facilitate diffusion of other cultural elements. Formal educational institutes have played a very important role in diffusion of science and technology (Ardila et al., 2010).

16.2.2 Culture and Neuropsychology

Every child resides in a culturally built specific social setup which comprises a specific set of knowledge system, norms, and socialization practices. The acquisition of specific knowledge and skills is dependent on a cognitive system that is greatly influenced by the ontogenetic and ecological context (Legare & Harris, 2016). Hence, neuropsychological assessment is meant to assess an individual's cognitive and behavioral processes more comprehensively by including psychological, emotional, interactive, and adaptive components. The available literature suggests that expression of emotions and interactive behaviors are not universal but vary considerably across cultures (Nigg, 2000).

Cognitive sciences are based on a primary assumption that all human beings, irrespective of their cultures and ethnicities, have evolved and developed same basic neural structures and neural networks. But the evidence shows that an individual's life experiences and environmental factors may configure the contents of this primary structure (Chua, Liu, & Nisbett, 2005; Goh & Park, 2005). In upcoming years, neuropsychologists must address the question of universality of human neural physiology in relation to cognitive and behavioral processes across different cultures. Therefore, cross-cultural neuropsychologists are recommended to adopt an interactive approach to assessment by focusing on the interaction of universality with cultural specific uniqueness. Evidently, the examination of cultural differences can significantly help to advance our understanding of the development and assessment of cognitive abilities in a cross-cultural context while considering the universality of human physiology and neuropsychology. The studies from neuropsychology and anthropology report different patterns of cognitive abilities across different ethnic and cultural groups (Gangestad & Simpson, 2016; Kan, Wicherts, Dolan, & van der Maas, 2013; Matsumoto & Juang, 2016).

Ardila (2018) has described the importance of why it is needed to understand cultural effects on executive cognitive skill. He describes two distinct types of executive functions: (i) metacognitive executive functions and (ii) emotional executive functions. Metacognitive functions include problem solving, abstract reasoning, planning, strategy development, and working memory. Emotional component coordinates cognitions and emotions. The two distinct executive components together explain how individuals satisfy basic impulses following socially and culturally acceptable manners.

Although some cognitive abilities including visual, perceptual, attentional processes and memory have been analyzed across different cultural setups, the topic that has been relatively overlooked in the area of cross-cultural cognitive neuropsychology is executive functions. Until the end of the twentieth century, neuropsychology had a laissez-faire attitude toward multiculturalism and cultural diversity. While it has been generally agreed that executive functions are central to all cognitive functions, they have not been sufficiently analyzed in relation to cultural and developmental factors. Cultural values, language diversity, and test-taking attitude, which have been studied by social psychologists for centuries, remained absent in the conscious body of neuropsychology. Although the discipline has now recognized the sociohistorical diversities, ithas not systematically incorporated ethnicity and cultural factors in assessment and rehabilitation.

Currently, neuropsychology is on the way to cultural awareness, but it has not reached the point where all aspects of neuropsychological assessment can be identified in its cultural context. Although some empirical work is available on cultural differences and cultural factors affecting executive functions test performance, even then, this is an area that is in a dire need of research. In the past, limited availability of neuropsychological assessment measures could have been partly blamed because either the clinicians and psychometricians did not have access to limited available measures or the instruments available were impractical. But currently, given the availability of user-friendly computer softwares, practical and sophisticated programs, and reasonably priced assessment measures, it is somewhat concerning why the traditional cognitive and neuropsychological assessment falls short of adequate assessment of attentional processes.

16.2.3 Popular Division of Culture: Individualism and Collectivism

Generally, social scientists and anthropologists classify all cultures into two major categories in two overlapping ways that are individualistic versus collectivistic cultures or Western versus Eastern cultures. Western cultures are described to be individualistic, while Asian cultures are described to be collectivistic. Both cultures are also considered as opposite ends of a single continuum. Individualistic cultures can be described as cultures where individuals have a preference for autonomy, give more weightage to their personal preferences, are independent from their in-groups, and pursue self-oriented goals. On the other way, in collectivistic cultures, people are interdependent within their groups (e.g., family group, school or gym class, friends group, community group, or a country group) and pursue group-oriented goals. People from the collectivistic cultures behave in a communal way by significantly considering their in-group norms. People from collectivistic cultures favor collectivistic self in contrast to people from individualistic culture who prefer individual self (Oyserman & Lee, 2008; Triandis, 2001). Cultural differences relative to relationships with others in society impact the concept of self, with East Asians defining the self in an interdependent manner in terms of social obligations in social networks, whereas Westerners see the self as unique and separate from others in an independent manner (Zhu, Zhang, Fan, & Han, 2007).

Social scientists have extensively studied social behaviors and psychological processes across individualistic and collectivistic cultures; the research regarding cultural differences in cognitive and executive function abilities across two contexts, however, is in its initial stage. Recently, Kelkar, Hough, and Fang (2013) studied executive functions across individualistic (Western) and collectivistic (Eastern) cultures and found a significant main effect of culture. They found that Western sample completed the four tasks on Functional Assessment of Verbal reasoning and Executive Strategies more rapidly as well as showed higher scores on category switching on verbal fluency test from Delis Kaplan Executive Functions System compared to Eastern counterparts. Conversely, performance of Eastern sample was faster on Trail Making Test than their Western counterparts. The researchers suggested that these cultural differences may be attributed to higher use of analytical cognitive strategies and rule-based categorization by Western samples and allocation of more holistic attentional resources by Eastern sample. Additionally, results from studies using neuroimaging techniques have also described that cultural differences not only modulate behavioral responses but also neural activity. Evidence shows that individuals from individualistic cultures represent larger cortical regions allocated to self-representation compared to those from collectivistic cultures (Zhu et al., 2007). This popular division of individualistic and collectivistic cultures provides the cultural neuropsychologist an avenue to understand the general tone of cultural differences in cognition, information processing, and executive abilities. In turn, the growing body of knowledge regarding cultural differences in cognitive and executive functions as well as in neural activation patterns will facilitate researchers to better understand and further contribute to the field of cultural neuropsychology.

16.3 Cultural Aspects Affecting Neuropsychological Test Performance

It is generally agreed that basic cognitive processes are universal. However, it is argued that cultural variations in cognitions may arise from the situations where these processes are applied rather than their existence in one group and absence in other groups (Ardila, 2018). Ardila (2018) has described five cultural factors that may affect test performance on executive functioning measures. These factors include patterns of abilities specific to a culture, cultural values, familiarity with the testing, language, and education.

Pattern of abilities in each culture depends on the ecological environment and learning opportunities. Culture along with ecological environment provides the guidelines as to what should pay attention to and what should be learned at different developmental stages and by different genders. Therefore, different cultures in the context of different ecological backgrounds may develop different patterns of abilities and so cognitive styles. Similarly, the content assessed by neuropsychological assessment measures at least in part depends on the learned abilities which are associated with ecological context and learning opportunities. *Cultural values* dictate as to what is situationally relevant, right, and worth to do and learn. Because a culture provides a base for thinking, acting, and feeling, cultural variations in cognitive test performance are evident. Ardila discusses that a standard neuropsychological testing involves a specific set of conditions which may not be equally relevant and familiar to all cultures or even may violate some cultural norms. These conditions involve: (i) *one-to-one relationship* of the testee with an unknown tester in an isolated room, which may not be equally at ease and appropriate in all cultures; (ii) *background authority* of the tester; (iii) *best performance* on any test is related to the importance of test stimuli to the testee; however, it is difficult to understand in all cultural groups, why it is important to perform best on a nonsense syllable digit span test or on draw a picture test; (iv) a special type of *formal communication and relationship* between testee and tester may not be equally acceptable in all cultures, particularly in those cultures which emphasize close interpersonal relationships; (v) many of the neuropsychological assessment measures are *speed tasks*, and given the fact that speed and quality are contradictory, the concept of speed in not equally important and worth emphasizing in all cultures; (vi) *internal or subjective issues*, which are highly variable and dependent on the cultural context; and (vii) *use of specific testing elements* which clearly vary across cultures so the reason of presenting figures, blocks, pictures is usually not equally clear to participants from all cultures.

Familiarity with the testing elements, testing settings, and strategies needed to complete the tasks is another important factor to be considered in cross-cultural assessment. For example, the Boston Naming Test includes naming a beaver and an acorn but the animal and plant are unfamiliar to people of South America and people from other regions. Also, figures representing snow can be very likely unfamiliar to people living in tropical regions. Similarly, cultural relevance of the test items and test elements is a related factor which makes it difficult to use the test items with other cultural groups even after translation. For example, the items to spell out words in Mini-Mental State Examination may not be used with people speaking languages which use phonological writing system (e.g., Russian and Italian). Similarly, picture arrangement test from Wechsler Intelligence Scale has a different level of familiarity and difficulty for different cultural groups. *Language* as an important cognitive system may affect test performance not only on verbal tests but also on nonverbal tests. Sapir Whorf's hypothesis states that different languages conceptualize the world differently. Also, language usage differs according to the cultural and educational background. Usually, the test instructions and test elements are written in a very formal and academic language which is generally not understandable for illiterate and even less educated people. The tester needs to put a lot of effort to make this formal language understandable for people from different cultural, language, and educational background.

Education plays a crucial role in neuropsychological test performance in several different ways. First, educational content contains some of the contents of cognitive tests and thus provides familiarity with the cognitive testing. Also, schooling provides opportunities to learn some of the learning strategies used in cognitive testing. Moreover, schooling develops a positive attitude toward cognitive or intellectual assessment in an individual. School as a subculture may reinforce certain cognitive abilities such as memory, visuospatial abilities, and perceptual discrimination (Ardila et al., 2010).

16.4 Executive Functions Test Performance Across Cultures

Currently, executive cognitive abilities such as working memory, inhibition, and executive control have been typically very much emphasized in neuropsychology, whereas underlying attentional abilities require much greater analyses as the differences in attentional abilities which may emerge from cultural differences are likely to influence higher regulatory abilities. Therefore, this section discusses assessment of basic cognitive functions of attention and memory as well as higher executive functions including executive attentional control, working memory, inhibition, and cognitive flexibility across cultures.

16.4.1 Cognitive Processes of Attention and Memory

Attention is a basic cognitive process underlying higher executive processes which guides human interaction with the environment by orienting their focus toward specific stimuli and by allowing specific stimuli to enter into the memory systems. Therefore, attention seems to be a primary process which carries cultural impact on other higher cognitive processes. Cross-cultural theories propose that cultural differences in complex mental and behavioral processes exist because primary attentional and psychological processes tend to vary across cultures. The literature describes that cultural variations tend to influence even those psychological processes which seem universal, for example attentional, perceptual, and mnemonic processes (Duffy & Kitayama, 2007; Hedden, Ketay, Aron, Markus, & Gabrieli, 2008; Masuda & Nisbett, 2001). More specifically, the literature suggests that people from Western cultures tend to pay attention to stimuli that are self-relevant and object-based, whereas Eastern individuals are more likely to attend contextual particulars and group-relevant stimuli (Chua et al., 2005; Hedden et al., 2008; Masuda & Nisbett, 2001). Moreover, it is argued that differences in attentional processes exist even at emotional level. Nisbett (2003) has reported that individuals from Asian cultures focus more attention to others' emotional status and emotional context because they believe that environmental context plays a major role in determining individuals' behavior than one's disposition. Further, Boduroglu, Shah, and Nisbett (2009) have also described cultural differences in attention, perception, and organization of knowledge. They found that East Asians compared to Americans are more holistic in their perception and they benefit more from displays covering a broader region. However, Americans are better than East Asians at indentifying a centrally presented target.

Related terms are sustained attention, selective attention, and divided attention. *Sustained attention* can be defined as the capacity to maintain focus over a long period of time. Behavioral manifestation of sustained attention is described as an ability to persist on tasks prolonging over time and having no immediate reward, as well as to resist distraction due to other stimuli. Real-life examples of sustained attention include maintaining attention in classroom listening to a lecture for a fairly long time period (Armengol, 2000). The concept of sustained attention can be tied to habituation. Developmental studies have assessed reflex orientation and habituation process using physiological measures such as galvanic skin response, heart rate, and respiration rate across age-groups. Importantly, the role of sociocultural processes cannot be overlooked in assessing the speed or accuracy of attentional processes. The concept of speed is given different weightage across cultures. Arnold and colleagues assessed cross-cultural effects on response speed. They administered Halstead Reitan battery to a sample comprising three groups of Mexicans, Mexican Americans, and Americans. They found that Mexican Americans were faster though not very accurate on spatial tactile memory test (Arnold, Montgomery, Castaneda, & Longoria, 1994). Additionally, in a multinational study, Levav and colleagues found reaction time differences on an auditory performance task and Trail Making Test across countries (Levav, Mirsky, French, & Bartko, 1998).

Historical roots of sociocultural bases of orienting and sustaining attention can be traced back to Vygotsky and Luria's work. Vygotsky emphasized the social organization of attention by explaining that complex psychological phenomenon of attention is shared between an adult and the infant. From the very beginning of life, the child develops in social environment where an adult directs and triggers child's attention to relevant aspects of environment and child responds by holding or pointing to it. In the succeeding stages, this socially organized psychological phenomenon is reorganized. When the child learns to speak, he can name and distinguish the specific object from the context by directing attention to it. In this way, the socially organized psychological process of attention is internalized and becomes self-regulatory and voluntary attention. Based on the Vygotsky's point of view, Luria emphasizes the social origins of voluntary attention because it bridges the gap between involuntary attention and voluntary attention. He further explains that social and voluntary attention, which develops around 4–5 years, differs from the orienting reflex and is more associated with the ability to ignore distractions (Luria, 1973). Commonly, Stroop test is used to assess sustained attention. Not surprisingly, language proficiency, another cultural variable, is a very important cognitive ability required for this test, but is often ignored as a cultural factor. Sociocultural effects on test performance on Stroop takes have also been examined. For example, in a study of Hispanic children from various socioeconomic strata, Armengol (2000) found that response latencies for Hispanic children from higher socioeconomic level were shorter. Further, Mexican and Hispanic children from lower socioeconomic strata were similar in performance but slower than Mexican children from higher socioeconomic level.

Selective attention refers to focusing attention, identifying, and recognizing particular stimuli that is embedded in distractors. Selective attention is assessed by cancellation tasks, in which the subject is required to circle a target letter or a symbol embedded in distractors. Importantly, selective attention is influenced by the number of shared features and similarity between the target and distractors as well as by the speed and accuracy of responses. *Divided attention* is also known as shifting attention or distributed attention. The concept is defined as an ability to shift and distribute attention between two tasks or between two components of the same task. Shifting attention is an important ability that facilitates the smooth conduction of daily activities, for example, in driving, an individual needs to distribute and shift attention between multiple components related to driving such as shifting gears, steering, taking turns, focusing on signals, etc. This ability is also important in academic setting where the student is required to divide attention between listening to lectures and taking notes. Shifting attention is described to be strongly associated with attention and other executive function components (Miyake, Friedman, Emerson, Witzki, & Howerter, 2000). Moreover, the researchers (e.g., Rushworth, Passingham, & Nobre, 2002) differentiate between attention shifting and response shifting based on whether the respondent is required to shift attention across stimuli or to shift motor response.

Accordingly, cultural variations in *memory* have also been studied in cultural studies. Masuda and Nisbett (2001) have studied cultural variations in memory across American and East Asian cultures. They have reported that East Asians are more likely to remember and report the background information accurately compared to

Americans. Also, compared to Americans, they are less likely to recognize the target object when the background information has been changed or removed, although both groups have reported similar scores on memory measures of central objects with stable background. The researchers have related differences in contextual details across Asian and American groups to cultural differences in collectivistic versus individualistic contexts of these groups, where East Asians are more interdependent within their social groups compared to Americans who are more independent.

Moreover, the learning of semantic information is based on culture-specific experiences; thus, the content of semantic information also differs across cultures (Yoon et al., 2004). Cross-cultural variations have been reported in sorting out semantic information across American and East Asian groups (Unsworth, Sears, & Pexman, 2005). East Asians have been reported to more likely sort information by relationships or similarities compared to Americans who preferred to sort by categories.

16.4.2 Executive Attentional Control

Attentional control can be described as an executive ability to ignore irrelevant information or distracters and to focus on required task. Researchers have suggested that attentional control is an important component of executive functions (e.g., Iguchi, Hoshi, Tanosaki, Taira, & Hashimoto, 2005) and is very close to working memory. Engle, Kane, and Tuholski (1999) discuss that working memory is a form of controlled attention because it involves the capacity to bring into, keep, and manipulate memory representations in a conscious focus and control, particularly, in the presence of distracters. Empirical evidence also supports that attentional control task performance is reported to discriminate between preschool children with low and high working memory span (Espy & Bull, 2005).

Cross-cultural studies have found difference in attentional control across Asian and American cultures. As discussed above, the study by Lan and colleagues found significant differences in attentional control component of executive functions between Chinese and American children with Chinese children outperforming their American counterparts (Lan, Legare, Ponitz, Li, & Morrison, 2011). This difference in attentional control abilities may be explained by socialization trainings and cultural practices. In Asian countries, more emphasis is placed on self-control during preschool and school years. Observational studies in classroom settings from Asian cultures report intensive self-control trainings such as teaching skills to follow instructions, focus on subject matter, be seated and wait for their turns, whereas in American classrooms, teachers allow free choice and self-expression. Additionally, Chinese children are frequently given proactive self-regulatory directions regarding what to do and what not to do, while American children are usually given reactive directions after children's misbehavior (e.g., Lan et al., 2009).

16.4.3 Working Memory

Working memory is a limited capacity conscious processing system, which receives most often auditory and visual information from sensory store and allows us to hold information in mind for few seconds. It is conceptualized as an executive function composed of short-term memory domain and central executive system (Baddeley, 2002). Ability to maintain information (i.e., item span) as well as to mentally manipulate information chunks comes under the rubric of working memory. The working memory capacity is particularly important in completing complex tasks such as calculating numbers and symbols (Espy et al., 2004). Working memory is often assessed from forward and backward digit span tasks. Accordingly, Armengol argues that backward digit span is clinically more sensitive measure compared to forward digit span. Developmental psychologists have extensively studied the development of attention span as well as mental operations active during working memory and concluded that child's capacity to store and mentally manipulate number of items in working memory increases with age (Armengol, 2000).

Findings from cross-cultural studies regarding working memory are inconclusive as few studies found differences in working memory across countries, but many of these studies could not find cross-cultural differences in working memory. For example, a study compared samples of children aged 6–11 years from four countries including Sweden, Spain, China, and Iran on executive functions and working memory tasks. The researchers found Chinese children to score better than Swedish, Spanish, and Iranian Children on working memory task as per teacher reports and parent reports (Thorell, Veleiro, Siu, & Mohammadi, 2013). Conversely, in a cross-cultural study based on two adolescent samples from Russia and Kyrgyzstan, researchers found no significant differences in working memory between two groups (Ismatullinaa, Voronina, Shelemetievab, & Malykhas, 2014). Moreover, Lan et al. (2011) could not find significant differences in working memory between Chinese and American individuals but they found that working memory uniquely predicted academic performance with some interesting patterns regarding tasks requiring complex processing. The cross-cultural psychologists argue that syllable length which typically varies across languages can affect digit span and thus working memory capacity. Therefore, more studies are needed from different linguistic contexts on working memory capacity to rule out whether language differences across different cultures correlate with working memory.

16.4.4 Inhibition

Inhibition is a higher regulatory executive cognitive skill which involves inhibiting prepotent/overlearned behavioral and cognitive responses in favor of novel responses. One major issue in the assessment of inhibition is that researchers are unsure of the extent to which working memory ability is involved in inhibition. As many of the inhibition measures also involve working memory component and necessitate subjects to keep information rule in mind while completing the task (e.g., Simon says task), whereas other measures are pure measures of inhibition (e.g., Stroop test and DKEFS color word interference test). Furthermore, inhibition task may also involve effective and motivational component such as tasks involving delayed gratification. Many studies have found that subjects with strong working memory capacity perform better on inhibition task (e.g., Kane, Bleckley, Conway, & Engle, 2001).

Cross-cultural studies have been conducted on the development of inhibition. For example, Sabbagh and colleagues compared the performance of Chinese preschoolers with US preschoolers on multiple executive functions: task tapping inhibition, cognitive flexibility and impulsivity. They found that Chinese children outperformed their US counterparts on all executive functioning measures including inhibition (Sabbagh, Xu, Carlson, Moses, & Lee, 2006). Moreover, Lan et al. (2011) assessed cultural differences in inhibition across Asian and Western context. They compared two groups of Chinese and American children on three measures of executive functions including working memory, attentional control, and inhibition. They found Chinese children outperform on measures of inhibition and attentional control with large effect sizes, compared to their American counterparts. Further, they found in the same study that inhibition uniquely predicted counting but not calculation. However, they found that the relationship between three executive functions was similar across two cultures. Importantly, the researchers reported that Asian children did not outperform uniformly across all executive function measures. Performance of Asian children was outstanding on inhibition and attentional control task but comparable on working memory task compared to Americans.

16.4.5 Cognitive Flexibility

Mental flexibility is a neuropsychological skill that is defined as a flexible adaptation of attention to focus on different aspects of the goal and to think about different and alternative perspectives. From the perspective of cultural adaptation, flexible cognitions explain the adaptive adjustment of attention, cognitions, and action policies in response to changing ecological and task demands (Deák, 2004). This mental ability allows individuals to readjust traditional and commonly practiced solutions by flexibly switching to innovative, advanced, and more productive solutions. Mental flexibility in coordination with other executive abilities including inhibition, working memory, and attentional regulation enables successful representation of complex behaviors such as problem solving, goal-directed planning, and conscious learning (Barkley, 2012). Developmental studies describe that this mental ability develops dramatically from 3 to 6 years. From 3 years of age, children from high socioeconomic status as commonly assessed in earlier literature show improvement in cognitive flexibility assessed from verbal rule switching in card sorting task and changing semantic cues to understand novel word meaning (Deák, 2000).

From cross-cultural perspective, earlier studies have found Asian children outperforming American children on measures of inhibition and cognitive flexibility (e.g., Lan et al., 2011). Potential explanation for this cultural variation in cognitive flexibility may include socialization training at home and at school. However, prevailing evidence from empirical studies is usually based on educated samples from relatively high socioeconomic background and from Western cultures. Recently, Legare, Dale, Kim, and Deák (2018) have compared two samples of children within age range of 3–5 years with different cultural backgrounds. They have selected one English-speaking sample of monolinguals from the USA who belong to high socioeconomic status and have highly educated parents and have been attending preschool. The other sample of multilinguals has been selected from South African ethnic background from a comparatively lower socioeconomic background that never attended preschool. They found that children from both ethnic groups showed comparable improved performance with increasing age on word learning task of cognitive flexibility, whereas only US children showed age-related improvement on rule switching test. Three-year-old children from both samples showed comparable performance on rule switching task, while older children from US sample showed improved cognitive flexibility than their South African counterparts. The researchers proposed that Westernized, educated, industrialized, and rich children who attend preschools under the guidance of educated teachers have rich experiences of learning, using, and manipulating symbols and sometimes of symbol–response mapping. Differential exposure of educational trainings which entail explaining abstract rules and categorization strategies may explain improved rule switching in Westernized and educated samples of children.

16.5 Cultural Effects on Nonverbal Test Performance

Until recently, it has been a very popular idea that nonverbal tests of mental abilities are culture free because they do not involve language and literacy skills. As a matter of fact, there is a range of intellectual and cognitive tests in practice that are supposed to be culture-free or culture-fair, merely because they do not include verbal and linguistic elements (Crampton & Jerabek, 2000). However, the recent evidence from contemporary literature in anthropology and cross-cultural psychology contradicts this assumption and extends that the development of nonverbal cognitive skills is also influenced by cultural values and practices (see Rosselli & Ardila, 2003 for a review).

Visual and perceptual abilities are basic cognitive abilities underlying higher executive functions. Cross-cultural researchers have also studied variations in perceptual abilities across different cultures. It is clear that although verbal element is nearly absent in nonverbal tasks, visuo-perceptual and spatial abilities are clearly involved. Evidence based on earlier studies in anthropology and cross-cultural cognitive psychology has shown that perceptual, spatial, and constructive skills are significantly correlated with cultural practices and environmental conditions (Smith, Fischer, Vignoles, & Bond, 2013). Therefore, it is suggested that nonverbal tests, which are currently used in cognitive and neuropsychology, are not necessarily more valid than verbal assessments for cross-cultural assessment. Additionally, training and demand history are also cultural variables that are described to be related to good visuo-perceptual abilities (Hegarty & Waller, 2005). Similarly, professionals from each discipline with a specialized training history are able to well recognize the relevant visuo-perceptual presentations compared to un-trained individuals. For example, a dactylographist compared to common individuals can easily differentiate different fingerprints; a neurologist can easily recognize symptoms of some neurological disorder; an artist can easily assess three-dimensional pictures etc.

Regarding spatial abilities, Mulenga, Ahonen, and Aro (2001), as discussed above, found that Zambian children performed better on visuospatial tests (such as design copying) than U.S children. Indeed, visuo-constructive and visuospatial test scores may be lower or higher in diverse cultural groups, but the important point is that they differ due to the specific cultural and ecological demands. However, in cross-cultural neuropsychology, spatial abilities and related disturbances in comparison with perceptual abilities have been very rarely assessed (Ardila & Keating, 2007). Ardila and Keating suggest that future neuropsychologists are required to develop norms for a broader range of perceptual measures across a variety of cultural and ecological contexts.

Moreover, specific nonverbal abilities which are quite commonly used in cross-cultural studies such as drawing a map and copying a figure are also not essentially universal. Such abilities can be perceived as meaningless to individuals from various cultures. For example, Ardila and Moreno (2001) studied samples of Colombian Aruaco Indians on the Rey-Osterrieth Complex Figure and Draw-a-Map test. They found that Aruaco Indians' performance on these nonverbal tasks was very low, whereas their performance on verbal fluency test was in normal range. In another study, Bossuroy, Wallon, Falissard, and Moro (2014) found differences on techniques used to draw figures on the Rey-Osterrieth Complex Figure by school children from diverse cultural backgrounds in France. They found that children of African origin drew more figures in vertical dimension (26%) compared to Westerners (5%). Additionally, Zambian children were reported to perform better on visuospatial tests than American children (Mulenga et al., 2001). Therefore, it is concluded that Cultural influences are not only limited to performance on verbal cognitive tasks but also likely to affect nonverbal test performance.

16.6 Current Status of Neuropsychological Assessment in Asian Region

Although history of cognitive testing dates back to the development of first cognitive test by Binet and Simon in the early twentieth century, followed by the development of cognitive tests and test batteries, the growth of neuropsychology is particularly reflected during the last 2–3 decades as evident by the growing number of papers and neuropsychological assessment scales published. However, majority of these tests have been developed and standardized with the Western population. Consequently, the aspects of a test which are specific to one culture may not be relevant to other cultural groups. Unfortunately, until the last decade, the literature was very rare regarding development and adaptation of cognitive and neuropsychological assessment scales in parts of the world including the Asian countries, where English was not spoken as a native language. Multiple reasons may explain it. First, maybe due to language disparity, there were a little motivation and effort to adapt language tests with non-English-speaking population. Second, the field of neuropsychology is a relatively younger field of psychology compared to other fields, and the early literature regarding this newly born filed was published in Western countries and was not readily available to Asian psychologist. On the other hand, the empirical research might have been done by Asian scholars but possibly could not gain access to the world's standard publishers and journals due to language problems. The literature might have been published in local journals which could not be viewed widely. Recently, a growing trend of research in neuropsychological assessment has been seen in Asia. From the last three decades, the neuropsychologists from Asian countries have started translating and adapting the Western neuropsychological scales. More recently, they have started developing the new scales.

During early stage of assessment, neuropsychological tests were translated and adapted from Western countries. Previously, it was thought that issue of cross-cultural validity was applicable only to verbal and language tests and had no clear relevance to nonverbal tests because a language element was missing in these tests. As the translation of nonverbal tests involves translation of verbal instructions only which is deemed easier and time saving, most of the researchers from Asian countries have translated the instructions and then used the nonverbal performance tests taken from Western cultures. However, in the past, due to the prevailing misunderstanding of cross-cultural validity of nonverbal tests, translation of instructions of nonverbal tests had been done but the adaptation of these tests had not been carried out. However, with the recent developments in the field of cross-cultural neuropsychology, it has been realized that the assumption of cross-cultural validity of nonverbal test does not always hold true, particularly on tests that involve elements of visuo-spatial abilities, perceptual abilities, and drawing abilities (Ardila & Moreno, 2001; Mulenga et al., 2001). For example, in a study, performance of Hong Kong Chinese was not comparable to that of native English speakers on Trail Making Test and its analogue Color Trail Test (Lee, Cheung, Chan, & Chan, 2000). The authors proposed that though the tests seemed to be generally fair across both cultures, the equivalence between two tests may likely be language specific. Additionally, cultural and ecological environment may also facilitate and thus correlate with specific basic cognitive skills and in turn higher executive functions.

Although translation and adaptation are easier and time saving, they raise questions of cross-cultural validity. On the other hand, test construction is more advanced and productive in several ways. First, test construction leads to the development of ecologically valid and sensitive tests which would incorporate the cultural needs, values, and learning experiences of local population in addition to the language effects. Second, the scholar has more freedom in test construction than in adaptation because one is free from constraints imposed by test items, format, and administration procedure of existing test that is standardized with another population. Third, whereas adaptation procedure involves cross-cultural validation of the translated and adapted test, this effort is not required for newly constructed test. Fourth, with the advancement of neuroimaging techniques, our understanding of brain–behavior relationship is increasing rapidly. Therefore, the development of new theories and refinement of existing theories require new ecologically valid and sensitive assessment tools for Asian cultural groups which may incorporate early language experiences and socialization trainings given the evidence that differences in early language experiences, ecological needs and socialization practices across Asian and Western cultures may determine the differential ways the child process information across two cultures (e.g., Kelkar et al., 2013).

Currently, with the advancement of field of cross-cultural neuropsychology and in turn greater recognition of cultural differences across Asians and Westerners on test performance, Asian researchers have started developing new tests and establishing cultural norms, with the aim of constructing culturally relevant and ecologically valid tools to be used with Asian samples. Among Asian countries, China, Japan, Hong Kong, and Korea have the most evident contributions in the field of neuropsychological test adaptations and development. Chan and Shum (2003) reviewed the literature and provided a general picture of neuropsychological assessment related to test development and test adaptation in Asian countries over the last two decades. The reviewers reviewed the literature from many Asian countries including China, Hongkong, Thailand, Japan, Malaysia, Korea, Singapore, Taiwan, Philippines, and India. The researchers reported the growing trend of neuropsychological assessment with an average 0f 1.8 number of published papers in 1980s to 16 in 2000. Notably, nearly 75% of 123 studies reviewed were conducted in Japan, China, and India. Rest of the studies were conducted in Korea and Hong Kong (20%), and Singapore, Thailand, and Taiwan (remainder 5%). They reported that nearly 40% of these studies were concerned with cognitive test adaptation and test construction. Out of the reviewed studies, 37% were concerned with test adaptation with the aim of assessing psychometric properties and validity and to establish norm for the local population for adapted tests from Western cultures. Only a small percentage of studies (around 3%) were intended to develop test. However, further screening of the reviewed studies based on the validity criteria set by the reviewers yielded eight valid tests including five adapted tests and three locally developed tests from four countries including China, Japan, Hong Kong, and Korea. The screening criteria were as follows: (i) proper procedure for test development or translation/adaption, (ii) validity in case of development and cross-cultural comparison in case of test adaptation, and (iii) norms collection on a sample of more than 50 individuals. Further, with regard to the cognitive domains assessed by these tests, four tests assessed dementia (one locally developed and three adapted tests), three tests assessed memory (two locally developed and one adapted tests), and the remaining one test assessed executive functioning. The general overview provided by Chan and Shum concludes that several researchers from Asian countries are now working on developing ecologically valid tests and adapting test for local communities.

Later on, Hsieh and Tori (2007) collected norms from young, middle, and older Chinese adults on a neuropsychological test battery. Afterward, Yang et al. (2012) collected norms from Chinese rural elderly on six cognitive tests assessing general cognitive functions, memory, language, and executive function. More recently, Fatima and colleagues from Pakistan translated instructions of nonverbal tests taken from Delis Kaplan Executive Functions System and then used these tests in multiples studies with Pakistani samples (e.g., Fatima & Sharif, 2017; Fatima & Sheikh, 2014, 2016; Fatima, Sheikh, & Ardila, 2016). But due to unavailability of cultural norms for Pakistani samples, the researchers used raw scores in these studies. Moreover, Niino et al. (2017) validated the Brief International Cognitive Assessment for Multiple Sclerosis on Japanese patients of multiple sclerosis and healthy controls. Regarding test development, Mahmood and Bashir (2018) have developed a neurocognitive assessment battery and validated it on a Pakistani sample of stroke patients. Further, a Neuropsychological Evaluation Screening Tool was developed in India by Chopra, Kaur, Pandey, and Nehra (2018).

The overview of neuropsychological assessment in Asian countries points to the reality that Asian neuropsychologists have grasped the idea that Asian and Western populations have different cultural experiences, learning opportunities, and socialization trainings embedded in individualistic versus collectivistic context which may lead to differential processing of cognitive information. However, efforts regarding neuropsychological test development still lag behind the test adaptation. Therefore, future researchers from Asia are recommended to broaden their vision from adaptation of Western tests toward the development and construction of original tests with better ecological validity for local communities.

References

Ardila, A. (2007). The impact of culture on neuropsychological test performance. In B. P. Uzzell, M. Pontón, & A. Ardila (Eds.), *International handbook of cross cultural neuropsychology* (pp. 23–44). Mahwah: Lawrence Erlbaum Associates.

Ardila, A. (2018). *Historical development of human cognition: A cultural-historical neuropsychological perspective*. Springer Nature Singapore Private limited.

Ardila, A., Bertolucci, P. H., Braga, L. W., Castro-Caldas, A., Cole, M., Judd, T., et al. (2010). Cognition without reading: Neuropsychology of illiteracy. *Archives of Clinical Neuropsychology, 25*(8), 689–712.

Ardila, A., & Keating, K. (2007). Cognitive abilities in different cultural contexts. In B. Uzzell, B. Ponton, & A. Ardila (Eds.), *International handbook of cross-cultural neuropsychology*. Mahwah: Lawrence Erlbaum Associates.

Ardila, A., & Moreno, S. (2001). Neuropsychological evaluation in Aruaco Indians: An exploratory study. *Journal of the International Neuropsychological Society, 7,* 510–515.

Armengol, C. G. (2000). Developmental and cross cultural issues in the assessment of attention and executive functions. *Revista Espanola de Neuropsicologia, 2*(3), 3–20.

Arnold, B. R., Montgomery, G. T., Castaneda, I., & Longoria, R. (1994). Acculturation and performance of Hispanics on selected Halstead-Reitan neuropsychological tests. *Assessment, 1,* 239–248.

Baddeley, A. D. (2002). The psychology of memory. In A. D. Baddeley, B. A. Wilson, & M. Kopelman (Eds.), *Handbook of memory disorders* (2nd ed., pp. 3–15). Hove: Psychology Press.

Barkley, R. (2012). *Executive functions: What they are, how they work, and why they evolved.* Guilford Press.

Boduroglu, A., Shah, P., & Nisbett, R. E. (2009). Cultural differences in allocation of attention in visual information processing. *Journal of Cross Cultural Psychology, 40*(3), 349–360.

Bossuroy, M., Wallon, P., Falissard, B., & Moro, M. R. (2014). The impact of cultural background on structural figure perception: Cultural biases in the reproduction of the Rey-Osterrieth complex figure. *Journal of Cognition and Culture, 14*(3–4), 273–285.

Chan, A. S., & Shum, D. (2003). Recent development of cognitive and neuropsychological assessment in Asian countries. *Psychological Assessment, 15*(3), 257–267.

Chopra, S., Kaur, H., Pandey, R. M., & Nehra, A. (2018). Development of neuropsychological evaluation screening tool: An education-free cognitive screening instrument. *Neurology India, 66*(2), 391–399.

Chua, H. F., Liu, J., & Nisbett, R. E. (2005). Culture and diverging views of social events. *Personality and Social Psychology Bulletin, 31,* 925–934.

Crampton, A., & Jerabek, I. (2000). *Culture-fair IQ test.* Montréal: Plumeus Inc.

Deák, G. O. (2000). The growth of flexible problem solving: Preschool children use changing verbal cues to infer multiple word meanings. *Journal of Cognitive Development, 1*(2), 157–191.

Deák, G. O. (2004). The development of cognitive flexibility and language abilities. In R. Kail (Ed.), *Advances in child development and behavior* (Vol. 31, pp. 271–327). San Diego: Academic Press.

Duffy, S., & Kitayama, S. (2007). Mnemonic context effect in two cultures: Attention to memory representations? *Cognitive Science, 31,* 1009–1020.

Engle, R. W., Kane, M. J., & Tuholski, S. W. (1999). Individual differences in working memory capacity and what they tell us about controlled attention, general fluid intelligence, and functions of the prefrontal cortex. In A. Miyake & P. Shah (Eds.), *Models of working memory. Mechanisms of active maintenance and executive control* (pp. 101–134). Cambridge University Press.

Espy, K. A., & Bull, R. (2005). Inhibitory processes in young children and individual variation in short-term memory. *Developmental Neuropsychology, 28,* 669.

Espy, K. A., McDiarmid, M. M., Cwik, M. F., Stalets, M. M., Hamby, A., & Senn, T. E. (2004). The contribution of executive functions to emergent mathematic skills in preschool children. *Developmental Neuropsychology, 26,* 465–486.

Fatima, S., & Sharif, I. (2017). Executive functions, parental punishment, and aggression: Direct and moderated relations. *Social Neuroscience, 12*(6), 717–729.

Fatima, S., & Sheikh, H. (2014). Socioeconomic status and adolescent aggression: The role of executive cognitive function as a mediator. *American Journal of Psychology, 127*(4), 419–430.

Fatima, S., & Sheikh, H. (2016). Adolescent aggression as predicted from parent-child relationships and executive functions. *American Journal of Psychology, 129*(3), 283–294.

Fatima, S., Sheikh, H., & Ardila, A. (2016). Association of parent-child relationships and executive functioning in South Asian adolescents. *Neuropsychology, 30*(1), 65–74.

Gangestad, S. W., & Simpson, J. A. (Eds.). (2016). *The evolution of mind: Fundamental questions and controversies.* New York: Guilford Publications.

Goh, J. O., & Park, D. C. (2005). Culture sculpts the perceptual brain. *Progress in Brain Research, 178,* 95–111.

Harris, M. (1983). *Culture, people, nature: An introduction to general anthropology* (3rd ed.). New York: Harper and Row.

Hedden, T., Ketay, S., Aron, A., Markus, H. R., & Gabrieli, J. (2008). Cultural influences on neural substrates of attentional control. *Psychological Science, 19,* 12–17.

Hegarty, M., & Waller, D. A. (2005). Individual differences in spatial abilities. In P. Shah & A. Miyake (Eds.), *The Cambridge handbook of visuospatial thinking* (pp. 121–169). Cambridge: Cambridge University Press.

Hsieh, S. J., & Tori, C. D. (2007). Normative data on cross-cultural neuropsychological tests obtained from Mandarin-speaking adults across the life span. *Archives of Clinical Neuropsychology, 22,* 283–296.

Iguchi, Y., Hoshi, Y., Tanosaki, M., Taira, M., & Hashimoto, I. (2005). Attention induces reciprocal activity in the human somatosensory cortex enhancing relevant- and suppressing irrelevant inputs from fingers. *Clinical Neurophysiology, 116,* 1077.

Ismatullinaa, V., Voronina, I., Shelemetievab, A., & Malykhas, S. (2014). Cross-cultural study of working memory in adolescents. *Procedia—Social and Behavioral Sciences, 146,* 353–357.

Kan, K. J., Wicherts, J. M., Dolan, C. V., & van der Maas, H. L. (2013). On the nature and nurture of intelligence and specific cognitive abilities: The more heritable, the more culture dependent. *Psychological Science, 24*(12), 2420–2428.

Kane, M. J., Bleckley, M. K., Conway, A. R. A., & Engle, R. W. (2001). A controlled-attention view of working-memory capacity. *Journal of Experimental Psychology: General, 130,* 169–183.

Kelkar, A. S., Hough, M. S., & Fang, X. (2013). Do we think alike? A cross-cultural study of executive functioning. *Culture and Brain, 1*(2–4), 118–137.

Lan, X., Legare, C. H., Ponitz, C. C., Li, S., & Morrison, F. J. (2011). Investigating the links between the subcomponents of executive function and academic achievement: A cross-cultural analysis of Chinese and American preschoolers. *Journal of Experimental and Child Psychology, 108*(3), 677–692.

Lan, X., Ponitz, C. C., Miller, K. F., Li, S., Cortina, K., Perry, M., et al. (2009). Keeping their attention: Classroom practices associated with behavioral engagement in first grade mathematics classes in China and the United States. *Early Childhood Research Quarterly, 24,* 198–211.

Lee, T. M. C., Cheung, C. C. Y., Chan, J. K. P., & Chan, C. C. H. (2000). Trail making across languages. *Journal of Clinical and Experimental Neuropsychology, 22,* 772–778.

Legare, C. H., Dale, M. T., Kim, S. Y., & Deák, G. O. (2018). Cultural variation in cognitive flexibility reveals diversity in the development of executive functions. *Scientific Reports, 8,* 16326.

Legare, C. H., & Harris, P. L. (2016). The ontogeny of cultural learning. *Child Development, 87*(3), 633–642.

Levav, M., Mirsky, A. F., French, L. M., & Bartko, J. J. (1998). Multinational neuropsychological testing: Performance of children and adults. *Journal of Experimental and Clinical Neuropsychology, 20,* 658–672.

Lewis, M. P. (2009). *Ethnologue: Languages of the world* (16th ed.). Dallas, TX: SIL International.

Luria, A. R. (1973). *The working brain.* London: Penguin Books.

Mahmood, S. N., & Bashir, U. (2018). Development and validation of neuro-cognitive assessment battery for stroke patients (NCABS) in Pakistan. *Pakistan Journal of Medical Sciences, 34*(5), 1164–1171.

Masuda, T., & Nisbett, R. E. (2001). Attending holistically versus analytically: Comparing the context sensitivity of Japanese and Americans. *Journal of Personality and Social Psychology, 81,* 922–934.

Matsumoto, D., & Juang, L. (2016). *Culture and psychology.* Scarborough, Canada: Nelson Education.

Miyake, A., Friedman, N. P., Emerson, M. J., Witzki, A. H., & Howerter, A. (2000). The unity and diversity of executive functions and their contributions to complex "frontal lobe" tasks: A latent variable analysis. *Cognitive Psychology, 41,* 49–100.

Mulenga, K., Ahonen, T., & Aro, M. (2001). Performance of Zambian children on the NEPSY: A pilot study. *Developmental Neuropsychology, 20,* 375–384.

Nigg, J. T. (2000). On inhibition/disinhibition in developmental psychopathology: Views from cognitive and personality psychology and a working inhibition taxonomy. *Psychological Bulletin, 126*(2), 220–246.

Niino, M., Fukazawa, T., Kira, J., Okuno, T., Mori, M., Sanjo, N., & Matsui, M. (2017). Validation of the brief international cognitive assessment for multiple sclerosis in Japan. *Multiple Sclerosis Journal—Experimental, Translational and Clinical,* 1–8.

Nisbett, R. E. (2003). *The geography of thought: How Asians and Westerners think differently and why*. New York: The Free Press.

Oyserman, D., & Lee, S. W. (2008). Does culture influence what and how we think? Effects of priming individualism and collectivism. *Psychological Bulletin, 134,* 311–342.

Rosselli, M., & Ardila, A. (2003). The impact of culture and education on nonverbal neuropsychological measurements: A critical review. *Brain and Cognition, 52,* 226–233.

Rushworth, M. F. S., Passingham, R. E., & Nobre, A. C. (2002). Components of switching intentional set. *Journal of Cognitive Neuroscience, 14,* 1139–1150.

Sabbagh, M. A., Xu, F., Carlson, S. M., Moses, L. J., & Lee, K. (2006). The development of executive functioning and theory of mind: A comparison of Chinese and U.S. preschoolers. *Psychological Science, 17*(1), 74–78.

Smith, P. B., Fischer, R., Vignoles, V. L., & Bond, M. H. (2013). *Understanding social psychology across cultures: Engaging with others in a changing world.* London: Sage.

Thorell, L. B., Veleiro, A., Siu, A. F., & Mohammadi, A. (2013). Examining the relation between ratings of executive functioning and academic achievement: Findings from a cross-cultural study. *Child Neuropsychology, 19*(6), 630–638.

Triandis, H. C. (2001). Individualism–collectivism and personality. *Journal of Personality, 69,* 907–924.

Unsworth, S. J., Sears, C. R., & Pexman, P. M. (2005). Cultural influences on categorization processes. *Journal of Cross-Cultural Psychology, 36*, 662–688.

Yang, L., Unverzagt, F. W., Jin, Y., Hendrie, H. C., Liang, C., Hall, S. K., et al. (2012). Normative data for neuropsychological tests in a rural elderly Chinese cohort. *Clinical Neuropsychology, 26*(4), 641–653.

Yoon, C., Feinberg, F., Hu, P., Gutchess, A. H., Hedden, T., Chen, H. M., et al. (2004). Category norms as a function of culture and age: Comparisons of item responses to 105 categories by American and Chinese adults. *Psychology and Aging, 19,* 379–393.

Zhu, Y., Zhang, L., Fan, J., & Han, S. (2007). Neural basis of cultural influence on self representation. *Neuroimaging, 34,* 1310–1316.

Index

A. Ardila et al. (eds.), *Dysexecutive Syndromes*,
https://doi.org/10.1007/978-3-030-25077-5

MIX
Papier aus verantwortungsvollen Quellen
Paper from responsible sources
FSC® C105338

If you have any concerns about our products,
you can contact us on
ProductSafety@springernature.com

In case Publisher is established outside the EU,
the EU authorized representative is:
Springer Nature Customer Service Center GmbH
Europaplatz 3, 69115 Heidelberg, Germany

Printed by Libri Plureos GmbH
in Hamburg, Germany